Nutritional Intervention in the Aging Process

Nutritional Intervention in the Aging Process

Edited by

H. James Armbrecht
John M. Prendergast
Rodney M. Coe

With 68 Illustrations

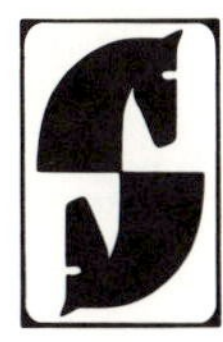

Springer-Verlag
New York Berlin Heidelberg Tokyo

H. James Armbrecht, Ph.D., GRECC, St. Louis VA Medical Center, and St. Louis University School of Medicine, St. Louis, Missouri 63104, U.S.A.

John M. Prendergast, M.D., GRECC, St. Louis VA Medical Center, and St. Louis University School of Medicine, St. Louis, Missouri 63104, U.S.A.

Rodney M. Coe, Ph.D., GRECC, St. Louis VA Medical Center, and Department of Community Medicine, St. Louis University School of Medicine, St. Louis, Missouri 63104, U.S.A.

Library of Congress Cataloging in Publication Data
Main entry under title:
Nutritional intervention in the aging process.
1. Aging—Nutritional aspects. 2. Aged—Nutrition. I. Armbrecht, H. James. II. Prendergast, John M. III. Coe, Rodney M.
QP86.N855 1984 613.2'0880565 84-5488

Typeset by Publishers Phototype International Inc., Carlstadt, New Jersey.
Printed and bound by Halliday Lithograph Corporation, West Hanover, Massachusetts.
Printed in the United States of America.

9 8 7 6 5 4 3 2 1

ISBN 0-387-96025-2 Springer-Verlag New York Berlin Heidelberg Tokyo
ISBN 3-540-96025-2 Springer-Verlag Berlin Heidelberg New York Tokyo

Contents

113458

Preface

There has been much popular and scientific interest in the fields of nutrition and aging in recent years. As the importance of proper nutrition in children and young adults becomes more fully understood, it is natural to wonder if proper nutrition could play a similar role in later life. Recent research has indicated that nutrition can potentially intervene in the aging process in at least two ways. First, studies in animals and humans have shown that nutrition can be used to improve functional status, which, in turn, is related to perceived quality of life. Second, nutritional manipulation has been used to extend maximal life span in laboratory animals. How these interesting findings apply to the human situation remains to be explored.

The purpose of this book is twofold. The first is to present recent advances in our basic knowledge of how nutrition and aging interact with each other. The second is to discuss some applications of this knowledge to the care of the elderly patient.

The interaction between aging and nutrition is complex because each may act on the other in either a synergistic or antagonistic fashion. Aging may alter the nutritional status of the elderly by affecting the way nutrients are absorbed and utilized by the body. Aging may also influence food intake and, therefore, nutritional status by decreasing the palatability of food. The environment of the elderly may change so they are less likely to eat well-balanced meals.

On the other hand, nutrition may increase length and quality of life. Intriguing animal studies have demonstrated that dietary restriction and antioxidant consumption may result in longer maximal life span. Proper nutrition may improve functional status by preserving bone integrity, cardiovascular and immune functions, and memory.

Discussions of these issues are presented in four sections. Part I is an overview of the effects of aging on nutrition; its five chapters review evidence of the influence of age-related changes on nutritional status. The concerns range broadly from general social and cultural factors to specific psychophysiologic ones and biochemical processes in the metabolism of vitamins, proteins, and lipids. Papers in the second section reverse the focus and examine evidence for the effects of nutritional manipulation on the dimensions of longevity as a facet of aging. These five presentations discuss dietary restriction and metabolism, nervous system structure, and membrane functions. Part III examines the effects of nutritional manipulation on functional abilities with respect to osteoporosis, diabetes mellitus, immune disorders, environmental chemicals, and memory. The final section shifts to clinical applications of nutritional knowledge for assessment and management of elderly patients in different environmental settings.

One of the challenges in treating the elderly is to avoid negative interactions between nutrition and aging. Poor nutrition resulting from physiologic and psychosocial factors may lead to an acceleration of the aging process and the aggravation of age-related diseases. Increased aging and disease can, in turn, lead to a further decline in nutritional status. This downward spiral can be difficult to reverse. We hope that this book will help to generate new ideas for preventing that downward spiral. Although it may be years before it can be used to extend maximal life span, nutritional intervention can play a significant role today in maintaining the functional status and, thus, the quality of life for the elderly.

We wish to express our appreciation for financial and administrative support for the conference that led to this publication, which was provided to the St. Louis Geriatric Research, Education, and Clinical Center (GRECC) by a continuing education grant from the Veterans Administration Office of Academic Affairs through the Office of Geriatrics and Extended Care; from the VA's South Central Regional Medical Education Center (RMEC); and St. Louis University School of Medicine. Support was also received from Ayerst Laboratories, Mead Johnson Laboratories, the National Dairy Council, Norwich-Eaton Pharmaceuticals, and Ross Laboratories.

Preparation of this volume has been greatly helped by the cooperation of individual contributors who submitted their manuscripts so promptly; by the GRECC office staff: Cheryl Duff who efficiently handled the many administrative tasks associated with the conference and this publication, and Sharon Smith and Sandy Melliere, who both provided technical assistance and moral support. We also thank the staff of Springer-Verlag.

While many have taken part in this project, we alone assume responsibility for this final product, which we hope will be informative and stimulate further research on nutritional interventions.

H.J. Armbrecht

J.M. Prendergast

R.M. Coe

Contributors

H. James Armbrecht, PhD GRECC, St. Louis VA Medical Center and St. Louis University School of Medicine, St. Louis, Missouri 63104 U.S.A.

Louis V. Avioli, MD Washington University School of Medicine, and, Jewish Hospital of St. Louis, St. Louis, Missouri 63110 U.S.A.

Charles H. Barrows, Jr., ScD Laboratory of Cellular and Comparative Physiology, Gerontology Research Center, NIA, Baltimore City Hospital, Baltimore, Maryland 21224 U.S.A.

Arthur Cherkin, PhD GRECC, Sepulveda VA Medical Center, and, UCLA School of Medicine, Los Angeles, California 90024 U.S.A.

Rodney M. Coe, PhD GRECC, St. Louis VA Medical Center, and, St. Louis University School of Medicine, St. Louis, Missouri 63104 U.S.A.

Bernard B. Davis, MD GRECC, St. Louis VA Medical Center, and, St. Louis University School of Medicine, St. Louis, Missouri 63104 U.S.A.

Carol J. Dye, PhD St. Louis VA Medical Center, and, Washington University, and, St. Louis University, St. Louis, Missouri 63104 U.S.A.

Margaret A. Flynn, PhD University of Missouri School of Medicine, Columbia, Missouri 65212 U.S.A.

Virginia M. Herrmann, MD St. Louis University School of Medicine, St. Louis, Missouri 63104 U.S.A.

S. Jill James, PhD GRECC, Wadsworth VA Medical Center, Los Angeles, California 90073 U.S.A.

Gertrude C. Kokkonen, BS Laboratory of Cellular and Comparative Physiology, Gerontology Research Center, NIA, Baltimore City Hospital, Baltimore, Maryland 21224 U.S.A.

Takashi Makinodan, PhD GRECC, Wadsworth VA Medical Center, and, UCLA School of Medicine, Los Angeles, California 90024 U.S.A.

Edward J. Masoro, PhD University of Texas, San Antonio, Texas 78284 U.S.A.

Douglas K. Miller, MD St. Louis University School of Medicine, St. Louis, Missouri 63104 U.S.A.

John M. Prendergast, MD GRECC, St. Louis VA Medical Center, and, St. Louis University School of Medicine, St. Louis, Missouri 63104 U.S.A.

Gustav Schonfeld, MD Lipid Research Center, Washington University School of Medicine, St. Louis, Missouri 63110 U.S.A.

John W. Shepard, Jr., MD GRECC, St. Louis VA Medical Center, and, St. Louis University School of Medicine, St. Louis, Missouri 63104 U.S.A.

Alan B. Silverberg, MD St. Louis University School of Medicine, St. Louis, Missouri 63104 U.S.A.

R. Strong, PhD GRECC, St. Louis VA Medical Center, and, St. Louis University School of Medicine, St. Louis, Missouri 63104

Albert Y. Sun, PhD Sinclair Comparative Medicine Research Farm, University of Missouri, Columbia, Missouri 65212 U.S.A.

Grace Y. Sun, PhD Sinclair Comparative Medicine Research Farm, University of Missouri, Columbia, Missouri 65212 U.S.A.

Deborah W. Vaughan, PhD Boston University Medical School, Boston, Massachusetts 02118

Ladislav Volicer, MD Boston University Medical School, and, Bedford VA Medical Center, Bedford, Masachusetts 02118 U.S.A.

Christopher D. West, PhD Harvard Medical School, and, Boston University Medical School, Boston, Massachusetts 02118 U.S.A.

W. Gibson Wood, PhD GRECC, St. Louis VA Medical Center, and, St. Louis University School of Medicine, St. Louis, Missouri 63104 U.S.A.

Vernon R. Young, PhD Massachusetts Institute of Technology, Cambridge, Massachusetts 02139 U.S.A.

Terry V. Zenser, PhD GRECC, St. Louis VA Medical Center, and, St. Louis University School of Medicine, St. Louis, Missouri 63105 U.S.A.

Part I

Effect of Aging on Nutrition

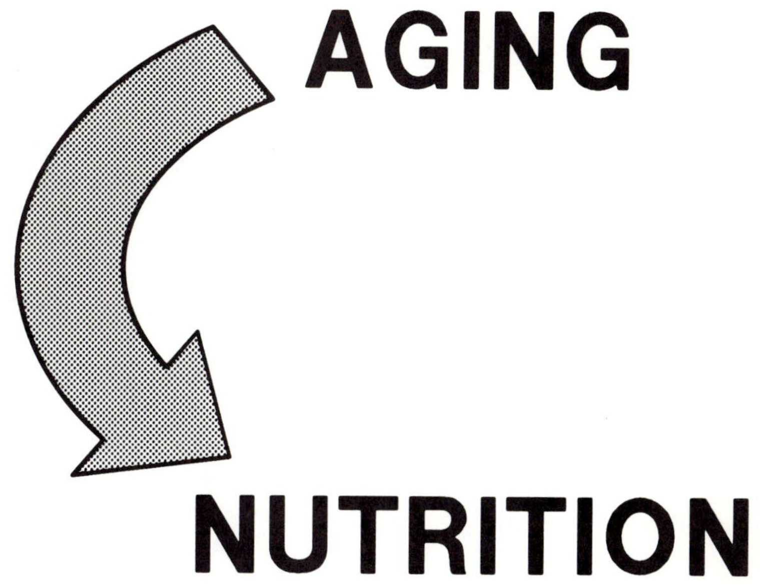

1

Sociologic Factors that Influence Nutritional Status in the Elderly

Rodney M. Coe and Douglas K. Miller

It is almost axiomatic that food serves more than one purpose. In addition to meeting biologic needs and satisfying a hunger stimulus, food also serves important social functions, both symbolic and real. However, the interaction between the cultural context of the elderly and the biopsychosocial processes of aging often results in malnutrition. Therefore, before reviewing the effects of selected sociologic factors, it may be useful to examine the data on the scope of malnutrition among the elderly.

The evidence on the nutritional status of noninstitutionalized elderly is equivocal. Some early reports cite widespread malnutrition or at least undernutrition (1). O'Hanlon and Kohrs have reviewed reports of 28 national and local surveys of nutrient intake in elderly persons living in communities (2). Almost all surveys report inadequate intake of various nutrients, some as much as one third below recommended standards. Food energy and calcium were most frequently found to be below standards. The mean caloric intake was below standards in all of the national surveys. On the other hand, Cape has summarized the results of several surveys in the United Kingdom and Europe, which show the prevalence of actual malnutrition among the elderly to be quite low (3). A principal finding in several community studies was that lower nutrient intake and true malnutrition were confined mostly to the 10% of elderly who were housebound because of chronic illness or disability. Thus, from most studies of this sort, it is not clear if the decline in nutrient intake (and subsequent malnourishment) is a consequence of disease or aging or both. Recent surveys conducted in the United States also tend to show low prevalence of overt malnutrition, although deficient intake of specific dietary needs is still found. In a study of 270 middle-income, healthy men and women aged 60 and over, Garry et al reported that dietary intake over a three-day study period met all or nearly all of the 1980 Recommended Dietary Allowances (4). The major exceptions were vitamin D and calcium intake in women. A local study of a sample of noninstitutionalized elderly in St. Louis, which employed self-reports and anthropometric measures, also found a low percentage (12%) of elderly who could be considered at nutritional risk, either over- or undernourished (5).

Despite these uncertainties, there are good reasons for continued interest in nutrition and the aged by the medical community. First, as everyone knows, the elderly, most often defined as persons aged 65 and over, are increasing rapidly both in absolute numbers and as a proportion of the total population. Persons over age 75 are the fastest growing segment (6). At the same time, older people tend to have the most days of hospital care, the most visits to physicians and the most admissions to nursing homes (7). Therefore, almost all physicians will see more and more patients in their practices.

Second, the onset and course of many of the chronic diseases that are so prevalent among the elderly are associated with poor nutritional status. Schlenker et al (8) have shown the importance of nutritional integrity in the maintenance of good health, while Mayer (9) has noted that good nutrition may actually delay the onset of some diseases. This suggests that adequate nutrition could be a valuable modality in a program of health maintenance (10) as well as treatment (11).

Third, evidence is mounting that the elderly are at especially high risk for nutritionally related problems (12). Part of the risk is in adequate intake of required nutrients, which has been shown in a number of reports (13,14). Another, perhaps more significant dimension of risk of nutrition-related problems includes social and psychologic factors prevalent among the elderly (15). Garetz described the interaction between clinical depression and both undernutrition and overeating. He noted particularly that social factors, such as poverty, social isolation, and role losses, were common etiologic agents (16). Grotkowski and Sims emphasized the association between adequate dietary intake and higher socioeconomic status, knowledge of nutrition, and positive attitudes toward good nutrition (17). Watkin has summarized the results of several such studies by pointing to the complex interaction between nutritional status and factors of physical health, dental health, sensory decrements associated with aging, and social variables of isolation and low income (18). It is on these social dimensions that further comments are focused here.

Social Factors in Food Choice and Consumption

Many social factors can influence human behavior. Furthermore, these factors are not mutually exclusive, but interact with each other, thus making analysis of their effects more complex. This is certainly the case for understanding behavior with respect to food choice and consumption patterns of the elderly. For purposes of illustration, four social dimensions have been selected for which there is some research evidence concerning their influence on food choice: (1) cultural factors; (2) role changes; (3) socioeconomic status; and (4) environmental characteristics.

Cultural Factors

All of us are conditioned to believe and to behave in accordance with our cultural norms and the specific rules of behavior of our subgroups. Our beliefs, attitudes, and behaviors are learned through a process called *socialization,* by which the individual becomes a participating member of particular ethnic, religious, occupational, and other groups. These memberships influence food choices (19,20). For example, culture defines what foods are edible. This becomes readily apparent when one makes cross-cultural comparisons involving cannabalistic rites of some primitive tribes. Even in our own Western culture, some foods are still proscribed by specific religious beliefs. Cultural factors also define when food is to be eaten and in what social context. Compare, for example, the stereotyped fast-food lunch, eaten alone and standing up that often characterizes urban office workers in our culture with the leisurely, family-oriented lunch followed by a siesta that is common in many Latin American homes.

Food also has culturally derived symbolic meanings (21). Food consumption most often occurs in a group context, particularly that of the family, and symbolizes congeniality and security. Food is also used as reward and punishment to induce or extinguish certain behaviors in children, prisoners, or other dependent persons. Withholding or granting candy or desserts to obtain desired behavior from a child and punishing prisoners with "bread and water" are prime examples. Similarly, in nursing homes, hospitals, and other institutional settings, perhaps even in private homes where the older adult is not the head of the household, granting or withholding food to control behavior of the elderly person has been reported (22). In the case of adults, use of food in this way symbolizes the loss of autonomy and exacerbates the impact on an already overstressed self-concept.

Culture is a principal source of beliefs about food and food consumption. Examples are food fads for "delaying aging" and for maintaining health through a "balanced" intake of hot and cold foods. The fact that people think they *ought* to delay the aging process, let alone that they believe they can do so through eating or avoiding certain foods, is itself a reflection of culturally approved values that emphasize youth, beauty, vigor, and energy. The specific fads vary from one part of the country to another and change over time. However, it is commonly believed that a specific disease is caused by a faulty diet and that processed foods have no nutritional value, or at least that "organically" grown foods are of superior nutritional value (23). Perhaps more common is the belief in vitamin supplements although there is still much controversy among professionals about their efficacy. Despite warnings about potential toxic effects of megavitamin therapy (especially self-prescribed), the elderly continue to spend money on vitamin supplements. Hale et al reported on a study of nearly 3,200 elderly who had been seen in a health screening program in which 46% of the women and 34% of the men regularly used vitamin supplements (24). The investigators concluded that many elderly were spending limited funds for vitamins that could better be used to improve the quality of their diets.

Using herbs and spices for their medicinal value is another example of a cultural influence. Stare has pointed out that these beliefs and associated behaviors persist despite evidence to the contrary, in part, because of the low level of knowledge about nutrition found among the population and because of advertising by health food stores in commercial publications and "testimonials" of users (25). The implications for the physician's role as educator are clear.

Role Changes

Social scientists employ the concept of *life course* to analyze behavioral changes during the life cycle of persons as individuals and as members of groups (26). In general, the process involves gradual accumulation of social roles and increasing integration into one's social networks as the individual moves from infancy and childhood through adolescence and young adulthood. At some time during "middle age" and accelerating in later maturity and old age, the process is reversed. Some roles are lost or changed and the person is "detached" from parts of his or her social network. Some obvious examples are the "empty nest," brought on by adult children becoming independent and establishing their own households; retirement from the occupational force, which often means loss of roles that were a major source of personal identity and feelings of worth; death of a spouse, often requiring profound psychologic adjustment along with significant role changes; death of lifelong friends and siblings, which can have a similar impact (22,27,28).

An important corollary of these role changes is increasing isolation of the elderly individual and the risk of depression (16), anxiety (29), and other mental health problems. There is considerable evidence to show that isolation produces psychologic deficits that can strongly influence eating patterns, and thus influence intake of nutrients (30), as well as affect life satisfaction (31) and self-esteem (32). There is an obvious correlation between isolation and the culturally derived meaning of eating as a social function of celebration, intimacy, and security, none of which would be fulfilled for the depressed elderly person who is living alone.

Socioeconomic Status

Socioeconomic status is a general concept that embraces several dimensions. It does indicate level of income and other financial resources and, therefore, enhances or constrains the individual's purchasing power (33). For example, persons on low fixed incomes are often left with few options after rent and utilities are paid. Food choices and amounts eaten are often the only "flexible" part of their spendable income budget. The elderly must then skimp on food or buy less nutritious foods. As a consequence, they become malnourished and at increased risk of infection and other health problems (12).

Educational achievement is also an important element in socioeconomic status. For the contemporary cohort of elderly, educational experiences were generally limited, which is associated with less knowledge about nutrition and greater acceptance of food fads (17), both of which are associated with poor nutrient intake. Socioeconomic status also reflects our value system with its emphasis on achievement and productivity. Success on these dimensions, which is not often attributed to the very old, is a key element in self-esteem. The stereotype of the elderly as unproductive and not achieving is part of the negative perspective on aging and the aged and affects the way in which the elderly view themselves, individually and as a group. Low self-esteem, as just noted, is associated with deficits in nutritional intake.

Environmental Conditions

Finally, some environmental factors related to accessibility to food should be mentioned. Disproportionate numbers of elderly and poor remain in old neighborhoods and inner-city areas as a consequence of population shifts in urban areas. One result is reduced availability of food stores and other services that offer wide choices at reasonable prices. In fact, many stores remaining in these areas are small and privately owned, with fewer choices of food and generally higher prices (22). Many elderly do not have their own means of transportation to overcome these limitations. Thus, ready access to a source of food is diminished.

Another dimension of urban living for the elderly is reduced mobility owing to fear of criminal assault (28). There are many reports of elderly individuals who do not get out of their locked apartments or houses for days or even weeks for food shopping, recreation, or even going to the physician without assistance from family members. Under especially adverse environmental conditions, this kind of immobility can contribute to fatal or near-fatal episodes. In a recent investigation of the results of a heat wave, some nutrition-related items (alcoholism, prescribed drugs, dehydration) were found to be risk factors for nonfatal and fatal episodes (34).

Impact on the Elderly

What are the effects of these sociologic factors on the patterns of food consumption and nutritional status of the elderly? The combined effects appear to place the elderly individual at "nutritional risk" (12). Common to all the factors is self-concept or self-esteem. One word of caution here is that there is greater variation among the elderly than among young adults on almost every dimension—physical, mental, and social. Thus, any characterization of "the elderly" will have many exceptions, the differences in findings of community surveys on nutritional risk having already been noted. Nonetheless, there is some value in a general description.

Self-esteem is the perception that a person has of himself or herself, derived as an interpretation of the positive and negative behaviors of others toward that person. The concept of self-esteem also assumes that the individual cannot long endure a negative self-concept and maintain physical and mental health (35). Much behavior that we call "coping" is directed toward maintaining the integrity of the self-concept.

As noted earlier, standards for food choices, preparation, and consumption are all derived from one's culture. The ability to conform to these cultural standards is an important part of one's self-esteem, symbolic of belonging to a group and being valued by its other members. Natural events in the life cycle of individuals can sometimes make conformity to cultural standards and participation in group life more difficult through role loss and systematic detachment or disengagement from social contacts. The harmful effects of detachment on the self-concept of the elderly individual have been documented, especially for the elderly in nursing homes where increasing "depersonalization" is associated with increased depression and psychotic behavior (36). Depersonalization through increased isolation and detachment from social networks is seen in other settings as well (37). Add to this the fact that a disproportionate number of elderly are poor or at least have severe limitations on expendable income, often living in areas that limit their access to food supplies. In addition, the factor of increasing age itself is associated with decreased nutritional intake, as shown in cross-sectional studies (38). Some recent longitudinal studies have shown that advancing age is associated with decreased intake of some nutrients, eg, calories and cholesterol, which may actually be healthful (39,40). These factors, alone and in combination, have a negative impact in varying degrees on the self-concept of the elderly individual.

From this review of selected research, it is possible to identify some key factors that trigger a degree of nutritional risk. The factors that appear most important for predicting nutritional risk include the following:

1. *Social factors*
   a. Age—risk increases directly with advancing age
   b. Living alone—represents an extra burden to those recently bereaved or who have experienced a significant life event
   c. Lack of effective support network, either family or neighbors
   d. Low income—severe limitations are placed on choices
2. *Psychologic factors*
   a. Depression
   b. Mental deterioration
   c. Impaired self-concept
3. *Physical factors*
   a. Functional dependence
   b. Sensory impairment
   c. Limited mobility

An elderly person who can be characterized as isolated, poor, depressed, with a poor self-image and some mental deterioration, and who is functionally dependent in one or more activities of daily living (ADL), through natural causes or environmental constraints, may be considered to be a "high-risk" individual for nutritionally related disorders.

Many of these same factors also are present in a research project now being conducted in St. Louis (41). One goal of this project is to develop an easily administered measure of nutritional risk that predicts the likelihood of disability and subsequent utilization of health services. Data for the study are from a survey of a random sample of 400 noninstitutionalized elderly individuals in the city of St. Louis. Preliminary analysis shows that the 16-item index of nutritional risk correlates strongly with utilization of physician and hospital services. The index has been shown to be reliable and valid in terms of face and concurrent validity. Known-groups validity was examined by comparing those at high risk with those at low risk according to the nutritional-risk index. In the absence of any statistical norms, the midpoint of the scale or above was arbitrarily chosen as high risk (12% of the sample). Analysis of variance tests showed significant differences between the groups on measures of physician visits, emergency room use, days of hospitalization, and ratings of emaciation. Differences on other dimensions such as body-mass index, tricep skinfold thickness, and ratings of obesity were in the predicted direction but did not reach statistical significance. Validation of the index with known laboratory measures of malnutrition is being planned. The predictive ability will be evaluated in terms of 6- and 12-month follow-ups of the original sample.

Implications for the Practitioner

Hanson has suggested that physicians employ a concept of "social nutrition" in assessing elderly patients (42). This is implemented in a more detailed history, especially of factors associated with food choices and consumption patterns. The physician should inquire about the social setting of mealtimes and opportunities for contact with others. Some specific questions for this expanded history might include: Do you live alone? With whom do you usually eat your meals? Do you have a refrigerator and stove? Who helps you with food shopping and preparation? Do you have an illness that limits what you usually eat?

Hanson suggests also that physicians make use of their superior status and give "psychotherapeutic permission" as a means for encouraging elderly patients to maintain a balanced diet suitable to their particular health status. The physician should remember, however, that therapeutic recommendations are most often followed and patient compliance will increase when the recommended action is compatible with the patient's existing beliefs.

Finally, Hanson believes that the physician should become an advocate for social nutrition for elderly patients by learning about community-based resources for nutrition. Most urban communities have several resources such as senior citizen centers where meals are served, meals-on-wheels programs, home health agencies that have dietary counselors, and churches and some civic groups that provide food. The insightful physician can influence the nutritional status and, therefore, the general well-being of elderly patients by helping them to practice these aspects of "social nutrition."

References

1. Conference Report: Malnutrition and hunger in the United States. *JAMA* 1970; 29:65–76.
2. O'Hanlon P, Kohrs MB: Dietary studies of older Americans. *Am J Clin Nutr* 1978; 31:1257–1269.

3. Cape RDT: Nutrition and the elderly, in Cape RDT, Coe RM, Rossman I (eds): *Fundamentals of Geriatric Medicine.* New York, Raven Press, 1983; pp 295–308.
4. Garry PJ, Goodwin JS, Hunt WC, et al: Nutritional status in a healthy elderly population: Dietary and supplemental intakes. *Am J Clin Nutr* 1982; 36:319–331.
5. Coe RM, Wolinsky FD, Miller DK, et al: Nutritional status among the elderly in a hospital service area. St. Louis University School of Medicine (mimeo), 1983.
6. Siegel JS: Prospective trends in the size and structure of the elderly population. *Curr Popul Rep* 1979; [P-23] No. 28.
7. Soldo BJ: America's elderly in the 1980's. *Popul Bul* 1980; 35:1–48.
8. Schlenker ED, Feurig JS, Stone LH, et al: Nutrition and health of older people. *Am J Clin Nutr* 1973; 25:1111–1119.
9. Mayer J: Aging and nutrition. *Geriatrics* 1974; 29:57–59.
10. Glick SM: Preventive medicine in geriatrics. *Med Clin North Am,* 1976; 60:1325–1332.
11. Todhunter EN, Darby WJ: Guidelines for maintaining adequate nutrition in old age. *Geriatrics* 1978; 33:49–51, 54–56.
12. Winikoff B: Nutritional Patterns, Social Choices and Health, in Mechanic D (ed): *Handbook of Health, Health Care, and the Health Professions.* New York, Free Press, 1983, pp 81–98.
13. *Preliminary Findings of the First Health and Nutrition Survey, U.S., 1971–72; Dietary Intake and Biochemical Findings.* National Center for Health Statistics. Government Printing Office, 1974.
14. *Ten State Nutrition Survey, 1968–70, V. Dietary.* National Center for Health Statistics. Atlanta, Center for Disease Control, 1972.
15. Davidson CS, Livermore J, Anderson P, et al: The nutrition of a group of apparently aging persons. *Am J Clin Nutr* 1962; 10:181–199.
16. Garetz FK: Breaking the dangerous cycle of depression and faulty nutrition. *Geriatrics* 1976; 31:73–75.
17. Grotkowski ML, Sims LS: Nutritional knowledge, attitudes, and dietary practices of the elderly. *J Am Diet Assoc* 1978; 72:499–506.
18. Watkin DM: Modern nutrition for those who are already old, in Hsu J, Davis R (eds): *Handbook of Geriatric Nutrition.* Park Ridge, NJ, Noyes Publications, 1981, pp 312–327.
19. Beeuwkes AM: *Studying the Food Habits of the Elderly.* National Research Council bulletin no. 111. National Academy of Sciences, Washington, DC, 1960.
20. Patten SE: Nutrition and the elderly: A cultural perspective. *Geriatrics* 1982; 37:141–147.
21. Saxson SV, Etten MJ: Psychological aspects of nutrition in aging, in Hsu J, Davis RD (eds): *Handbook of Geriatric Nutrition.* Park Ridge, NJ, Noyes Publications, 1981, pp 19–42.
22. Edwards SJ: Nutrition and lifestyle, in Feldman EB (ed): *Nutrition in the Middle and Later Years.* Boston, John Wright PSG, 1983, pp 1–16.
23. Davis AK, Davis RL: Food facts, fads, fallacies and folklore of the elderly, in Hsu J, Davis RL (eds): *Handbook of Geriatric Nutrition.* Park Ridge, NJ, Noyes Publications, 1981, pp 328–349.
24. Hale WE, Stewart RB, Cerda JJ, et al: Use of nutritional supplements in ambulatory elderly population. *J Am Geriatr Soc* 1982; 30:401–403.

25. Stare FJ: Nutrition–sense and nonsense. *Postgrad Med* 1980; 67:147–152.
26. Atchley RC: *Social Forces in Later Life.* Belmont, CA, Wadsworth, 1980.
27. Wilson AJE: Sociological aspects of nutrition and aging, in Hsu J, Davis RL (eds): *Handbook of Geriatric Nutrition.* Park Ridge, NJ, Noyes Publications, 1981, pp 43–55.
28. Sherwood S: Sociology of food and eating: Implications for action for the elderly. *Am J Clin Nutr* 1973; 26:1108–1110.
29. Howell SC, Loeb MB: Adult stress and diet. *Gerontologist* 1969; 9:46–52.
30. Natow AB, Heslin J: *Geriatric Nutrition.* Boston, CBI Publishing, 1980.
31. Harrill IC, Erbes C, Schwartz C: Observations on food acceptance by elderly women. *Gerontologist* 1976; 16:349–355.
32. Learner RM, Kivett VR: Discriminators of perceived dietary inadequacy among the rural elderly. *J Am Diet Assoc* 1981; 78:330–337.
33. Davis AK: Nutritional hazards of retirement, in Hsu J, Davis RL (eds): *Handbook of Geriatric Nutrition.* Park Ridge, NJ, Noyes Publications, 1981, pp 296–311.
34. Kilbourne EM, Choi K, Jones TS, et al: Risk factors for heatstroke: A case control study. *JAMA* 1982; 247:3332–3336.
35. Goffman E: *The Presentation of Self in Everyday Life.* New York, Anchor, 1959.
36. Coe RM: Institutionalization and self conception, in Rose AM, Peterson WA (eds): *Older People and Their Social World.* Philadelphia, F.A. Davis, 1965, pp 225–244.
37. Henry J: *Culture and Madness.* New York, Random House, 1963.
38. Brewster L, Jacobson MF: *The Changing American Diet.* Washington, DC, Center for Science in the Public Interest, 1978.
39. Elahi VK, Elahi D, Andres R, et al: A longitudinal study of nutritional intake in men. *J Gerontol* 1983; 38:162–180.
40. Garcia PA, Battese GE, Brewer WD: Longitudinal study of age and cohort influences on dietary patterns. *J Gerontol* 1975; 30:349–356.
41. Wolinsky FD, Coe RM, Miller DK, et al: Measurement of global and functional dimensions of health status in the elderly. *J Gerontol* 1984; 39:88–92.
42. Hanson RG: Considering "social nutrition" in assessing geriatric nutrition. *Geriatrics* 1978; 33:49–51.

2

Age-related Changes in Taste and Smell that Affect Nutritional Adequacy

Carol J. Dye

At any age, the perception of the taste and the odor of food has several important and basic contributions to the nutritional process for the individual. These chemical senses serve selective protective and stimulative functions for nutrition. The choice of food substances to be ingested is determined to a great extent by preferences for and aversions to foods. These choices are based on the learned pleasantness or unpleasantness a food has acquired to the senses of taste and smell. And these choices have been observed to become stubbornly resistant to change even in the face of modified nutritional needs at different stages in the life span. Young (1) indicated this in his statement: "new habits (in food consumption) tend to form in agreement with body needs, but established habits tend to persist as regulators of food selection even when the selections are out of the tune with bodily needs." Cultural influences (2), cohort effects, (3,4), and specific familial experiences all serve to determine taste and odor preferences and aversions. By later life, these are well-ingrained determinants of nutritional behavior, and planning for changes in nutritional status in older adults that will be maintained necessarily includes gathering a detailed nutritional history that considers each of these factors.

In addition to this selective function, the chemical senses have a protective function for nutrition. They guard the individual against food poisonings. But, beyond contributing to the *choice* of foods, the attractiveness of food, based on its perceived taste and smell, is important in determining the amount of saliva secreted in the mouth, the flow of pancreatic juices, gastric contractions, and intestinal motility (5–7). Therefore, the taste and smell of food contributes significantly to its digestion and utilization within the body.

As will be seen, there are seemingly age-related variations over the life span in gustatory and olfactory sensitivity and in the tastes and smells that are favored. All these variations, plus the cohort and other influences indicated above, contribute in significant ways to the ease and enthusiasm with which good nutrition can be accomplished. These factors pose special problems and challenges to the nutritionist (in the home or institution) to keep the proper foods appealing so that they will be chosen for consumption in the appropriate frequency and amount by the older adult. To help the nutritionist, specific guidelines from research documenting cohort and cultural effects in the development of preferences and aversions in taste and smell are helpful, as are data on age changes in gustatory and olfactory sensitivity. While there is a body of information in this area, it is limited and there is some variation in results, probably due in part to the greater difficulty in performing research in these areas. Experimental methods have varied and appropriate experimental controls are still under discussion (8). The smaller amount of research data for the chemical senses as compared to the others, probably results from the view that these senses are less important for the adequate functioning of the individual although the number of reported health care problems based on chemical sense disorders appears significant (9).

Age Changes in Taste Affecting Nutrition

Generally the results of studies of threshold sensitivity in taste over the age span show that older adults require greater concentrations than younger persons of almost any solution or food substance to be able to detect its presence. In an early study, Richter and Campbell (10) explored sucrose thresholds in rats and humans and found increases in thresholds with age for both populations. In their human subjects (aged 19 to 85 years), the threshold for the oldest group was almost three times that of the younger subjects. Subsequent studies supported Richter and Campbell's finding for the other so-called basic taste substances, ie, salty, acid (or bitter), sour (or tart) (8,11–18). Two studies explored the relative changes in the four basic taste substances within the same groups of adults over the life span. Cooper et al (19) studied individuals aged 15 to 89 and found that, while thresholds clearly rise with age, they do not do so at the same rate or to the same extent. In this study, the difference between young and old subjects for sour was just as significant, sweet and salty were significantly different between age groups and at a higher point of threshold, while bitter showed the highest threshold and the greatest change with age. Interestingly, Balogh and Lelkes (20) found that older adults were most sensitive to bitter of all tastes. They suggested that this was due to the age increases in protrusion and size of papillae on the back of the tongue that are most involved in sensing this taste. In a more recent study of thresholds of eight substances (sweet, salty, three acid, and three bitter tastes), Murphy (21) found that thresholds for the two age groups were not significantly different for one of the sour (HCl) and two of the bitter substances (caffeine and quinine). For the other substances tasted, there were significant differences between young and old individuals in threshold. This study seems to indicate that different food tastes vary in their potencies and properties, even though they are thought to belong to a basic taste group, and that they are affected by aging in different ways, a model supported by Schiffman and her colleagues (22).

The decrease in taste sensitivity with age is also seen when actual foods are utilized as stimuli. For example, Schiffman (23) found that compared to younger adults (18 to 22 years of age), older adults (67 to 93 years of age), were less able to recognize foods and complained more often of the foods' lack of flavor. The food substances included in the study (fruits, vegetables, meat, fish, nuts, dairy products, and grains) were steamed and blended to provide a similar texture before presentation to subjects, who were requested to guess the name of the stimuli. Older adults were correct far less often than their younger counterparts, but there was great interstimuli variation in the difference between younger and older subjects. Additionally, far more older adults complained of the weakness in taste of these 20 foods than younger adults, although the interstimuli differences between the two age groups were quite variable and the percent of group complaining ranged widely (3% to 52% within the older group and 0% to 48% within the younger group). Again, from this study, it would seem that the specific stimulus sampled is important in determining age differences and that it is difficult to make general statements about groupings of foods and age differences.

The age differences in taste thresholds are important for nutrition in that foods not tasted are not likely to be chosen for consumption. However, preferences for tastes will also shape food choice and nutrition. While some studies document age differences in preferences, it has not been determined how cohort effects might have operated to produce the differences seen or if these might be age changes as well. One early study by Laird and Breen (24) found preferences among the elderly for less sweet, ie, tarter (more acidic) tastes. Desor et al (25) studied choice of four suprathreshold solutions of sweet and salty tastes within a group of 9- to 15-year-olds and adults (no age given). In the older group, Desor found no specific preference for any of the concentrations of sucrose or lactose.

There was a decreasing preference for salt as concentration increased. The children in this study showed an increased preference for the sweetest tastes and a majority of these subjects favored the less salty concentrations.

Clearly, more information needs to be gathered on food preferences in later life. Studies should be done utilizing designs that can determine the cohort effects and the age changes in preferences. If preferences are determined early in life, successive cohorts within the population are likely to show their own patterns of food choice and nutritionists will have to recognize the changes as they work with successive cohorts of elderly. It may be, too, that age differences in sensitivity and preference are determined by lifelong habits in food consumption. Some evidence for this hypothesis comes from an interesting study of Indian laborers who regularly consumed relatively large amounts of sour foods (26). As a result, their ratings of the pleasantness of sour and bitter tastes were quite unlike Western preferences. The Indians rated more intense concentrations of quinine and citric acid as pleasant. The author hypothesized that this preference stemmed from genetic factors or dietary history.

Age Changes in Sense of Smell Affecting Nutrition

Changes in olfactory thresholds may also rise with age although the data for this sensory process are less clear than for gustation. Some studies that include a wide variety of odorants indicate a decline in olfactory sensitivity with age (27,28). Schiffman and Pasternak (29) explored the ability of young and old subjects to discriminate between pairs of food odors and found this ability greatly diminished in the elderly. In hedonic ratings of the food odors, elderly subjects indicated a preference for fruity odors. Stevens and colleagues (30) indicated that, despite large individual differences, older adults (65 to 83 years) rated odors as being only about half as intense as did younger adults (18 to 25 years). Stevens et al commented on the individual variation of the older subjects, hypothesizing the presence of age and concomitant pathologic conditions where there is a decrease in acuity. Two studies focused on the importance of health as a factor determining apparent age changes in olfactory sensitivity. Chalke et al (31) studied the ability of people over 65 years of age who were in apparent good health to detect town gas. In order to determine the basis for accidental poisoning, this group was compared with inpatients and outpatients at a hospital. The ability to perceive the gas decreased with increasing age, but poor health in individuals at any age was found to also cause a decrease in this ability.

In another study, Rovee et al (32) showed no changes with age in intensity ratings of suprathreshold concentration of *n*-propul alcohol. The physically superior older adults assessed in this study showed an increased sensitivity to odorants compared to the younger group (subject group ranged from 20 to 90 years of age). Engen (33) reported in another study done by Engen and Zweban that no significant differences were shown between younger and older subjects in sensitivity to a smoky odor (guaiacol). Individual differences were so large that any attempt to sort out subjects into age groups based on performance would have been difficult.

Several studies provide information as to preferences in odors over the age span. Moncrieff had subjects rank order 132 odors from liked to disliked (3,4). In a group of 550 persons (children under 15 years of age to adults), older adults were found to enjoy and favor fruity smells more than the odors of flowers that children preferred. Choice of sophisticated flower smells increased in the thirties and reached a plateau at that point. Moncrieff's important determination was that most of the changes in preferences were found to occur during the decades of the thirties, with little change in these preferences taking place in later life.

In a study of perception of a nonfood odor, Springer and Dietzman (28) presented objectionable traffic odors to a group of individuals aged 15 to over 65. The older group rated these odors as less objectionable, which seemed to indicate less sensitivity to these odors in older adults. However, the authors point out that individuals in poor health of any age rate these odors as less objectionable. Perhaps in this case again, health was more important than age in determining the results. In a very recent study, Murphy (34) explored the pleasantness of suprathreshold menthol solutions, a commonly used odorant, in a group of 18- to 26-year-olds and in an over-65-year-old group. Her results indicated than older adults perceived the menthol concentrations to be less intense than younger adults and the older adults' ratings of the pleasantness of several suprathresholds showed less differentiation in ratings between the various solutions than the younger adults. These results seem to confirm the notion of lessened sensitivity to tastes with age. One additional result was found. Within the older adult group, there was less of a familiarity response after repeated contact with this odorant: the menthol was not experienced as irritating or less appealing over time by these older adults as frequently as by younger adults.

Implications of Age Changes in Taste and Smell for Nutrition

The practical implication of the age changes in gustatory threshold seems to be that normal older adults will probably need to take in more of many substances, such as salt and sugar, to make food taste as it once did and tasty in any sense. This provides complications for the clinician who works to control diabetes, hypertension, and other illnesses. On the other hand, the rise in these thresholds may help in attaining good nutrition in old age also. For example, since the threshold for bitter does increase, the older adult may not object to being given a protein supplement, which makes the food taste more bitter (30). But perhaps age changes in *threshold levels* in tasted substances should not be the only guide to nutrition. Perhaps gustatory preferences, olfactory variables, and other factors determining appeal are more important in the selection of foods. For example, while the data for threshold sensitivity in taste in old age indicate that additional sugar is needed for the older person to be able to perceive the same level of sweetness in food, the information on food preference indicates that older adults may actually prefer less sweet, perhaps tarter, tastes. Preferences then would seem to provide some protection against exaggerated consumption of sugars. One of the challenges here is to find and utilize alternative substances that provide suitable levels of flavors and give appealing tastes to foods. These may take the form of substituting alternative forms of sugars, such as fructose, that provide greater sweetness than the more commonly utilized sucrose (35,36). Sugar substitutes may also be considered. However, since the elderly experience less growth in intensity with increased concentration, they may be at risk for adverse dose effects if they rely on artificial sweeteners to increase the sweetness level of foods considerably (37).

The practical implications of the results of the studies on olfaction are somewhat less clear than those on taste, especially since the health variable has been demonstrated to be so important in determining loss of olfactory capacity over the age span. If the older adult does indeed experience a loss of olfactory ability, then the enjoyment and attractiveness of food is reduced since smell contributes to taste. On the other hand, if health is the crucial variable in determining the decline in the olfactory sense, then it would be important to determine which illnesses affect smell to the greatest extent and which olfactory sensations are affected. Another important implication comes from the results of the Murphy study (34) pertaining to the familiarity factor. She indicated that older adults better tolerate odors over a period of time. As a result, it would seem that older adults might be satisfied with repetitious meals that provide satisfying olfactory sensations, despite the nutritional value involved.

The "true" taste or "flavor" of food is based upon taste, odor, visual appeal, palatability, social setting in which it is served, and individual variables such as level of satiety (38). The smell of food, of course, is a very important part of its appeal, perhaps a more important component of its attractiveness than taste. Almost everyone has experienced the blandness of food during a bad head cold that impairs olfactory functioning.

Interestingly, some foods seem to have contradictory tastes and smells. Chocolate and some vegetables have bitter tastes but very pleasant odors that apparently are more important for their consumption. In later life, as both senses become impaired, there may be less appeal to these foods, since the bitter taste may become a more predominant part of the experience of eating (30). Perhaps the most important direction to focus greater efforts in making food more appealing is enhancement of its appeal through odorants. For example, the addition of herbs and spices in appropriate quantities could increase the pleasant anticipation of food and its overall appeal.

Issues in Studies of Taste and Smell

The Influence of Health Status

The studies on olfaction raise an important issue that was not evident in the studies in the gustatory area, ie, the role of concomitant health status factors in determining apparent age changes in sensitivity. While the studies in olfaction noted the importance of poor health in determining apparent age changes, those in gustation did not. Yet this variable may be a subtle underlying factor determining loss of taste sensitivity. And, if health factors effect a decline in taste and olfaction, nutritionists need to carefully individualize diets for older adults, taking this additional variable of health status into account in planning the preparation of appealing food. These health status variables, as they affect food consumption in the populations of older adults in hospitals, are especially important since it is necessary to maintain the body systems to fight illness. Perhaps the decline in gustation and olfactory senses, resulting in loss of adequate nutrition in later life, precipitates illness.

On a very basic level, health may determine survival of taste buds. Counts of taste buds over the life span generally indicate that the number of functioning taste buds per papillae declines (39,40). Taste buds per papillae have been averaged at 324 for the age group 4 to 20 years and at 88 for people 70 years and over. The loss of taste buds may result from many factors, including primary degeneration of the papillae (41), changes in salivary flow (42), and other oral environmental factors (20). Whether any of these changes are caused by a basic aging process, poor health, or even nutritional status has been opened to question (43). Indirect evidence of the possible influence of health on taste sensitivity was hypothesized by Dye and Koziatek (44). These authors compared their results to three other earlier studies of sucrose thresholds over the life span that utilized the same experimental procedures. Over the four decades in which they were done, these studies (10,19,44,45) showed a progressive reduction in threshold for the older adult population, while there was essentially no change in the thresholds of the younger adults. The authors interpreted this to be due to the cohort effects of health status over the decades studied. With successive decades, older adults were probably in better physical condition and consequently had better oral conditions for survival of taste buds.

One easily identified health variable that might influence acuity of taste and smell in later life is smoking. In an early study on aging effects in taste, Kaplan et al (46) indicated the importance of smoking in diminishing acuity. More recent studies have also documented the negative influence of smoking on the gustatory (47) and olfactory senses (48). Usually, however, most studies do not control for this factor. Those that do require subjects not to smoke for at least one hour before assessment, but there is no certainty that this experimental requirement diminishes the effect of a lifetime of smoking in tested taste perception thresholds.

Actually, there is evidence that many diseases occurring over the entire life span alter the sense of taste and smell (49,50). Those occurring most frequently in old age include multiple sclerosis (51,52), cancer (53,54), diabetes mellitus (55), and hypertension (56). Since the probability of disease (in fact, multiple diseases) is greater in later life, the possibility of experiencing ageusia, hypogeusia, dysgeusia, anosmia, hyposmia, or dysosmia is also increased for the aged. In a recent report on disorders of taste and smell (9), it has been estimated that as many as two million adults have such disorders and that these symptoms were the basis for 435,000 visits to physicians' offices in a combined two-year period (1975 to 1976). These were combined data for adults of all ages. It could be hypothesized, of course, that older adults are probably overrepresented in these numbers on utilization.

Not only do diseases cause alterations in perceptions of tastes and smells, but the drugs taken to control the disease also cause alterations in the chemical senses. These are of a wide variety, ranging from those for the treatment of the serious and chronic diseases indicated above to such simple agents as toothpaste (49). In fact it has been shown that even one aspirin causes taste perception to have greater sensitivity to bitter tastes (57).

Yet another relationship of illness to the senses of taste has been described by Garb and Stunkard (58). These authors studied the tendency of individuals to develop learned aversions to foods that were experienced in close proximity in time to illnesses such as gastrointestinal upsets and other conditions. Comparing young children (6 to 12 years) with adults (over 60 years of age) they found 30% and 6% prevalence rates in taste aversion in these respective groups. The differences between the age groups were hypothesized to originate from the reduced sensitivity in taste among older adults. The development of aversions documented by these authors was essentially one trial learning that occurred with the pairing of the conditioned (food) and unconditioned stimuli (illness) separated by as much as six hours and with the aversions lasting as long as 50 years. Additionally, taste aversions have been documented as a response to chemotherapeutic drugs. Bernstein and Webster (59) demonstrated the development of aversions to specific flavors of ice cream consumed before drug treatment in cancer patients (17 to 77 years of age, mean age = 52 years). Again, in one trial learning, there was a significant reduction in preference for those flavors. In this study, nausea from the drug treatment was not a necessary condition for producing the aversion.

Influence of Age Changes in Body Composition and Utilization of Nutrients on Taste and Smell

Older adults show mineral deficiencies that influence sensory acuity for taste. It is not certain whether this condition results from aging changes influencing the utilization of these nutrients or from fewer economic resources, causing the choice of less expensive foods that lack sufficient minerals. Older adults consume fewer animal proteins that contain the more biologically available proteins and minerals. This tends to be true even in congregate settings that serve the elderly, since budget considerations are important in these settings also.

Zinc is one of these minerals that has been documented to be at reduced levels in the body in later life. Zinc deficiency results in impaired taste acuity in children (60) and is hypothesized to cause similar deficiencies in older adults (60). An appropriate question here is if the diet of the older adult is supplemented with zinc, does taste acuity improve and ultimately affect nutrition by better choice of foods? Gregor and Geissler (62) attempted to answer this question in a group of 49 institutionalized aged. In a double blind study, diet was supplemented for several minerals, as well as for zinc, in excess of the RDA for a period of 95 days. This regimen failed to produce significant improvements in taste acuity, although hair zinc levels increased significantly in the experimental group. Perhaps the ability of increased zinc intake to affect taste acuity is lost after a period during which the zinc level declines. Perhaps other minerals are involved in interaction with zinc in determining taste acuity in the older adult. Henkin and colleagues (63–65) indicated that zinc, while an important determinant, is only one among many substances causing changes in sensory acuity.

Summary

Many research studies and a number of issues have been reviewed as they are likely to influence nutrition for the older adult. Clearly, there are many factors that complicate the attainment of adequate nutrition, if the taste and the smell of foods are among the determinants of food choice. It is also clear that more research needs to be done to clarify some of the existing results. Much more research is needed in the area of the interaction of the sensation of odors and tastes, as these senses determine food choice and consumption in later life. Most important, studies need to be done (1) to explore the connection between gustatory and olfactory status and the actual choice of foods for consumption in later life, and (2) to solve some of the problems of loss of sensitivity and decline in pleasure from foods so as to enhance the quality of later life.

References

1. Young PT: The role of affective processes in learning and motivation. *Psychol Rev* 1959; 66:104–125.
2. Snapper I: The etiology of different forms of taste behavior, in Kare MR, Maller O (eds): *The Chemical Senses and Nutrition.* Baltimore, Johns Hopkins Press, 1967, pp 337–346.
3. Moncrieff RW: Changes in olfactory preference with age. *Rev Laryngol Otol Rhinol (Bord)* 1966; 86:895–904.
4. Moncrieff RW: Odour Preferences. New York, John Wiley, 1966.
5. Mower GD, Mair RG, Engen T: Influence of internal factors on the perceived intensity and pleasantness of gustatory and olfactory stimuli, in Kare MR, Maller O (eds): *The Chemical Senses and Nutrition.* New York, Academic Press, 1977, pp 104–121.
6. Naim M, Kare MR: Taste stimuli and pancreatic function, in Kare MR, Maller O (eds): *The Chemical Senses and Nutrition.* New York, Academic Press, 1977, pp 145–163.
7. Nicolaidis S: Early systemic responses to orogastric stimulation on the regulation of food and water balance: Functional and electrophysiological data. *Ann NY Acad Sci* 1969; 157:1176–1203.
8. Grzegorczyk PB, Jones SW, Mistretta CM: Age-related differences in salt taste acuity. *J Gerontol* 1979; 34:834–840.
9. *Report of the Panel on Communicative Disorders to the National Advisory Neurological and Communicative Disorders and Stroke Council,* US Dept. of Health, Education, and Welfare publication No. NIH 79-1914. Washington, DC, Public Health Service, 1979.
10. Richter CP, Campbell KH: Sucrose taste thresholds of rats and humans. *Am J Physiol* 1940; 128:291–297.
11. Bourliere PF, Cendron H, Rapaport A: Action de l'acide acetylsalicylique sur la sensibilité au gout amer chez l'homme (Action of aspirin on the sense of bitter taste in man). *Rev Fr Études Clin Biol* 1959; 4:380–382.
12. Glanville EV, Kaplan AR, Fischer R: Age, sex, and taste sensitivity. *J Gerontol* 1964; 19:474–478.
13. Moore LM, Nielson CR, Mistretta CM: Sucrose taste thresholds: Age-related differences: *J Gerontol* 1982; 37:64–69.
14. di Lumia V: Sulla sensibilita gustativa dell'uomo in eta senile (On the taste sensitivity of men in old age). *Arch Fisiol* 1959; 59:69–84.
15. di Lumia V: Richerche sulla sensibilita gustativa differenziale per il sapore acido in soggetti di diversa eta (Research on the differential taste sensitivity for sour taste in subjects of various ages). *Arch Fisiol* 1961; 60:240–246.

16. di Lumia V: Richerche sulla sensibilita gustativa differenziale per il sapore amaro in soggetti di diversa eta (Research on the differential taste sensitivity for bitter taste in subjects of various ages). *Arch Fisiol* 1961; 60:387–394.
17. di Lumia V: Richerche sulla sensibilita gustativa differenziale per il sapore dolce in soggetti di diversa eta (Research on the differential taste sensitivity for sweet taste in subjects of various ages). *Arch Fisiol* 1961; 60:232–239.
18. di Lumia V: Richerche sulla sensibilita gustativa differenziale per il sapore salato in soggetti di diversa eta (Research on the differential taste sensitivity for salty taste in subjects of various ages). *Arch Fisiol* 1960; 59:279–287.
19. Cooper RM, Bilash T, Zubek JP: The effect of age on taste sensitivity. *J Gerontol* 1959; 14:56–58.
20. Balogh K, Lelkes K: The tongue in old age. *Gerontol Clin* 1961; 3(suppl): 38–54.
21. Murphy C: The effect of age on taste sensitivity, in Han SS, Coons DH (eds): *Special Senses in Aging: A Current Biological Assessment.* Ann Arbor, Michigan, Institute of Gerontology, 1979, pp 21–33.
22. Schiffman SS, McElroy AE, Erickson RP: The range of taste quality of sodium salts. *Physiol Behav* 1980; 24:217–224.
23. Schiffman SS: Food recognition by the elderly. *J Gerontol* 1977; 32:586–592.
24. Laird DA, Breen WJ: Sex and age alterations in taste preferences. *J Am Diet Assoc* 1939; 15:549–550.
25. Desor JA, Green LS, Maller O: Preference for sweet and salty in 9- to 15-year-old and adult humans. *Science* 1975; 190:686–697.
26. Moskowitz HR: Cross-cultural differences in simple taste preferences. *Science* 1975; 190:1217–1218.
27. Kimbrell GMcA, Furchgott E: The effect of aging on olfactory threshold. *J Gerontol* 1963; 18:364–365.
28. Springer KJ, Dietzmann HE: Correlation studies of diesel exhaust odor measured by instrumental methods to human odor panel ratings. Presented at the Odor Conference of the Korlinska Institute, Stockholm, Sweden, 1970.
29. Schiffman SS, Pasternak M: Decreased discrimination of food odors in the elderly. *J Gerontol* 1979; 34:73–79.
30. Stevens JC, Plantinga A, Cain WS: Reduction of odor and nasal pungency associated with aging. *Neurobiol Aging* 1982; 3:125–132.
31. Chalke HD, Dewhurst JR, Ward CW: Loss of sense of smell in old people. London, *Public Health,* 1958; 72:223–230.
32. Rovee CK, Cohen RY, Shlapack W: Life span stability in olfactory sensitivity, *Developmental Psychology* 1975; 11:311–318.
33. Engen T: Taste and smell, in Birren JE, Schaie KW (eds): *Handbook of the Psychology of Aging.* New York, Van Nostrand Reinhold, 1977, pp 554–561.
34. Murphy C: Age related effects on the thresholds, psychophysical function and pleasantness of menthol. *J Gerontol* 1983; 38:217–222.
35. Moskowitz HR: The sweetness and pleasantness of sugars. *Am J Psychol* 1971; 84:387–405.
36. Stone H, Oliver SM: Measurement of the relative sweetness of selected sweeteners and sweetener mixtures. *J Food Sci* 1969; 34:215–222.
37. Schiffman SS, Lindley MG, Clark TB: Molecular mechanisms of sweet taste: Relationship of hydrogen bonding to taste sensitivity for both young and elderly. *Neurobiol Aging* 1981; 2:173–185.

38. Cabanac M: Physiological role of pleasure. *Science* 1971; 173:1103–1107.
39. Arey LB, Tremaine MJ, Monzingo FL: The numerical and topographical relations of taste buds to human circumvallate papillae through the life span. *Anat Rec* 1935; 64:9–25.
40. El-Baradi AF, Bourne GH: Theory of tastes and odors. *Science* 1951; 113:660–661.
41. Harris W: Fifth and seventh cranial nerves in relation to the nervous mechanism of taste sensation: A new approach. *Brit J Med* 1952; 1:831–836.
42. Burket LW: Oral pediatrics and geriodontics, in Burket LW (ed): *Oral Medicine, Diagnosis and Treatment,* ed 2. Philadelphia, Lippincott, 1952, pp 429–446.
43. Baum BJ: Current research on aging and oral health: An assessment of currrent status and future needs. *Special Care in Dentistry* 1:105–109.
44. Dye CJ, Koziatek DA: Age and diabetes effects on threshold and hedonic perception of sucrose solutions. *J Gerontol* 1981; 36:310–315.
45. Langan MJ, Yearick ES: The effects of improved oral hygiene in taste perception and nutrition of the elderly. *J Gerontol* 1976; 31:413–418.
46. Kaplan AR, Glanville EV, Fischer R: Cumulative effect of age and smoking on taste sensitivity in males and females. *J Gerontol* 1965; 20:334–337.
47. Smith SE, Davies PDO: Quinine taste thresholds: A family study and a twin study. *Ann Hum Genet* 1973; 37:227–232.
48. Dunn JD, Connetto-Muniz JE, Cain WS: Nasal reflexes: Reduced sensitivity to CO_2 irritation in cigarette smokers. *J Appl Toxicol* 1982; 2:176–178.
49. Schiffman SS: Taste and smell in disease: Part I. *N Eng J Med* 1983; 308:1275–1279.
50. Henkin RI: Abnormalities of taste and olfaction in various disease states, in Kare MR, Maller O (eds): *The Chemical Senses and Nutrition.* Baltimore, Johns Hopkins Press, 1967, pp 95–113.
51. Cohen, L: Disturbance of taste as a symptom of multiple sclerosis. *Br J Oral Surg* 1964; 2:184–185.
52. Pinching AJ: Clinical testing of olfaction reassessed. *Brain* 1977; 100:377–388.
53. DeWys WD, Walters K: Abnormalities of taste sensation in cancer patients. *Cancer* 1975; 36:1888–1896.
55. Halter J, Kalkosky P, Woods S, et al: Afferent receptors, taste perception and pancreatic endocrine function in man. *Diabetes* 1975; 24:414.
57. Fallis N, Lasagna L, Titreault L: Gustatory thresholds in patients with hypertension. *Nature* 1962; 196:74–75.
57. Bourliere PF, Cendron H, Rapaport A: Modification avec l'age des seuils gustatifs de perception et de reconnaissance aux saveurs salée et sucrée chez l'homme (Effects of age on the gustatory thresholds of perception and recognition of salty and sweet tastes in man). *Gerontologie* 1958; 2:104–112.
58. Garb JL, Stunkard AJ: Taste aversions in man. *Am J Psychiatry* 1974; 131:1204–1207.
59. Bernstein IL, Webster MM: Learned taste aversion in humans. *Physiol Behav* 1980; 25:363–366.
60. Hambidge KM, Hambidge C, Jacobs M, Baum JD: Low levels of zinc in hair, anorexia, poor growth and hypogeusia in children. *Pediatr Res* 1972; 6:868–874.

61. Gregor JL: Dietary intake and nutritional status in regard to zinc of institutionalized aged. *J Gerontol* 1977; 32:549–553.
62. Gregor JL Geissler AH: Effect of zinc supplementation on taste acuity of the aged. *Am J Clin Nutr* 1978; 31:633–637.
63. Henkin RJ, Schechter PJ, Hoye R, Mattern CFT: Idiopathic hypogeusia with dysgeusia, hyposmia and dysosmia. *JAMA* 1971; 217:434–440.
64. Henkin RI, Bradley DF: Hypergeusia corrected by Ni^{++} and Zn^{++}. *Life Sci* 1970; 9:701.
65. Henkin RI, Schechter PJ, Raff MS, et al: Zinc and taste acuity: A clinical study including a lazer microprobe analyses of the gustatory receptor area, in Pories WJ, Strain WH, Hsu JH, Woosley RL (eds): *Clinical Applications of Zinc Metabolism.* Springfield, IL, CC Thomas, 1974, p 204.

3

Impact of Aging on Protein Metabolism

Vernon R. Young

In this short review, selected aspects of protein and amino acid metabolism, with particular reference to the human subject, will be covered. Other researchers (1–3) have recently presented more extensive treatments of the effects of aging on the more basic aspects of protein metabolism, and my colleagues and I have discussed various aspects of human protein metabolism and nutrition. We will begin with a brief reference to findings made in studies in experimental animals and in vitro model systems. An overview of the major findings of human studies will be presented, and some of the possible nutritional implications of these observations will be discussed.

Protein Synthesis in Nonhuman Systems

A recent review by Richardson and Birchenall-Sparks (1) concluded that, in a majority of studies, an age-related decline in tissue protein synthesis had been observed. A partial summary of their compilation of the published data is given in Table 3-1, showing that with various model systems the synthesis of mixed proteins in such organs as the liver, brain, and pancreas is lower in the aged rat. These observations are concerned with mixed proteins, but information or synthesis rates of specific proteins is less extensive. Indeed, some studies in rats have suggested increased rates of albumin synthesis by hepatocytes obtained from aged

Table 3-1. Partial Summary of Recent Studies Concerning Aging and Protein Synthesis in Rats*

Sex	*Strain*	*Tissue*	*System*	*Ages (mo)*	*Change (%)*	*Reference*
Male	SD	Liver	Cell-free	6–30	75↕	Bolla & Greenblatt (7)
Female	Wistar	Liver	Cell-free	10–30	48↕	Cook & Beutow (8)
Male	F344	Liver	Hepatocytes	2–18	44↕	Coniglio et al (9)
Male	F344	Brain	Cell-free	6–32	56↕	Ekstrom et al (10)
Male	SD	Pancreas	Slices	2–30	50↕	Kim et al (11)

*From a more extensive tabulation by Richardson and Birchenall-Sparks (1) rats (12). Further discussion of these studies is given in more extensive accounts by Rothstein (3) and Richardson (1,2). However, it might be of interest to discuss briefly the possible basis for alterations in tissue protein synthesis.

A number of steps are involved in protein synthesis, including the activation of amino acids and formation of aminoacyl–tRNA, formation of the initiation complex, and elongation and termination of polypeptide chain synthesis. Various components of the protein synthetic apparatus may be affected by advancing old age, and reports have appeared showing reduced aggregation and activity of polyribosomes and changes in rates of the initiation and elongation phases of protein synthesis (see references 1 and 3 for review articles).

In a series of recent studies, we explored the effect of aging on rat skeletal muscle protein synthesis using a cell-free system (13). We observed that the activity of crude polyribosomes from hindlimb skeletal muscle was reduced by 40% in aging animals (22 to 24 months) and by 20% in the mature (12 months) animal compared to young (2 months) rats (Table 3-2). Also, in a poly(U)-directed incorporation system, the ribosomes from aged and mature animals showed a decrease in activity, and from sucrose density gradient analysis there appeared to be a loss of heavy polyribosomes in aged and mature animals. The pH5 enzyme fraction from aged and mature animals was found to be less efficient than that from young rats in support of protein synthesis, suggesting a decreased activity of soluble factors. Thus, the conclusion from these studies was that aging leads to a progressive decline in the efficiency of muscle protein synthesis and this decline is associated with changes in both the ribosomal and soluble fractions of the cellular machinery.

In a follow-up study, we further investigated the age-related reduction

Table 3-2. Activity of Crude Ribosomes and of "Washed" Polyribosomes from Skeletal Muscle of Rats at Various Ages*

	Synthetic Protein Activity	
Age (mo)	*Ribosomes†*	*Washed Polyribosomes‡*
Young (1–2)	193	110
Mature (12)	163	105
Aged (22–24)	124§	114

*Summarized from Pluskal et al (13) and Burini et al (14).

†^{14}C incorporation from ^{14}C-leucine/μg RNA/30^{minute}

‡^{14}C incorporation from ^{14}C-leucycl tRNA/μg RNA/30^{1}, using a common elongation factor preparation from young rats.

§P<.001 from young group.

in muscle protein synthesis activity discussed above, which was based on a crude polyribosome/pH5 system. We (14), therefore, exposed crude ribosomes to a potassium chloride washing procedure in order to remove the nonribosomal factors from the muscle polyribosomes. Then, using a common source of enriched elongation factor fraction from young animals, it was not possible to demonstrate any significant difference in protein synthesis between the 0.5 mol/L KCl washed-polyribosomes isolated from the various age groups of rat muscle (Table 3-2). However, using a cell-free system containing young salt-washed polyribosomes, we found that the addition of 0.5 mol/L KCl-wash fractions from mature and aged salt wash fractions stimulated in vitro protein synthesis less than did the material obtained from young animals. From these studies, the decline in protein synthesis efficiency during aging in rat muscle may be attributed to a reduced capacity of protein factors to promote the initiation/elongation phase of polypeptide synthesis.

Although the cell and subcellular events leading to and the molecular mechanisms responsible for age-dependent changes in protein synthesis remain to be clarified, it is nevertheless pertinent to assess the physiologic significance of a reduced rate of in vitro protein synthesis, if indeed this synthesis reflects the status of protein metabolism in vitro.

Unfortunately, it is not yet possible to make a satisfactory statement about the significance of the reduction in protein synthesis with advancing age. However, rapid rates of protein synthesis and breakdown (turnover) are associated with conditions of rapid growth and repletion, or they occur in response to stressful states such as infection and injury (15). Rapid rates of turnover (synthesis and breakdown) are thought to confer on the organism an ability to adapt successfully to changes in the internal and external environments. Hence, it might be speculated that lower rates of protein synthesis and protein breakdown might diminish the capacity of the body for adaptation to unfavorable circumstances, such as in response to physical trauma or to infectious agents. Also, rapid rates of protein turnover may prevent accumulation of abnormal or defective proteins (3) and may also facilitate redistribution within the body of nitrogen and amino acids under conditions of nutritional deprivation. However, it is clear that a more complete survey, using animal model systems, of the dynamic status of protein synthesis with reference to age and the capacity of cells to meet specific physiologic and biochemical functions should be undertaken.

In the final context, we wish to know how these various studies in nonhuman systems predict the status of protein metabolism in the organs and whole body of human subjects. This requires direct investigations in humans, and the following section will mainly be a discussion of the observations that my colleagues and I have made in our laboratories at Massachusetts Institute of Technology.

Protein Metabolism in the Aging Human

Quantity of Protein in the Body

It is pertinent to assess the size and distribution of the body protein mass and how these body composition parameters might change during the advancing adult years.

Briefly, cross-sectional and longitudinal studies have shown that there is a progressive decline in total body potassium (16–18) with increasing adult age in humans. This may be interpreted to indicate a decrease in total body protein mass (Table 3-3). Thus, it is apparent that body nitrogen increases rapidly from birth through childhood and early maturity, approaching a maximum by about the third decade and decreasing thereafter. This may occur somewhat more rapidly in men than in women (17). These changes in total body protein mass have nutritional implications, because the physiologic requirement for protein is usually considered to be that intake necessary just to achieve a "maintenance" of total body protein (nitrogen) content. The decline in total body nitrogen (protein) in the older subject (Table 3-3) may be the consequence of parallel changes in the protein content of many organs or a relatively greater change only in selected organs. Table 3-4 presents a summary of some observations on differences in the weight of individual muscles in young and aged animals. As shown here, in old age, there are decreases in total muscle mass with marked differences in the degree of change among different muscles. Also, about 85% of total body potassium and 50% of body nitrogen in the adult is located in the skeletal musculature. Thus, changes in total body potassium during human aging are probably caused by atrophy of skeletal muscles.

Although data on age-related changes in the mass of muscles of human subjects are limited, autopsy studies (23) of hospitalized patients suggest that total muscle mass undergoes a relatively greater percentage decline in old age than does that of other organs, such as the liver and heart. Fur-

Table 3-3. An Approximation of Total Body Nitrogen in Humans at Different Ages.*

	Body Nitrogen	
Age Group	*g*	*g·kg^{-1} body wt*
Newborn (full-term)	66	19
Child (10 yr)	615	19
Adult (25 yr)	1,320	18
Elderly (65–70 yr)	1,070	15

*From Young et al (5).

Table 3-4. Some Observations on Skeletal Muscle Weights in Old Versus Young Rats and Mice*

Species	*Age Comparison*	*Muscle*	*Weight Change*	*Fiber Number*	*Reference*
Rat	4 mo *v* 2 yr	Soleus	—	Decreased	Gutmann and Hanzlikova (19)
Mouse (M)	137 *v* 750 d	Soleus	Little change	Little change	Rowe (20)
Mouse (F)	137 *v* 750 d	Soleus	Little change	Decreased	Rowe (20)
Mouse (M)	137 *v* 750 d	Anterior tibialis	26% decrease	No change	Rowe (20)
Rat (M&F)	200 *v* 800 d	Gastrocnemius	22%–29% decrease	—	Neumaster & Ring (21)
Rat	450 *v* 900 d	Gastrocnemius	Decreased	—	McCafferty & Eddington (22)
		Soleus	Little change	—	

*From Young et al (5).

ther supporting this hypothesis is a decline in urinary creatinine excretion, assumed to be an index of muscle mass (24) in aged people (25). We observed a correlation between urinary creatinine and body cell mass in adult humans, and lower rates of creatinine output in older subjects (26), again suggesting that muscle atrophy accounts for a major portion of the decline in total body potassium and cell mass during aging in humans.

Dynamic Aspects of Protein and Amino Acid Metabolism

The protein content of cells, and of the body as a whole, is determined by the balance between the rate of incorporation of amino acids into proteins (protein synthesis) and their subsequent release via protein breakdown. In order to begin to explore the possible metabolic basis for changes in organ and whole body protein mass, we have undertaken an initial series of studies designed to quantify the movement of amino acids into and their release from whole body proteins. To do this, we have resorted to use of tracer approaches, the details of which have been described in a previous review (6).

Based on these approaches, we have examined two aspects of whole body amino acid metabolism in relation to human aging. The first is the quantitative metabolism of leucine in healthy young adult and elderly individuals. This series of experiments was conducted in subjects after they had undergone an overnight fast; they were, therefore, examined in the postabsorptive state of amino acid metabolism (27). In Table 3-5, the re-

Table 3-5. Rate of Protein Synthesis and Breakdown (Expressed as Leucine Kinetics and Estimated with the Aid of [1-^{13}C]-Leucine) in Young Adult and Elderly Male and Female Subjects During the Postabsorptive State*

	Young Adult		*Elderly*	
	Male	*Female*	*Male*	*Female*
No subjects	10	5	6	4
Mean age (yr)	25	22	75	76
Mean wt (kg)	77	61	74	61
Protein synthesis as leucine incorporation/kg/h	80 ± 4†	99 ± 8	72 ± 8	68 ± 6
Protein breakdown as leucine release/kg/h	101 ± 3	120 ± 8	97 ± 10	85 ± 7

*Summarized from Robert et al (27).

†Values for protein synthesis and protein breakdown are mean ± SEM and expressed as μmol/L leucine/h.

Table 3-6. Comparison of Rates of Whole Body Protein Synthesis, Determined with the Aid of ^{15}N-Glycine, in Young Men and Elderly Males

Parameter	*Young Men*	*Elderly Men*
Age (yr)	21 ± 1*	72 ± 2
Body wt (kg)	77 ± 5	69 ± 4
Body cell mass (kg)	37.6 ± 3.3	25.9 ± 1.4
BCM† (% body wt)	48 ± 1	38 ± 1
Creatinine excretion		
(g/d)	2.1 ± 0.2	1.3 ± 0.1
(mg/kg BCM/d)	55 ± 0.6	50 ± 1.6
Whole body protein synthesis (g)		
per kg/d	3.1 ± 0.2	3.1 ± 0.2
per kg BCM	6.5 ± 0.3	8.1 ± 0.6
per g creatinine	118 ± 6	165 ± 16
Whole body protein breakdown		
g/kg/d	3.0 ± 0.2	2.7 ± 0.2

*Mean ± SEM for 5 young and 6 elderly men. From Gersovitz M, Munro HN, Young VR: Unpublished data.

†BCM = Body cell mass determined from whole body ^{40}K.

sults for body leucine flux are summarized for a group of healthy young adults and elderly subjects. These data show little major difference between the two age groups when leucine metabolism is assessed in the postabsorptive state.

However, the dynamic aspects of amino acid metabolism vary throughout the day (28) and are particularly responsive to the variable intake of amino acids released from proteins during the ingestion and subsequent utilization of meals (29). Thus, it would be of interest to establish the average status of whole body protein turnover for the entire 24-hour period, which includes both the absorptive and postabsorptive phases of amino acid metabolism. This represents the second aspect of whole body amino acid metabolism that we have explored.

To accomplish this, we estimated rates of body protein synthesis and breakdown, using the ^{15}N-glycine method of Picou and Taylor-Roberts (30), which may provide an integrative estimate of total daily protein turnover. The results of our small series of cross-sectional studies (Table 3-6) reveal only small but possibly statistically significant differences in these rates between young adult and older subjects, when the results are expressed per unit of body weight (26,31). These results are in agreement with those reported by Golden and Waterlow (32) using a similar approach.

Because of differences in body composition between young and elderly adults, we also examined rates of whole body protein synthesis and breakdown in relation to indices of body composition. Creatinine was used as an index of muscle mass, and body cell mass was determined by whole body ^{40}K. The results of our more recent studies are also summarized in Table 3-6 and show that whole body protein synthesis and breakdown rates, per unit of creatinine excretion, tend to be higher in the elderly than in young adults. These findings may reflect a lower contribution by muscle to whole body protein synthesis and breakdown in the elderly as compared with young adults.

To explore this possibility, we have estimated the rate of muscle protein breakdown. We (33) have discussed the ways by which this might be accomplished and none is without its significant limitations. The approach that we have chosen is based on measurement of urinary N^{τ}-methylhistidine (3-methylhistidine) excretion, and we (33) have reviewed the evidence indicating that the output of this amino acid can serve as a useful index of the rate of muscle protein breakdown in vivo, in both rats and human subjects. Although there are a number of major problems associated with the interpretation of 3-methylhistidine excretion in urine as a reliable index of muscle protein turnover, we consider that in well-nourished individuals of relatively normal body composition the measurement of urinary 3-methylhistidine output does offer a valuable assessment of the dynamics of muscle protein turnover in man. It therefore may be exploited to examine age-related alterations in protein metabolism in this organ.

Accordingly, the urinary excretion of N^{τ}-methylhistidine in groups of healthy young adult and elderly subjects, all consuming flesh-free diets that are free of a source of this amino acid, has been determined (26) and some recent data are summarized in Table 3-7. The urinary output of the amino acid is lower for elderly men than for young men. However, this reduction may be entirely caused by the decline in muscle mass because N^{τ}-methylhistidine output per unit of creatinine output does not differ between the two age groups (Table 3-7).

Estimates of the daily amount of muscle protein breakdown, based on these findings, are about 69 g in young men, or 0.9 g protein $kg^{-1} \cdot day^{-1}$, and 36 g, or 0.5 $g \cdot kg^{-1} \cdot day^{-1}$, in elderly males (Table 3-7). Furthermore, in relation to the rate of whole body protein breakdown, it can be seen from Table 3-7 that muscle accounts for approximately 30% of whole body protein turnover in young men as compared with 20% in elderly men. These data, therefore, agree with our previous findings (26) and indicate that during progression of the adult years there is a decline in the quantitative contribution made by skeletal muscles to whole body protein metabolism.

These observations in human subjects also extend the findings we observed in animals and in vitro, including cell-free model systems. How-

Table 3-7. Urinary N^{τ}-Methylhistidine Excretion and Derived Estimates of Muscle Breakdown as Related to Adult Age*

	Young Men	*Elderly Men*
N^{τ}-Methylhistidine		
μmol/L/d	287 ± 33†	151 ± 9
μmol/L/kg BCM	7.6 ± 0.3	5.6 ± 0.2
μmol/L/g Cr	137 ± 6	118 ± 6
Muscle protein breakdown		
g/day	69 ± 8	36 ± 2
g/kg BCM‡	1.8 ± 0.06	1.4 ± 0.04
g/g Cr	33 ± 1.4	28 ± 1.6
% whole body	30 ± 2	20 ± 1

*From Gersovitz M, Munro H, Young VR: Unpublished data.

†Mean ± SEM for 5 young men and 6 elderly men.

‡BCM = Body cell mass determined by whole body ^{40}K.

ever, studies in man are still highly preliminary, and it will require considerable additional research to establish the true effects of advancing adult age on human whole body amino acid and protein metabolism. Furthermore, the nutritional significance of the changes in body protein metabolism with increased aging is uncertain.

We have speculated that the fall in muscle protein synthesis might lead to changes in the efficiency with which the dietary protein intake meets the requirement for protein (6). Also, because muscles contribute to the adaptations in whole body energy and amino acid metabolism during restricted dietary energy and protein intake (34,35), a reduced contribution by muscle to body protein metabolism might diminish the capacity of the elderly individual to respond successfully to unfavorable dietary situations or to other stressful conditions, such as infection or physical injury. An adequate response to these conditions requires mobilization of amino acids from the peripheral tissues to maintain protein synthesis in vital organs such as liver.

It must be emphasized that these conclusions about changes in whole body protein synthesis and breakdown during passage of the adult years are to be taken as tentative. The present data are based on cross-sectional studies in small groups of subjects and the methods used to quantify rates of whole body and muscle protein turnover have significant limitations. New and improved noninvasive methods for quantifying dynamic aspects of whole body protein and amino acid metabolism in vivo are necessary in order to validate and to clarify further the picture of the status of protein metabolism during aging in people.

Metabolism of Specific Proteins

In contrast to a more extensive, although somewhat confusing, data base on the turnover of whole body and mixed organ proteins in aged experimental animals (1–3), there are relatively few data available in human subjects on the dynamic aspects of metabolism of specific proteins, making it possible to discuss only briefly the effects of increasing age on the metabolism of albumin. Findings in aged rats suggest that they synthesize albumin at a faster rate than do young rats (12), although not all studies agree with this conclusion (1).

Albumin is a protein of interest in the biochemical evaluation of protein nutritional status in humans. Hence, we (36) have developed a stable isotope procedure for the estimation of albumin synthesis, in relation to human aging, that involves labeling with ^{15}N-glycine administered orally every three hours as a donor of ^{15}N for liver-free arginine. This method follows the nitrogen enrichment of the guanidine group of albumin-bound arginine and monitors ^{15}N-urea in the urine at isotopic steady state, as an index of the enrichment of the liver-free arginine pool. The progressive labeling of the arginine in serum albumin can be related to the level of ^{15}N enrichment of urinary urea to provide a measure of the albumin synthesis rate. Elsewhere, we have discussed in detail the various assumptions applied in the application of this model (36).

Young adults were given an adequate protein intake, and albumin synthesis was determined to proceed at 186 mg·kg^{-1}·day^{-1} (36). This value falls within the range obtained by the previous and more widely used ^{14}C-carbonate method and is in good agreement with the fractional catabolic rate as measured with radioiodinated albumin, approximating 200

Table 3-8. Parameters of Whole Body Albumin Metabolism in *Young Adult Men* Studied with ^{15}N-Glycine as Precursor of the Guanidine N or Albumin-Based Arginine, and Receiving Diets Adequate or Low in Protein*

Parameter	*Diet*		*P*
	Adequate	*Low Protein*	
Serum albumin (g/dL)	4.5 ± 0.12*	4.58 ± 0.05	NS
Intravascular albumin (g/kg body wt)	1.86 ± 0.04	2.22 ± 0.08	<.01
Albumin synthesis			
% d^{-1}	3.97 ± 0.58	2.98 ± 0.31	<.05
mg·kg^{-1}·d^{-1}	186 ± 30	140 ± 15	<.025
% whole body protein synthesis	6.16 ± 1.22	4.57 ± 0.64	<.05

*Summarized from Gersovitz et al (36).

†Mean ± SEM for 5 young men.

Table 3-9. Parameters of Whole Body Albumin Metabolism in Elderly Men, Studied with ^{15}N-Glycine as Precursor of the Guanidine N or Albumin-Bound Arginine, and Receiving Diets Adequate or Low in Protein*

	Diet		
Parameter	*Adequate*	*Low Protein*	*P*
Serum albumin (g/dL)	4.22 ± 0.07†	4.12 ± 0.13	NS
Intravascular albumin (g/kg body wt)	1.79 ± 0.15	1.90 ± 0.11	NS
Albumin synthesis			
%d^{-1}	3.35 ± 0.46	3.09 ± 0.49	NS
mg•kg^{-1}•d^{-1}	149 ± 22	147 ± 36	NS
% whole body synthesis	4.84 + 0.68	5.56 + 1.51	NS

*Summarized from Gersovitz et al (36).

†Mean ± SEM for six elderly men.

mg·kg^{-1}·day $^{-1}$. Furthermore, our stable isotope method was also found to be sensitive in detecting a reduction in the rate of albumin synthesis when young adults received a low protein diet for seven days (Table 3-8).

Using this ^{15}N-glycine approach in elderly subjects, we found that there was a lower concentration of albumin in the plasma of subjects in this age group compared with young adults, but the fractional synthesis of the albumin pool was only slightly and insignificantly lower in the elderly. Of possible greater interest was the fact that this value was not affected by differences in dietary protein level, in contrast to the impact of protein intake in the young men (Table 3-9). This implies that only the younger subjects are able to respond to increased protein intake. In this context, Munro et al (37) have pointed out that albumin synthesis in rats shows no consistent responses to increased consumption of protein when the animals already are receiving an adequate intake of protein, but they become responsive when serum albumin concentration is first lowered by depletion.

From these findings, we have concluded that there is an upper rate of albumin synthesis, limited by a set-point beyond which a more generous amino acid supply cannot stimulate it further (36). Clearly, these observations should be extended, in view of the fact that serum albumin levels are measured to evaluate nutritional status and to judge the effectiveness of nutritional therapies in aged hospitalized patients.

Protein and Amino Acid Requirements

Studies of body protein and amino acid metabolism, such as those discussed above, are intended to provide a sounder basis for improving methods in assessment of the nutritional requirements in human subjects. Much of the published data about amino acid metabolism has been reviewed by Irwin and Hegsted (38,39), and several other reviews have concentrated on the elderly as the population group of interest (4–6). Here, a brief summary will be given of some of the major issues and problems regarding quantitative definition of the protein and amino acid requirements in older humans.

Requirements for Indispensable (Essential) Amino Acids

Table 3-10 gives a listing of the nutritionally indispensable amino acids in human nutrition. Compared with studies of amino acid requirements in infants and young adults, there have been few definitive investigations of the essential amino acid requirements in the elderly (see reference 6 for review). The present data base leads to contradictory conclusions; there is wide individual variation among subjects studied and there are significant experimental errors and confounding factors involved in the nitrogen balance technique, which has been used to determine the requirement for specific amino acids (6).

We have explored an alternative approach to the nitrogen (N) balance technique for estimating amino acid requirements in adults, including the elderly. It is based on measurement of the concentration of free amino acids in blood plasma, and we have discussed our observations at length (6). Briefly, however, using this technique, we estimated the tryptophan requirement in healthy, elderly subjects to be approximately 2 mg/kg body weight per day, a value slightly lower than the values of 3 and

Table 3-10. Classification of Amino Acids, as Indispensable or Dispensable Dietary Constituents, According to Their Role in the Maintenance of Nitrogen Equilibrium in Adults

Essential *(Indispensable)*	*Nonessential* *(Dispensable)*
Valine	Glycine
Leucine	Alanine
Isoleucine	Serine
Threonine	Cystine
Methionine	Tyrosine
Phenylalanine	Aspartic acid
Lysine	Glutamic acid
Tryptophan	Proline
Histidine	Arginine
	Citrulline

4 mg/kg determined for young men and children, respectively, by the same plasma amino acid procedure. Similarly, we estimated the threonine requirement to be about 7 mg/kg/day in elderly women, or similar to that for young men. However, in view of the differences in body composition between young adult and elderly individuals, our findings imply that the threonine requirement *per unit of total body protein* may increase with age, because lean body mass is less in proportion to total body weight in the older subject, as compared with young adults. This conclusion also applies to the valine requirement, based again on an interpretation of the plasma valine response curve (see reference 6 for review).

It is evident that information about requirements for individual essential amino acids in the aging human is still fragmentary and that the available data are contradictory. Furthermore, we have also questioned the reliability of the current estimates for healthy adults (40). Thus, an expansion of careful studies of amino acid metabolism and requirements would be highly desirable.

Requirement for Total Nitrogen (Protein)

The minimum physiologic needs for total protein in adult humans have been determined generally using one of two N balance methods (41): (a) the factorial approach and (b) the N balance response curve method to determine directly the intake required to just maintain body N balance.

In the factorial approach, the losses of "obligatory" N via urine and feces are measured and summated, together with additional corrections for N losses via the integument and other minor routes (42). The aim of this method is to determine the total nitrogen loss occurring from the body when the subject receives, for a brief period, a protein-free but otherwise adequate diet. The minimum dietary protein requirement is then computed to be that amount of high-quality protein necesssary just to balance these endogenous N losses. We have compared and contrasted the estimates of protein needs in young adults and elderly subjects as judged by this approach (43,44). It appears that the needs for either age group may not be adequately assessed by this methodology since the levels of total protein intake predicted as being adequate fall a long way below levels that are present in fully adequate but low protein diets (41).

Thus, a more direct method for assessing the minimum physiologic needs for dietary protein should be undertaken and this can be accomplished from the N balance response to graded protein intakes (41). Several recent investigations in the elderly have made an attempt to standardize correlates of nitrogen balance in order to arrive at a reliable estimate of the protein requirement for this age group. We (45) have measured nitrogen balances in response to graded levels of egg protein

Table 3-11. Nitrogen Balances in Elderly Men and Women Given 0.9 g Egg Protein/kg/d for 30 Days*

	Elderly Men		*Elderly Women*	
Number	7		8	
Age (yr)	72–82		74–99	
Wt (kg)	51–89		48–69	
Energy intake (kcal/kg)†	32 ± 3		29 ± 5	
Nitrogen balance‡ (mg N/kg/d)				
days: 6–10	−7.4 ± 3†		−0.8 ± 1.9	
16–20	1.5 ± 3.8			
26–30	0.4 ± 3.4	(3)§	−2.3 ± 2.8	(4)

*Results extracted from Gersovitz et al (47).

†Mean ± SD.

‡Mean ± SEM.

§Number in parentheses indicates number of subjects showing persistent negative balance during last 15 of 30 d.

intake by elderly men and women. However, this N-balance study was based on relatively short dietary periods. Therefore, the conduct of nitrogen balance studies of longer duration seemed desirable in order to assess whether there is a short-term adaptation to a given level of dietary protein intake that may complicate interpretation of N-balance results obtained in relatively brief diet periods. Accordingly, we have conducted a study to evaluate the current recommended daily protein allowance, as proposed by the Dietary Allowances Committee of the U.S. Food and Nutrition Board (46) for older men and women by exploring the response of body protein metabolism to this level of dietary protein during a 30-day metabolic study period. An additional purpose of this investigation concerned the age ranges of the present U.S. dietary protein allowances for older adults, which are presently proposed for those aged 51 years and older without specific allowances for groups within this broad category.

A summary of results for N balances obtained in this study is given in Table 3-11. Our results indicate that 0.8 g egg protein/kg/day may not be sufficient to support an adequate body N balance in many elderly females, even after a 30-day adaptation period (47).

These findings differ from two other recent studies in elderly human subjects. However, in the first of these studies (48), elderly subjects, as well as a control group of young adults, were given an energy intake of 40 kcal/kg/day. This was probably in excess of the actual energy requirements of the older subjects and would have led to an underestimation of protein needs (41). In the second study (49), N equilibrium in elderly males was achieved at an intake of 0.8 g protein/kg body weight, but the subjects had received a protein-free diet for 17 days immediately prior to the test period. Because an initial period of dietary protein deprivation will influence N balance responses when protein is subsequently reincorporated into the diet, it is likely that the body N retention achieved in elderly subjects, in this second study by Zanni et al (49), was probably more favorable than would have occurred in initially well-nourished subjects.

In view of the growing proportion of elderly in populations of technically advanced nations, it would be prudent to improve upon the limited data and state of knowledge concerning protein and amino acid needs for this age group.

Effects of Stressful Stimuli on Protein Requirements

It is important to emphasize that the results of the studies discussed above, concerning protein allowances in the elderly, apply to "healthy" individuals. However, altered gastrointestinal function, the changes in metabolism that accompany aging, and the existence of infections and other chronic diseases all may have a profound influence on the nutritional status and protein requirement of the elderly population. For example, the qualitative effects of acute infection on dietary protein utilization and requirements have been well described (50) for some infections. A listing of characteristics of the metabolic responses to infection is given in Table 3-12. Thus, any infection or other stressful stimulus of physical and psychologic origin results in the development of a negative nitrogen balance through the cumulative effect of several different mechanisms (Table 3-12). Therefore, in Table 3-13, an approximation is

Table 3-12. Characteristics of the Catabolic Response to Infection*

A. Most prominent metabolic response to a generalized febrile infection of any cause.
B. Caused by increased metabolic requirements of body tissues in the presence of a generally inadequate dietary intake
C. Modulated by complex hormonal influences.
D. Consistent features include:
   Onset time following that of fever
   Muscle wasting and weight loss
   Negative balances of nitrogen and other nitracellular elements
   Persistence into convalescence
E. Minimized by effective control of illness
F. Magnified during severe, uncontrolled, complicated, or recurrent illness
G. Followed by wasting and malnutrition if infection becomes chronic

*Based on Beisel (50).

Table 3-13. Protein Needs in Specific Diseases*

1. Normal Adult:
   a. for N equilibrium: 0.55 g/kg, raised to 0.8 g/kg by protein quality correction (90%).
   b. customary intake: 1–2 g/kg.
2. Metabolic response to severe burn injury and trauma:
   a. Acute phase: 2–4 g/kg plus energy.
   b. Convalescence: 2+ g/kg.
3. Malabsorption and GI diseases:
   a. Malabsorption syndrome: 1 g/kg.
   b. Ulcerative colitis: 1–1.4 g/kg.†
   c. Ileocecostomy: 1–1.4 g/kg.†
4. Liver disease:
   a. Acute hepatic encephalopathy; very low.‡
   b. Recovered encephalopathy: 1–1.5 g/kg.
   c. Chronic encephalopathy: 0.5 g/kg.‡
5. Renal disease
   a. Uremia: 0.5 g/kg‡ (ketoanalogs).
   b. Nephrosis: 1–1.4 g/kg.†
6. Malignant disease:
   Increased protein and energy.

*From Munro and Young (51).

†In each condition, losses of protein can double minimal requirement.

‡Intake restricted on clinical grounds.

given of the changes in protein needs in some major disease states and, as shown here, the dietary protein requirement may be increased twofold. This topic deserves much more exploration, particularly in reference to a more adequate definition of the nutritional and dietary needs of the elderly population.

Summary

In this review some aspects of body protein and amino acid metabolism during aging, with particular reference to human subjects, have been explored. There is a slow loss of total body protein with aging, caused largely by a reduction in the size of the muscle skeletal mass. These changes are accompanied by a shift in the overall pattern of whole body protein synthesis and breakdown, with muscle mass being estimated to account for about 30% of whole body protein turnover in the young adult, as compared with a lower value of about 20% or less in the elderly subject. Studies on albumin metabolism suggest that the regulation of albumin synthesis is altered with advancing old age in the human. Investigations on the dynamic aspects of metabolism of specific amino acids are limited, but those currently available do not yet reveal any major differences between young adult and older individuals when they are studied in the postabsorptive phases of amino acid metabolism. Additional investigations of the effects of various stimuli, especially nutritional factors, in young adult and elderly subjects should be undertaken to better characterize the impact of aging on the economy of human amino acid metabolism.

The determination of requirements for individual essential amino acids and for total protein has also been discussed, and it is evident that the data are limited and often contradictory. Elderly individuals are more likely to be affected by various biologic, environmental, and social factors that would tend to increase protein needs above those for younger adults. The reduction in energy intake, together with its possible consequences for reduced dietary protein utilization, will also tend to increase the protein need of elderly subjects, relative to that for active young adults. We have concluded that for food planning purposes, an appropriate protein allowance would be 12% to 14% of the total energy intake for the elderly age group (47,51).

References

1. Richardson A, Birchenall-Sparks MC: Age-related changes in protein synthesis. *Rev Biol Res Aging* 1983; 1:255–273.
2. Richardson A: The relationship between aging and protein synthesis, in Florini JR (ed): *Handbook of Biochemistry of Aging.* Florida, CRC Press, pp 79–101.
3. Rothstein M: *Biochemical Approaches to Aging.* New York, Academic Press, 1982, p 314.
4. Young VR, Uauy R, Winterer JC, et al: Protein metabolism and needs in elderly people, in Rockstein M, Sussman ML, (eds): *Nutrition, Longevity and Aging.* New York, Academic Press, 1976, pp 67–102.
5. Young VR, Winterer JC, Munro HN, Scrimshaw NS: Muscle and whole body protein metabolism with special reference to man, in Elias MF, Eleftheriou BE, Elias PK (eds): *Special Review of Experimental Aging Research.* Bar Harbor, Maine, EAR, 1976.
6. Young VR, Gersovitz M, Munro HN: Human aging in protein and amino acid metabolism and implications for protein and amino acid requirements, in Moment GB, (ed): *Nutritional Approaches to Aging Research.* Florida, CRC Press, 1982, pp 47–81.
7. Bolla RJ, Greenblatt C: Age-related changes in rat liver total protein and transferrin synthesis. *Age* 1982; 5:72–79.
8. Cook JR, Beutow DE: Decreased protein synthesis by polysomes, tRNA and aminocyl-tRNA synthetases isolated from senescent rat liver. *Mech Ageing Dev* 1981; 17:41–52.
9. Coniglio JJ, Liu DSH, Richardson A: A comparison of protein synthesis by liver parenchymal cells isolated from Fischer F344 rats of various ages. *Mech Age Dev* 1979; II:77–90.

10. Ekstrom ER, Liu DSH, Richardson A: Changes in brain protein synthesis during the life span of male Fischer rats. *Gerontology* 1980; 26:121–128.
11. Kim SK, Weinhold PA, Calkins DW, et al: Comparative studies of the age-related changes in protein synthesis in rat pancreas and parotid gland. *Exp Gerontol* 1981; 16:91–99.
12. Van Bezooijen CFA, Grell R, Knook DL: The effect of age on protein synthesis by isolated liver parenchymal cells. *Mech Ageing Dev* 1977; 6:293.
13. Pluskal MG, Moreyra M, Burini RC, et al: Protein synthesis studies in skeletal muscle of aging rats I. Alterations in nitrogen composition and protein synthesis using a crude polyribosome and pH5 enzyme system. *J Gerontol* 1984; (in press).
14. Burini RC, Pluskal MG, Wei I, et al: Protein synthesis studies in skeletal muscle of aging rats II. In vitro studies with 0.5M potassium chloride washed polyribosomes. *J Gerontol* 1984; (in press).
15. Waterlow JC, Garlick PJ, Millward DJ: Protein Turnover, in *Mammalian Tissues and in the Whole Body*. Amsterdam and New York, Elsevier North-Holland, 1978.
16. Allen TH, Anderson EC, Langham WH: Total body potassium and gross body composition in relation to age. *J Gerontol* 1960; 15:358.
17. Forbes GB, Reina JC: Adult lean body mass declines with age: Some longitudinal observations. *Metabolism* 1970; 19:653–663.
18. Steen B, Isaksson B, Svanborg A: Body composition at 70 and 75 years of age: A longitudinal population study. *J Clin Exp Gerontol* 1979; 1:185–200.
19. Gutmann E, Hanzlikova V: Motor unit in old age. *Nature* 1966; 209:921.
20. Rowe RWD: The effect of senility on skeletal muscles in the mouse. *Exp Gerontol* 1969; 4:119.
21. Neumaster TD, Ring GC: Creatinine excretion and its relation to whole body potassium and muscle mass in inbred rats. *J Gerontol* 1965; 20:379.
22. McCafferty WG, Edington DW: Skeletal muscle and organ weights of aged and trained male rats. *Gerontologia* 1974; 20:44.
23. Korenchevsky V: *Physiological and Pathological Aging*. New York, Hafner, 1961.
24. Graystone JE: Creatinine excretion during growth, in Cheek DB (ed): *Human Growth*. Philadelphia: Lea & Febiger, 1968 pp 182–197.
25. Rowe JW, Andres R, Robin JD, et al: The effect of age on creatinine clearance in men: a cross-sectional and longitudinal study. *J Gerontol* 1976; 31:155.
26. Uauy R, Winterer JC, Bilmazes C, et al: The changing pattern of whole body protein metabolism in aging humans. *J Gerontol* 1978; 33:663–671.
27. Robert JJ, Bier D, Schoeller D, et al: Effects of intravenous glucose on whole body leucine dynamics, studied with 1-^{13} C-leucine, in healthy young and elderly adults. *J Gerontol* 1984; (in press).
28. Garlick PJ, Clugston GA, Swick RW, Waterlow JC: Diurnal pattern of protein and energy metabolism in man. *Am J Clin Nutr* 1980; 33:1983–1986.
29. Motil KJ, Matthews DE, Bier DM, et al: Whole body leucine and lysine metabolism: Response to dietary protein intake in young men. *Am J Physiol* 1981; 240:E712–E721.
30. Picou D, Taylor-Roberts T: The measurement of total protein synthesis and

catabolism and nitrogen turnover in infants in different nutritional states and receiving different amounts of dietary protein. *Clin Sci* 1969; 36:283–296.

31. Winterer J, Steffee WP, Perera WDA, et al: Whole body protein turnover in aging man. *Exp Gerontol* 1976; 11:79–87.
32. Golden MHN, Waterlow JC: Total protein synthesis in elderly people: a comparison of results with ^{15}N-glycine and (^{14}C-) leucine. *Clin Sci* 1977; 53:227–238.
33. Young VR, Munro HN: N$^{\tau}$-methylhistidine (3-methylhistidine) and muscle protein turnover: an overview. *Fed Proc* 1978; 37:2291–2300.
34. Cahill GF, Jr: Starvation in man. *N Engl J Med* 1970; 282:668–675.
35. Young VR: The role of skeletal and cardiac muscle in the regulation of protein metabolism, in Munro HN (ed): *Mammalian Protein Metabolism.* New York, Academic Press, 1970; pp 585–674.
36. Gersovitz M, Munro HN, Udall J, et al: Albumin synthesis in young and elderly subjects using a new stable isotope methodology: response to level of protein intake. *Metabolism* 1980; 29:1075–1086.
37. Munro HN, Hubert C, Baliga BS: Regulation of protein synthesis in relation to amino acid supply. A review, in Rothschild MA, Oratz M, Schreiber S (eds): *Alcohol and Abnormal Protein Synthesis.* New York, Pergamon Press, 1975, pp 33–66.
38. Irwin MI, Hegsted DM: A conspectus of research on amino acid requirements of man. *J Nutr* 1971; 101:539–566.
39. Irwin MI, Hegsted DM: A conspectus of research on protein requirements of man. *J Nutr* 1971; 101:385–430.
40. Young VR, Meguid M, Mederith C, et al: Recent developments in knowledge of human amino acid requirements, in Stephen JML, Waterlow JC, (eds): *Nitrogen Metabolism in Man.* London, Applied Science, 1981, pp 133–153.
41. Young VR, Scrimshaw NS: Nutritional evaluation of proteins and protein requirements, in Milner M, Scrimshaw NS, Wang DIC, (eds): *Protein Resources and Technology: Status and Research Needs.* AVI, 1978, pp 136–173.
42. FAO/WHO. *Energy and Protein Requirements.* World Health Organization Tech. Rept. Ser. 522. Geneva, Switzerland, WHO, 1973.
43. Nancy R, Scrimshaw NS, Rand WM, et al: Human protein requirements in obligatory urinary and fecal nitrogen losses and the factorial estimation of protein needs in elderly men. *J Nutr* 1978; 108:97–103.
44. Scrimshaw NS, Perera WDA, Young VR: Protein requirements of man: obligatory urinary and fecal nitrogen losses in elderly women. *J Nutr* 1976; 106:665–670.
45. Uauy R, Scrimshaw NS, Young VR: Human protein requirements: Nitrogen balance response to graded levels of egg protein in elderly men and women. *Am J Clin Nutr* 1978; 31:779–785.
46. NAS/NRC: *Recommended Dietary Allowances,* ed 9, National Research Council. Washington, DC National Academy of Sciences, 1980.
47. Gersovitz M, Motil KJ, Munro HN, et al: Human protein requirements: assessment of the adequacy of the current recommended dietary allowance for dietary protein in elderly men and women. *Am J Clin Nutr* 1982; 35:6–14.
48. Cheng AHR, Gomez A, Bergan JG, et al: Comparative nitrogen balance study between young and aged adults using three levels of protein intake

from a combination of wheat-soy-milk mixture. *Am J Clin Nutr* 1978; 31:12–22.

49. Zanni E, Calloway DH, Zezulka AY: Protein requirements of elderly men. *J Nutr* 1979; 109:513–524.
50. Beisel WR: Infectious diseases, in Schneider H, Anderson CE, Coursin DB, Schneider H,(eds): *Nutritional Support of Medical Practice.* New York, Harper & Row, 1977, pp 350–366.
51. Munro HN, Young VR: Protein metabolism and requirements, in Extam-Smith AN, Caird FI (eds): *Metabolic and Nutritional Disorders in the Elderly.* Bristol, England, John Wright & Sons, 1980, pp 13–25.

4

Atherosclerosis and Plasma Lipid Transport with Aging

Gustav Schonfeld

Strong associations between coronary risk and lipoprotein concentrations in plasma have been well documented in several large epidemiologic studies (1). Low density lipoprotein (LDL) cholesterol concentrations are positively correlated with coronary risk, whereas high density lipoprotein (HDL) cholesterol concentrations are negatively correlated. Total plasma triglyceride or very low density lipoprotein (VLDL) cholesterol levels also are associated with coronary risk when the data are analyzed as univariate correlations. However, when multivariate analyses are performed, the association is lost in many, but not all, studies. Nevertheless, in spite of statistical ambiguities, professionals who deal with patients have interpreted the epidemiologic results as demonstrating that hypertriglyceridemia does signal the presence of increased coronary risk. If the question is examined from the other side and the prevalence of hyperlipoproteinemia among survivors of myocardial infarction or among individuals with angiographically significant atherosclerotic coronary disease is ascertained, a sizable proportion are found to have one or another form of hyperlipoproteinemia, and lesion severity is correlated with lipoprotein levels (2,3). Thus, epidemiologic evidence strongly supports a role for lipoproteins in atherosclerosis.

The other types of evidence linking lipoproteins with atherosclerosis are genetic and experimental. It is clear that several of the familial dyslipoproteinemias, including familial hypercholesterolemia and familial combined hyperlipidemia, are associated with premature severe vascular disease (4). LDL concentrations in plasma may be high and HDL concentrations low in both of these conditions. On the other hand, having high plasma levels of HDL, as in familial hyperalphalipoproteinemia, or low levels of LDL, as in familiar hypobetalipoproteinemia, seem to be protective and lead to longevity (5). Patients having familial dysbetalipoproteinemia, which is associated with unusual forms of VLDL in plasma, also clearly stand at an increased risk for decreasing atherosclerotic vascular disease. Experimental studies carried out in many species of animals have established a strong connection between dietary lipids, plasma lipoproteins, and arterial lesions. In these species diets produce both qualitative and quantitative changes in plasma lipoproteins, and concomitantly lesions appear in the arterial wall. Regression of both the hyperlipidemia and the lesions occurs when the high-fat, high-cholesterol "atherogenic" diets are discontinued.

Aging, too, is a risk factor for the development of coronary heart disease, ie, older people die at a greater rate than younger people and the elderly die more frequently of atherosclerotic vascular disease (1). It is likely that aging-related changes in several body organ systems are responsible. The development of arterial lesions and the associated clinical manifestations, such as angina pectoris or myocardial infarction, involve several factors including (a) the systems responsible for the absorption of dietary fats; (b) the production of lipoproteins and the "remodeling" of lipoproteins in plasma; (c) the cellular and fibrous elements of the arterial wall; and (d) the blood platelets and coagulation system. The major focus here is on lipoproteins.

Nomenclature and Composition of Lipoproteins

The lipoproteins that circulate in plasma have been classified by two commonly used nomenclatures, based on an operational method that separates lipoproteins from each other (Table 4-1). Electrophoresis yields bands of lipoproteins that migrate to the α_1, α_2, and β positions and a class that remains at the origin. These electrophoretic bands correspond to the α, pre-β, and β-lipoproteins and the chylomicrons respectively (6,7).

Another technique for separating lipoproteins is flotation in the preparative ultracentrifuge. Since lipoproteins contain both lipids and proteins, they are less dense and more buoyant than the rest of the plasma proteins; therefore, lipoproteins float in a gravitational field under conditions where lipid-free plasma proteins sediment. The rate of flotation depends on the size and density of the particles: large, less dense lipoprotein particles float more rapidly than small dense particles. Using this principle, lipoproteins of various densities can be made to float by adjusting appropriately the densities of the solvent (plasma) in which the lipoproteins are suspended.

Table 4-1. Lipoproteins: Nomenclature, Flotation Rates and Sizes

Ultracentrifugal Designation	*Density Ranges*	*Electrophoretic Mobility*	*Flotation Rates*	*Diameters (Å)*
			S°_{f}	
Chylomicrons	<1.006	Origin	400–10	750–12,000
α-VLDL	<1.006	α_2, pre-β	60–400	500–700
β-VLDL*	<1.006	β	60–100	500–600
IDL*	1.006–1.019	Between β and pre-β	12–60	300–500
LDL	1.019–1.063	β	0–12	225
Lp(a)	1.050–1.080	Pre-β	0–2	180
			f° 1.20	
HDL_2	1.063–1.125	α_1	3.5–9	100
HDL_3	1.020–1.090	α_1	0–2	150
HDL_c (HDL_1)	1.060–1.090	Between α_1 and α_2		200

*Present in plasma of experimental animals fed high fat–high cholesterol diets and in plasma of some subjects with various dyslipoproteinemias; not usually found in normal fasting plasma.

Although electrophoresis separates various lipoproteins from each other, it does not separate them from other plasma proteins of like electrophoretic mobility. On the other hand, ultracentrifugation does both; and therefore, it is the preferred procedure when the isolation and subsequent characterization of lipoproteins is desired. When ultracentrifugally isolated, chylomicrons remain at the origin, HDL migrate to the α_1 position, and LDL to the β position. Most VLDL migrate to the α_2 or pre-β position. These are called α-VLDL. But in some cases VLDL can migrate to the β position. These are called β-VLDL and are distinct from LDL (8). A minor class of lipoproteins, called Lp(a), is isolated by d 1.050 to 1.080 but migrates in the pre-β position. Since Lp(a) sediments at d 1.006 when other pre-β-lipoproteins float, it also has been called "sinking pre-β-lipoprotein" (9). The comparison of the ultracentrifugal and electrophoretic nomenclatures is given in Table 4-1, along with physical parameters derived by analytic ultracentrifugation and electron microscopy (6,7). Other lipoproteins present in small quantities or under special circumstances also are listed in Table 4-1. These latter lipoproteins are isolated by combinations of techniques, including ultracentrifugation, electrophoresis, and column chromatography. Lipid and protein compositions of lipoproteins are found in Table 4-2. Note that all lipoproteins contain all of the major classes of lipids but in differing proportions. All lipoproteins also contain proteins, but the proteins are more characteristic of individual lipoprotein classes (Table 4-3). The densities of lipoproteins are inversely related to their content of lipids relative to proteins, ie. the greater the lipid content, the less dense are the particles.

Apoprotein Chemistry

Originally apoproteins were named by their discoverers, who used a variety of designations based on operational criteria such as relative elution positions on column chromatography (eg D_1 to D_4 for the several apoCs), abundance of a given amino acid in the protein (eg, arginine-rich protein for apoE), or the identity of the amino acid at the carboxyl terminus (eg, R-gln for apoAI). In recent years the ABC nomenclature proposed by Alaupovic (10–12) has been adopted by most but not all workers.

The amino acid sequences of several apoproteins are known. ApoAI has a molecular weight (mol wt) of ~28,000; it normally exists in two forms, which differ slightly in their isoelectric points (13). ApoAII (mol wt ~17,500 (14) and apoAIV (mol ~46,000) (15) appear to be single proteins. Initially, apoB (mol wt ~250,000) was thought to be a single large protein, but recently it was found that apoB may consist of four proteins (16), all of which may share some structural features. The amino acid sequences of apoB are unknown. There are three apoCs: apoCI, CII, and

Table 4-2. Compositions of Lipoproteins

	Protein	*Phospholipid*	*Cholesterol Ester (% of Mass)*	*Free Cholesterol*	*Triglyceride*
Chylomicrons	2	3	3	2	90
α-VLDL	6	14	16	4	60
β-VLDL	12	15	32	16	25
IDL	18	22	32	8	20
LDL	21	22	42	8	7
Lp(a)	21	20	45	8	6
HDL_2	44	26	20	5	5
HDL_3	52	28	15	3	2
HDL_c (HDL_1)	19	43	—	37 —	1

Table 4-3. The Apoprotein Contents of Lipoproteins*

	ApoAI	*ApoAII*	*ApoAIV*	*ApoB*	*ApoCI*	*ApoCII*	$ApoCIII\frac{1}{0\text{–}2}$	*ApoD*	*ApoE*
Mesenteric lymph chylomicrons	15	5	10	10	—	55	—	1–2	4
Plasma chylomicrons	TR	TR	TR	25	—	65	—	—	10
Mesenteric lymph VLDL	16	5	—	10	—	35	—	—	6
Plasma VLDL	TR	TR	—	40	5	8	32	—	15
Plasma LDL	—	—	—	>95	TR	TR	TR	—	TR
Intestinal lymph HDL	65	~5	~5						15–25
Hepatic perfusate HDL	5–10	~5	4	10–20	—	10–15	—	—	17
Plasma HDL_1 (or HDL_c)	20	>5	10	—	—	10	—	—	50–60
Plasma HDL_2	70	10	TR	—	—	10	—	10	TR
ApoE HDL_2	20	2		—	—	10	—	—	60
ApoAI HDL_2	70	10	—	—	—	20	—	10	TR
Plasma HDL_2	55	25	—	—	—	10	—	10	TR

*Percent of total protein.

CIII. The amino acid sequences of each apoC are known. These are distinctive proteins with distinctive functions. ApoCI is a single protein (mol wt ~7,000) (17). ApoCII (mol wt ~9,000) (18) exists in two varieties distinguishable on isoelectric focusing as apoCII$_1$ and apoCII$_2$ (19). The chemical basis for the slight differences in isoelectric points are unknown. ApoCIII (mol wt~9,000) (20) is found in at least three isoelectric forms apoCIII$_{0,1,2,}$ etc. The differences are due to the sialic acid contents of the protein. ApoCIII$_0$ has none, apoCIII$_1$ has 1 mol of sialic acid per mole of protein, apoCIII$_2$ has 2 mol, etc (21). The degree of sialylation can be altered by dietary or hormonal manipulations (22). ApoD is a single protein (11,12). ApoE (mol wt ~35,000) (23), as will be seen, has two sources of heterogeneity. One is genetic, caused by substitutions in the primary amino acid sequence, and another results from varying degrees of sialylation (24,25).

Lipoprotein Structure

Most of the mature lipoproteins that circulate in plasma appear as spheres under the electron microscope (7). Chylomicrons and VLDL are secreted as spheres and HDL is secreted as a disc, which is converted to a sphere in plasma (36,37). The outer surface regions of lipoprotein particles are formed by hydrophilic molecules, the phospholipids, and apoproteins, while the inner or core regions contain the hydrophobic cholesterol esters and triglycerides. Unesterified cholesterol is found in the region between the surface and the core (27).

Apoprotein Functions

Apoproteins perform a variety of important metabolic functions related to specific domains on the three-dimensional structure of the individual proteins (Table 4-4). Since all apoproteins bind to lipids, they share one structural feature: domains containing amphipathic helices (28). The amino acid sequences of these regions are such that when the proteins fold into helices, the hydrophobic amino acids form one side or face of the helix and the polar amino acids form the other face. This accounts for the amphipathic designation. The hydrophobic face of the helix is thought to interact with the hydrophobic, fatty acid portion of phospholipids and the hydrophilic face with the polar region of the phospholipids.

In addition to the lipid-binding amphipathic helices, other functional domains have been identified on some apoproteins. For example, apoCII, which activates the enzyme lipoprotein lipase (see below), contains a helical region that enables the apoCII to interact with the lipopro-

Table 4-4. Metabolic Roles of Apolipoproteins

Name of Apolipoprotein	*Lipoprotein Association*	*Concentration in Plasma*	*Metabolic Role*
AI	HDL, CM*	110–120	LCAT activator
AII	HDL, CM	25–50	Unknown
AIV	CM, HDL, D<1.21	8	Unknown
B-100 74 26	VLDL	90	Transports lipids from liver as a structural part of VLDL, β-VLDL, and LDL; recognized by cellular LDL receptors
B-48	CM	5	Transports lipids from enterocytes of gut as CM
CI	CM, VLDL, HDL	4	? Activates LCAT
CII	CM, VLDL, HDL	4	Activator of lipoprotein lipase
$CIII_{0-2}$	CM, VLDL, HDL	12	Inhibits recognition of apoE by cellular lipoprotein receptors; inhibits activation of lipoprotein lipase by apoCII.
D	HDL, D<1.21	8	Transfers cholesterol esters between lipoproteins as part of apoAI-D-LCAT "transfer complex"
E	CM, VLDL, IDL, HDL	5	Recognized by cellular LDL and apoE receptors
Transfer proteins	HDL, D<1.21	—	Several proteins that transfer cholesterol esters, phospholipids, and triglycerides between lipoproteins in plasma.

*CM = chylomicrons.

teins, and it also contains another domain where apoCII interacts with the enzyme (29). ApoE, which serves as a recognition marker for the uptake of lipoproteins by several cell types, also contains at least two, and perhaps more, functional domains: an amphipathic helix for interacting with lipids on lipoproteins, a domain that contains the signal by means of which apoE is recognized by the apoE receptor on hepatocytes, and perhaps other domains for the recognition of apoE by the apoB,E receptors (30,31). Abnormalities in lipoprotein transport occur when the structures of critical domains of apoproteins or enzymes are altered by substitutions or deletions of amino acids.

Cellular Receptors

In addition to apoproteins, cellular receptors also are important in lipoprotein metabolism (Table 4-5). The apoB,E receptor is an intrinsic protein found in small coated pits in membranes of most mammalian cells (32). Its mol wt is ~164,000 (33). The protein specifically binds lipoproteins that contain either apoB or apoE. Binding is followed by the process of endocytosis, which internalizes the receptor–lipoprotein complex. Endocytotic vesicles fuse with lysosomes where the various components of lipoprotein particles are degraded, eg, apoproteins are hydrolyzed down to their amino acids and cholesterol esters are hydrolyzed to unesterified cholesterol and free fatty acids. The unesterified cholesterol finds its way to the microsomes, the site of endogenous cholesterol synthesis, and there inhibits further cholesterol synthesis. The apoE receptor is found on hepatocytes, where it binds chylomicron remnants (34). Receptors for β-VLDL (35) and the chemically altered lipoproteins are found on macrophages. The expression of the apoB,E receptor is under metabolic control. When cells contain adequate quantities of cholesterol, small numbers of receptors are expressed. Cells grown in the absence of exogenous cholesterol express large numbers of receptors. The other receptors do not seem to be under similar feedback regulation by cholesterol.

Relevant Enzymes

Enzymes also play critical roles in lipoprotein metabolism (Table 4-5). Lipoprotein lipase (LPL) is synthesized in virtually all parenchymal tissue (kidney, skeletal and heart muscle, adipose tissue). It is secreted by cells and finds its way by unknown mechanisms to the endothelial cells of the local capillary beds, where it is bound to glycoseaminoglycans located on

Table 4-5. Metabolic Roles of Cellular Lipoprotein Receptors and Enzymes

Lipoprotein Receptor	*Cell Type*	*Function*
B,E	All cells	Endocytosis of apoB and apoE containing lipoproteins; ie remnants, β-VLDL, IDL, LDL
E	Hepatocyte	Endocytosis of chylomicron remnants, β-VLDL, apoE-HDL
β-VLDL	Macrophage	Endocytosis of β-VLDL
Scavenger	Macrophage	Endocytosis of a variety of negatively charged molecules including altered LDL (eg, fructosyl-, malonimyl-, acetyl-LDL)
Dextran SO_4-LDL		Endocytosis of Dextran SO_4-LDL complexes
Enzyme	*Site of Activity*	*Catalytic Function*
Lipoprotein lipase (LPL)	Endothelial cells in all vascular beds	Hydrolyzes CM and VLDL TG to FFA, diglycerides, monoglycerides, and glycerol; hydrolyzes CM- and VLDL-phospholipids
Hepatic triglyceride lipase (HTGL)	Endothelial cells in hepatic and adrenal vascular beds	Hydrolyzes β-VLDL-triglycerides, IDL-triglycerides, and HDL-phospholipids
Lecithin cholesterol acyl transferase (LCAT)	Intravascular plasma	Esterifies cholesterol in plasma by transferring fatty acids from phospholipids to unesterified cholesterol. Phospholipids are converted to lysophospholipids in the process

the luminal surfaces of the cells. Heparin causes the release of the bound enzyme into plasma and the appearance of "postheparin lipase." The enzyme has a mol wt of ~65,000 and contains carbohydrate (36). Its synthesis requires the presence of insulin. LPL catalyzes the hydrolysis of triglyceride emulsions to glycerol and free fatty acids at low rates. The addition of apoCII to such emulsions accelerates the rates of hydrolysis ~20-fold (37). It is suggested that apoCII, interacting as it does with both the enzyme and the emulsion, orients the enzyme so as to assure optimum alignment between the catalytic site of the enzyme and its lipid substrate. Apparently, in the absence of apoCII, the orientation is random and catalytic efficiency is greatly impaired. In vivo it is thought that LPL catalyzes the hydrolysis of sufficient amounts of chylomicron and VLDL triglycerides to convert these large nascent particles to their remnants.

Another enzyme released into plasma by heparin is hepatic triglyceride lipase (HTGL), which has been found both in hepatic and adrenal membranes (38). HTGL and LPL differ from each other at least in their carbohydrate compositions (36). One current concept is that HTGL continues the work of LPL by catalyzing the hydrolysis of the triglyceride remnants to the point where ~80% to 90% of the triglycerides are gone. Another concept holds that HTGL hydrolyzes the fatty acid–glycerol ester bonds of phospholipids in HDL and thus may be instrumental in the interconversions or catabolism of HDL (57).

Lecithin cholesterol acyl transferase (LCAT) has been highly purified from human plasma. Its mol wt is ~70,000 (39). This enzyme is secreted by the liver into plasma where it catalyzes the transfer of a fatty acid from the 2-carbon position of the glycerol in phosphatidylcholine to the 3-carbon position in cholesterol. Thus the enzyme has both hydrolase and ligase activities. The preferred substrate for LCAT is nascent HDL, the disclike structure that contains primarily phospholipids, small amounts of unesterified cholesterol, apoAI, and apoE (40). LCAT activity is essential in converting nascent HDL to the mature spherical HDL that circulates in normal plasma.

Lipoprotein Metabolism

Chylomicrons and Chylomicron Remnants

Dietary triglycerides and phospholipids are partially hydrolyzed in the lumen of the gut and are absorbed into enterocytes along with cholesterol. There, the lipids are reesterified and assembled with several specific apoproteins (apos B,AI, and AIV) into chylomicron particles, which are secreted into the lacteals of the lamina propria (41). Intestinal lymph, containing chylomicrons, is collected in the cysterna chyli whence it enters the venous system via the thoracic lymphatic duct. As chylomicrons move from lymph to venous plasma, they undergo a series of changes (Fig. 4-1). First, they acquire apoC and apoE by transfer, probably from the HDL already in plasma (42). Then triglycerides and phospholipids are hydrolyzed by LPL, the enzyme located on the surfaces of endothelial cells of arteries and capillary beds (43). The enzyme interacts with the apoCII on the chylomicron surface and thus becomes properly oriented for optimal "solid phase" catalytic activity (37) (Fig. 4-1). The resultng lipolytic products, free fatty acids, glycerol, and lysophospholipids, are taken up by tissues as sources of energy or for cell membrane synthesis.

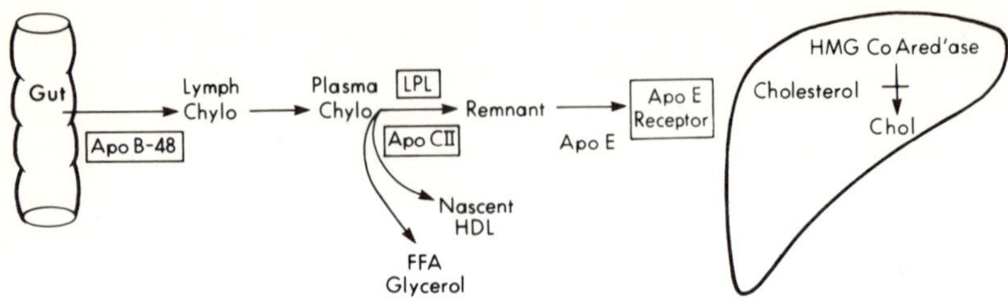

Figure 4-1. Metabolism of chylomicrons. Depicted are the secretion of chylomicron particles from gut, the intravascular events leading to the formation of chylomicron remnants, and the uptake of remnants by the liver via the apoE receptor (see text for details).

Along with triglycerides and phospholipids, chylomicrons also lose some cholesterol, and apo's AI, AIV, and C, but apoB is retained by the particles. Phospholipids and proteins are lost as complexes that have the appearance of lipid bilayer discs under the electron microscope, and are thought to be one of the precursors of plasma HDL (44). Therefore, these discs are called "nascent" HDL. (The conversion of nascent to "mature" HDL is described below.) The net result of the intravascular catalysis and the movement of lipids and apoproteins is the conversion of chylomicrons to chylomicron remnants, which are smaller than chylomicrons in size and relatively enriched in cholesterol and apoproteins.

Liver parenchymal cells possess on their surfaces specific receptors that "recognize" apoE on chylomicron remnants (Table 4-5) (34). This allows circulating remnants, as they are generated, to be removed from circulation by the liver via receptor-mediated endocytotic mechanisms (45). ApoCIII seems to inhibit remnant removal (46). An unknown proportion of remnants also may be removed via the "scavenger pathway" by macrophage cells, which are present in many tissues including arterial walls. These scavenger cells recognize a variety of altered lipoproteins via at least two separate receptors (47). The overloading of scavenger cells with lipoproteins results in the production of foam cells, which, if located in arterial walls, may represent the initial lesions of atherosclerosis.

In sum, chylomicrons deliver a large proportion of their dietary triglyceride components to a variety of tissues, whereas some triglyceride components and most dietary cholesterol wind up in the liver, transported there via chylomicron remnants. In liver, cholesterol can be used for maintenance of hepatocyte membranes and for bile acid production. Triglycerides and cholesterol also may be reexported in VLDL particles (see below). Hepatocytes do synthesize their own cholesterol, but the rate of synthesis is regulated by negative feedback mechanisms. The greater the amount of dietary cholesterol delivered by chylomicron remnants, the less cholesterol is synthesized.

α and β VLDL and LDL

In a fashion analogous to chylomicron production, VLDL is assembled in liver from lipids and apos B,E, and C (48). The lipids used in VLDL assembly are derived either from plasma lipoproteins (eg, chylomicron remnants), from free fatty acid–albumin complexes circulating in blood, or from lipids synthesized within hepatocytes (49). The VLDL secreted under ordinary conditions has α_2 migration on electrophoresis and may be called α-VLDL. VLDL, following its secretion into blood, again in analogy with chylomicrons (Fig. 4-1), undergoes a series of changes, resulting in the acquisition of apoC, the liberation of free fatty acids and glycerol, and the subsequent losses of phospholipids and apos C and E (50,51). Phospholipids and apoE are lost as discs, ie, nascent HDL. ApoB is retained with the VLDL particles. The operation of these processes in plasma gradually transforms α-VLDL to VLDL remnants, which behave as β-VLDL and IDL, and finally LDL.

Virtually all cells express receptors on their surfaces, which recognize apos B and E (38). Thus, the smaller lipoproteins generated from nascent VLDL are taken up by a variety of cells throughout the body including the liver itself (52), resulting in the intracellular delivery of cholesterol, which is used for membrane assembly in all cells and for corticosteroid or sex steroid synthesis in adrenals and gonads (53). As is true for liver, other cells also can synthesize their own cholesterol, and the rate of cholesterol synthesis is regulated by the availability of exogenous cholesterol. The amount delivered via LDL probably is sufficient to make LDL-cholesterol the most important source of cellular cholesterol for most cells. In the fasted state in normal subjects, chylomicron and VLDL remnants are present in very low concentrations, but under certain dietary conditions, and in unusual individuals, they may accumulate in plasma. The presence of these particles (remnants, β-VLDL, IDL) in plasma is defined as "dysbetalipoproteinemia." Under other conditions, when LDL clearance from plasma may be slowed, LDL protein may become chemically modified either within the circulation or in the arterial wall. Remnants and modified lipoproteins can be removed from biologic fluids via the scavenger pathway, and thus they may contribute to atherogenesis (54).

High Density Lipoproteins

As noted above, nascent HDL particles arise from the intravascular metabolism of chylomicrons and VLDL, and in addition, enterocytes and hepatocytes also secrete nascent HDL directly (26). Thus, nascent HDL originate from several sources. The conversion of nascent to mature HDL in plasma occurs by a process that involves the transport of cholesterol away from cells.

As cell membranes or senescent cells are replaced, their unesterified cholesterol components are picked up by circulating apoAI-containing lipoprotein complexes (55). One hypothesis proposes that the complex consists of apoAI, the enzyme lecithin-cholesterol acyl transferase (LCAT), and cholesterol exchange proteins, eg, apoD (56). The apoAI serves as cholesterol acceptor, LCAT catalyzes the esterification of unesterified cholesterol, and the cholesteryl ester transfer proteins facilitate the transfer of the newly formed cholesteryl esters to nascent HDL (56). Since cholesteryl esters are hydrophobic, they enter the hydrophobic inside "core" region of the lipid bilayer, expanding it—much as a collapsed balloon is expanded by air—until the flat discs become spheres (57). Unesterified cholesterol also may be transported out of cells by an apoE–phospholipid complex that is found in peripheral lymph and is probably secreted by a variety of cells. These complexes also are converted to mature HDL via the LCAT pathway. Since nascent HDL particles originating from intestine contain primarily apoAI (26), and those from liver and peripheral tissues contain mostly apoE, mature HDL also are heterogenous in their apoprotein compositions.

Mature HDL are removed from the circulation by liver via apoE and non-apoE receptors (45). Thus is cholesterol transported from peripheral to hepatic cells, whence it is excreted into bile. This "reverse cholesterol transport" provides a mechanism for the removal of cholesterol, which arises from cellular membrane turnover and cell death. Were the cholesterol not removed, increasing amounts of cholesterol crystals would accumulate all over the body with advancing age.

Atherosclerosis and Lipoproteins

One concept of atherogenesis widely held at the present time postulates that atherogenesis begins with an injury to the inner endothelial surface of the vessel wall. In response to the injury, cellular proliferation occurs along with some fibrous deposition and the injured vessel is repaired. Gradually the proliferated cells and fiber accumulated during healing disappear, the vessel wall is remodeled to resemble its former self, and no permanent lesion results. But if the injury is severe, recurrent, or chronic or if the cells and fibers do not regress, a permanent lesion may result (58,59). Mechanical, immunologic, and chemical injuries, among others, have been implicated in the initiation of atherosclerosis. Hyperlipoproteinemia appears among the chemical group of injurious agents. Injuries produced in animals with low plasma lipid levels tend to produce flat fibrotic lesions, while similar injuries in hyperlipidemic animals result in more complex lesions containing both intracellular and interstitial lipids (60,61). Thus, in addition to being implicated as one initiating agent among many, hyperlipidemia (62) also may serve to retard regression and therefore compound any injuries due to other causes. Hyperlipidemia consists of changes both in the plasma concentrations and structures of lipoproteins (63). The subtle structural changes may be detectable only by immunochemical or biologic assays (64,65), but frequently the result is that the lipoproteins are more easily taken up by cells (66). If sufficient lipid is taken up, the cells become lipid-laden foam cells—a frequent feature of atherosclerotic lesions. Thus, both qualitative and quantitative changes in lipoproteins are important in atherosclerosis.

Atherosclerosis and Aging

It is easy to imagine that arterial lesions accumulate with age as the number of injuries multiplies and as reparative processes may be impaired. It is not known in detail how lipoprotein metabolism is altered with age and whether lipoprotein structures are altered. It is known that VLDL- and LDL-cholesterol and triglyceride levels rise progressively with age (67). The fact that atherosclerosis increases with age most steeply in those populations whose plasma lipids rise most dramatically (67,68) suggests that lipoproteins play an important role in atherosclerosis throughout life. Unfortunately, much of the detailed information linking the relative hyperlipidemia of aging with the other intravascular and intrinsic vascular factors that contribute to the advancing atherosclerosis of the aged is lacking. Indeed, even the factors responsible for increasing lipid levels with aging have not been identified.

Summary and Conclusions

Epidemiologic studies have shown that among several risk factors for the development of coronary heart disease (CHD) are aging, smoking of cigarettes, hypertension, and hypercholesterolemia. Cholesterol in plasma is transported by several lipoproteins. Chylomicrons transport dietary fats from the gut to the liver. VLDL transport fats synthesized by the liver and dietary fats already present in liver to a variety of "peripheral" tissues, including adipose tissue, muscle, kidney, and skin. During the process of traversing the plasma from liver to the "periphery," VLDL are transformed to LDL, and it is actually LDL that delivers most of the cholesterol. High density lipoproteins transport excess cholesterol from peripheral tissues back to the liver for excretion from the body. Individuals who have high concentrations of LDL in their plasmas stand at increased risk for the development of CHD, whereas people with high concentrations of HDL stand at decreased risk. The most favorable combination is low LDL and high HDL. The incidence of CHD increases with age in both sexes. Cholesterol levels in the population also increase with age. Most of the increase is due to rises in LDL-cholesterol. HDL-cholesterol levels are much more stable. It is not clear what factors are responsible for rising LDL-cholesterol levels. Ingestion of a Western diet combined with age-related changes in the body's ability to metabolize cholesterol probably both contribute to the rising LDL-cholesterol levels with age. Both factors are suggested because LDL-cholesterol levels do not rise with age in populations that eat vegetarian diets. The rising LDL levels are at least in part responsible for the increasing incidence of CHD with age, and dietary changes to control LDL levels have been advocated by the American Heart Association and the American Medical Association.

References

1. Castelli WP, Doyle JT, Gordon T, et al: HDL cholesterol and other lipids in coronary heart disease. *Circulation* 1977, 55:768–772.
2. Tatami R, Mabuchi H, Udea K, et al: Intermediate density lipoprotein and cholesterol rich very low density lipoprotein in angiographically determined coronary artery disease. *Circulation* 1981; 64:1174–1184.
3. Cohn PF, Gabbay SI, Weglicki WB: Serum lipid levels in angiographically defined coronary artery disease. *Ann Intern Med* 1976; 84:241–245.
4. Stone NJ, Levy RI, Frederickson DR, et al: Coronary artery disease in 116 kindred with familial type II hyperlipoproteinemia. *Circulation* 1974; 69:476–488.
5. Glueck CJ, Gartside P, Fallat RW, et al: Longevity syndromes: Familial hypobeta and familial hyperalpha lipoproteinemia. *J Lab Clin Med* 1976; 88:941–957.
6. Frederickson DS, Levy RI, Lindgren FT: A comparison of heritable abnormal lipoprotein patterns as defined by two different techniques. *J Clin Invest* 1968; 47:2446–2457.
7. Forte GM, Nichols AV, Glaeser RM: Electron microscopy of human serum lipoproteins using negative staining. *Chem Phys Lipids* 1968; 2:396–408.
8. Mahley RW: Atherogenic hyperlipoproteinemia. *Med Clin North Am* 1982; 66:403–430.
9. Albers JJ, Cabana VG, Warnick GR, et al: Lp(a) lipoprotein: Relationship to sinking pre-beta lipoprotein, hyperlipoproteinemia, and apolipoprotein B. *Metabolism* 1975; 24:1047–1054.
10. Alaupovic P, Lee DM, McConathy WJ: Studies on the composition and structure of plasma lipoproteins. Distribution of lipoprotein families in major density classes of normal human plasma lipoproteins. *Biochim Biophys Acta* 1972; 260:689–707.
11. Kostner GM: Studies of the composition and structure of human serum lipoproteins. Isolation and partial characterization of apolipoprotein AIII. *Biochim Biophys Acta* 1974; 336:383–395.
12. McConathy WJ, Alaupovic P: Isolation and partial characterization of apolipoprotein D: A new protein moiety of the human plasma lipoprotein system. *FEBS Lett* 1973; 37(2):178–182.

13. Brewer HB Jr, Fairwell T, Larue A, et al: The amino acid sequence of human apoA-I, an apolipoprotein isolated from high density lipoproteins. *Biochem Biophys Res Commun* 1978; 80(3):623–630.
14. Brewer HB Jr, Lux SE, Ronan R, et al: Amino acid sequence of human apoLp-Gin-II (apoA-II), an apolipoprotein isolated from the high density lipoprotein complex. *Proc Natl Acad Sci USA* 1972; 69(5)1304–1308.
15. Beisiegel U, Utermann G: An apolipoprotein homolog of rat apolipoprotein A-IV in human plasma. *Eur J Biochem* 1979; 93:601–608.
16. Kane JP, Hardman DA, Paulus HE: Heterogeneity of apolipoprotein B: Isolation of a new species from human chylomicrons. *Proc Natl Acad Sci USA* 1980; 77:2465–2469.
17. Shulman RS, Herbert PN, Wehrly K, et al: The complete amino acid sequence of C-I (apoLp-Ser), and apolipoprotein from human very low density lipoproteins. *J Biol Chem* 1975; 259:182–190.
18. Jackson RL, Baker N, Gilliam EB, et al: Primary structure of very low density apolipoprotein C-II of human plasma. *Proc Natl Acad Sci USA* 1942; 74:1942–1945.
19. Havel RJ, Kotite L, Kane JP: Isoelectric heterogeneity of the cofactor protein for lipoprotein lipase in human blood plasma. *Biochem Med* 21:121–128.
20. Brewer HB Jr, Shulman R, Herbert P, et al: The complete amino acid sequence of alanine apolipoprotein (apoC-III), an apolipoprotein from human plasma very low density lipoproteins. *J Biol Chem* 1974; 249:4975–4984.
21. Vaith P, Assman G, Uhlenbruck G: Characterization of the oligosaccharide side chain of apolipoprotein C-III from human plasma very low density lipoprotein. *Biochim Biophys Acta* 1978; 541:234–240.
22. Patsch W, Schonfeld G: The degree of sialylation of apoC-III is altered by diet. *Diabetes* 1982; 30:530–534.
23. Rall SC Jr, Weisgraber KH, Mahley RW: Human apolipoprotein E—the complete amino acid sequence. *J Biol Chem* 1982; 257:4171–4178.
24. Zannis VI, Breslow JL: Human very low density lipoprotein apolipoprotein E isoprotein polymorphism is explained by genetic variation and posttranslational modification. *Biochemistry* 1981; 20:1033–1041.
25. Weisgraber KH, Rall SC Jr, Mahley RW: Human E apoprotein heterogeneity: Cysteine-arginine interchanges in the amino acid sequence of the apo-E isoforms. *J Biol Chem* 1981; 256:9077–9083.
26. Green PHR, Tall AR, Glickman RM: Rat intestine secretes discoid high density lipoprotein. *J Clin Invest* 1978; 61:528–534.
27. Small DM: Membrane and plasma lipoproteins-biolayer-to-emulsion and emulsion-to-bilayer transitions, in Bloch K, Bolis L, Tosteson DC (eds): *Membranes, Molecules, Toxins, and Cells.* Boston, John Wright PGS, 1981, pp 11–34.
28. Segrest JP: A molecular theory of lipid-protein interactions in the plasma lipoproteins. *FEBS Lett* 1974; 38:247–253.
29. Mantulin WW, Rohde MF, Gotto AM Jr, et al: The conformational properties of human plasma apolipoprotein C-II. *J Biol Chem* 1980; 255:8185–8191.
30. Rall SC Jr, Weisgraber KH, Innerarity TL, et al: Structural basis for receptor binding heterogeneity of apolipoprotein E from type II hyperlipoproteinemic subjects. *Proc Natl Acad Sci USA* 1982; 79:4696–4700.
31. Weisgraber KH, Innerarity TL, Mahley RW: Abnormal lipoprotein receptor-binding activity of the human E apoprotein due to cysteine-arginine interchange at a single site. *J Biol Chem* 1982; 257:2518–2521.

32. Goldstein JL, Anderson RGW, Brown MS: Coated pits, coated vesicles, and receptor mediated endocytosis. *Nature* 1979; 279:679–685.
33. Schneider WJ, Beisiegel U, Goldstein JL, et al: Purification of the low density lipoprotein receptor, and acidic glycoprotein of 164,000 molecular weight. *J Biol Chem* 1982; 247:2644–2673.
34. Mahley RW, Hui DY, Innerarity TL, et al: Two independent lipoprotein receptors on hepatic membranes of dog, swine, and man. *J Clin Invest* 1981; 68:1197–1206.
35. Mahley RW, Innerarity TL, Brown MS, et al: Cholesterol ester synthesis in macrophages: Stimulation by β-very low density lipoproteins from cholesterol-fed animals of several species. *J Lipid Res* 1980; 21:970–980.
36. Augustin J, Freeze H, Tejada P, et al: A comparison of molecular properties of hepatic triglyceride lipase and lipoprotein lipase from human post heparin plasma. *J Biol Chem* 1978; 253:2912–2920.
37. Bengtsson G, Olivecrona T: Lipoprotein lipase: Some effects of activator proteins. *Eur J Biochem* 1980; 106:549–555.
38. Jansen H, Birkenhager JC: Liver lipase-like activity in human and hamster adrenocortical tissue. *Metabolism* 1981; 30:428–430.
39. Albers JJ, Cabana VG, Barden Stahl YD: Purification and characterization of human plasma lecithin : cholesterol acyltransferase. *Biochemistry* 1976; 15:1084–1087.
40. Rose HG: High density lipoproteins: Substrates and products of plasma lecithin:cholesterol acyltransferase, in Day CE (ed): *High Density Lipoproteins.* New York, Marcel Dekker, 1981, pp 214–263.
41. Schonfeld G, Bell E, Alpers DH: Intestinal apoproteins during fat absorption. *J Clin Invest* 1978; 61:1539–1550.
42. Havel RJ, Kane JP, Kashyap ML: Interchange of apolipoproteins between chylomicrons and high density lipoproteins during alimentary lipemia in man. *J Clin Invest* 1973; 52:32–38.
43. Higgins JM, Fielding CJ: Lipoprotein lipase. Mechanism of formation of triglyceride rich remnant particles from very low density lipoproteins and chylomicrons. *Biochemistry* 1975; 14:2288–2292.
44. Tall AR, Small DM: Plasma high density lipoproteins. *N Engl J Med* 1978; 299:1232–1236.
45. Cooper AD, Yu PYS: Rates of removal and degradation of chylomicron remnants by isolated perfused rat liver. *J Lipid Res* 1978; 19:635–643.
46. Shelburne F, Hanks J, Meyers W, et al: Effect of apoproteins on hepatic uptake of triglyceride emulsions in the rat. *J Clin Invest* 1980; 65:652–658.
47. Goldstein JL, Ho YK, Brown MS, et al: Cholesteryl ester accumulation in macrophages resulting from receptor mediated uptake and degradation of hypercholesterolemic canine β-very low density lipoproteins. *J Biol Chem* 1980; 255:1839–1848.
48. Moore DJ, Ovtracht L: Structure of rat liver Golgi apparatus: Relationship to lipoprotein secretion. *J Ultrastruct Res* 1981; 74:284–295.
49. Schonfeld G, Pfleger B: Utilization of exogenous free fatty acids for the production of very low density lipoprotein triglyceride by livers of carbohydrate-fed rats. *J Lipid Res* 1971; 12:614–621.
50. Schonfeld G, Gulbrandsen CL, Wilson RB, et al: Catabolism of human very low density lipoproteins in monkeys. The appearance of human very low

density lipoprotein peptides in monkey high density lipoproteins. *Biochim Biophys Acta* 1972; 270:426–432.
51. Deckelbaum RJ, Eisenberg S, Fainaru M, et al: In vitro production of human plasma low density lipoprotein like particles. *J Biol Chem* 1979; 254:6079–6087.
52. Attie AD, Pittman RC, Steinberg D: Hepatic catabolism of low density lipoprotein: Mechanisms and metabolic consequences. *Hepatology* 1982; 2:269–282.
53. Gwynne JT, Mahaffee D, Brewer HB Jr, et al: Adrenal cholesterol uptake from plasma lipoproteins: Regulation by corticotropin. *Proc Natl Acad Sci USA* 1976; 73:4329–4333.
54. Fogelman AM, Haberland ME, Seager J, et al: Factors regulating the activities of the low density lipoprotein receptor and the scavenger receptor on human monocyte-macrophages. *J Lipid Res* 1981; 22:1131–1141.
55. Stein O, Goren R, Stein Y: Removal of cholesterol from fibroblasts and smooth muscle cells in culture in the presence and absence of cholesterol esterification in the medium. *Biochim Biophys Acta* 1978; 520:309–318.
56. Chajek T, Aron L, Fielding CJ: Interaction of lecithin : cholesterol acyltransferase and cholesteryl ester transfer protein in the transport of cholesteryl ester into sphingomyelin liposomes. *Biochemistry* 1980; 19:3673–3677.
57. Patsch JR, Gotto AM Jr, Olivecrona T, et al: Formation of high density lipoprotein-like particles during lipolysis of very low density lipoproteins in vitro. *Proc Natl Acad Sci USA* 1978; 75:4519–4528.
58. Ross R: Atherosclerosis: A problem of the biology of arterial wall cells and their interactions with blood components. *Arteriosclerosis* 1981; 1:293–311.
59. Schonfeld G: Lipoproteins, atherosclerosis, and the regression of lesions, in Joist JH, Sherman LA (eds): *Venous and Arterial Thrombosis.* New York, Grune & Stratton, 1979, pp 305–312.
60. Armstrong ML, Megan MB, Warner ED: Intimal thickening in normocholesterolemic Rhesus monkeys fed low supplements of dietary cholesterol. *Circ Res* 1974; 34:447–454.
61. Minick CR, Murphy GE: Experimental induction of atheroarteriosclerosis by the synergy of allergic injury to arteries and lipid rich diet. *Am J Pathol* 1973; 73:265–300.
62. Armstrong ML: Regression of atherosclerosis, in Paoletti R, Gotto AM Jr (eds): *Atherosclerosis Reviews,* vol 1. New York, Raven Press, 1976, pp 137–182.
63. Schonfeld G: Disorders of lipid transport—update 1983. *Prog Cardiovasc Dis* 1983; 27:89–108.
64. Schonfeld G, Patsch W, Pfleger B, et al: Lipolysis produces changes in the immunoreactivity and cell reactivity of very low density lipoproteins. *J Clin Invest* 1979; 64:1288–1297.
65. Gianturco SH, Brown FB, Gotto AM Jr, Bradley WA: Receptor mediated uptake of hypertriglyceridemic very low density lipoproteins by normal human fibroblasts. *J Lipid Res* 1982; 23:984–994.
66. Brown MS, Goldstein JL: Lipoprotein metabolism in the macrophage: Implications for cholesterol deposition in atherosclerosis, abstracted in *Annual Review of Biochemistry,* vol 52. Palo Alto, CA, Annual Reviews, 1983, pp 223–261.
67. Heiss G, Tamir I, Davis CE, et al: Lipoprotein–cholesterol distributions in se-

lected North American populations: The Lipid Research Clinics Program Prevalence Study. *Circulation* 1980; 61:302–315.

68. Connor WE, Cerqueira MT, Connor RW, et al: The plasma lipids, lipoproteins, and diet of the Tarahumara Indians of Mexico. *Am J Clin Nutr* 1978; 31:1131–1142.

5

Changes in Calcium and Vitamin D Metabolism with Age

H. James Armbrecht

One of the major health problems faced by the elderly, particularly elderly women, is the bone disease osteoporosis (see Chapter 11). The causes of osteoporosis are multiple in nature and are still the object of intense investigation (1). However, it is known that osteoporosis is aggravated by two factors: (a) lack of calcium in the diet and (b) poor absorption of dietary calcium by the intestine (2,3).

Unfortunately, both of these factors are characteristic of the elderly population. Several nutritional surveys have reported that the elderly tend to consume diets deficient in calcium. A national nutritional survey has reported that women 45 years and older consume only half of the recommended daily allowance of calcium (4). The age-related decline in capacity for intestinal absorption of calcium has been documented in many clinical studies (3,5,6). In addition, the intestine loses its ability to adapt to a low-calcium diet (7). Young subjects (mean age = 28 years) adapted to a low calcium diet by absorbing 55% more calcium from a test dose than when they were fed a high calcium diet. However, old subjects (mean age = 68 years) fed the same low calcium diet showed only a 14% increase in calcium absorption compared to when they were fed a high calcium diet.

These findings raise two questions: Why is there an age-related decline in intestinal absorption of calcium and adaptation to a low calcium diet? What can be done to improve calcium absorption in the elderly?

Calcium Homeostasis

Since calcium homeostasis involves several organ systems and hormones, the decline in intestinal absorption of calcium with age may be the result of several factors. The regulation of serum calcium levels by bone and intestine has been extensively studied in young animals (Fig. 5-1). Total serum calcium must be maintained near 10 mg/100 ml for the proper function of nerve and muscle, and studies have shown that serum calcium is maintained at this level throughout the life span in man (8) and rat (9). If a young mammal is fed a low calcium diet, a slight decrease in serum calcium may result. This decreased serum calcium results in increased secretion of parathyroid hormone (PTH) by the parathyroid glands. Among other things, PTH alters vitamin D metabolism. PTH stimulates the renal conversion of 25-hydroxyvitamin D (25[OH]D) to 1,25-dihydroxyvitamin D (1,25[OH]$_2$D), a biologically active form of vitamin D. 1,25(OH)$_2$D then greatly stimulates the absorption of dietary

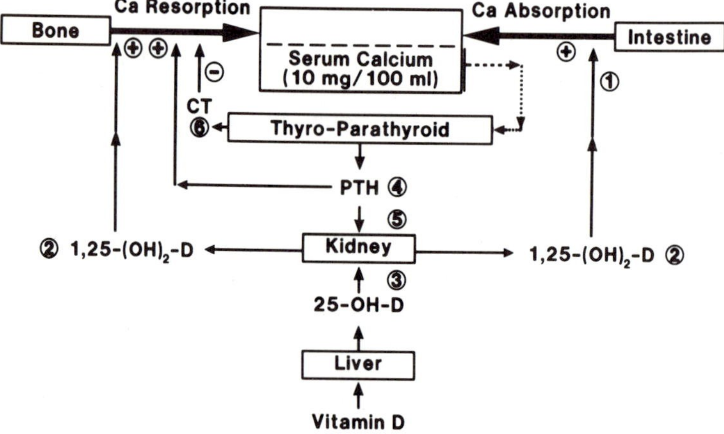

Figure 5-1. Regulation of serum calcium by vitamin D, PTH, and CT. Hypocalcemia results in increased secretion of PTH (step 4). PTH acts on the kidney (step 5) to stimulate renal production of 1,25(OH)$_2$D from 25(OH)D (step 3). The 1,25(OH)$_2$D in serum (step 2) acts on the intestine to stimulate calcium absorption (step 1) and on the bone to stimulate bone resorption. CT (step 6) may act to inhibit bone resorption. Positive (+) and negative (−) actions of each agent are noted by appropriate symbol. Modified from DeLuca HF (18).

calcium by the intestine. In addition, 1,25$(OH)_2$D and PTH together stimulate the resorption of calcium from bone. Decreased serum calcium also results in decreased secretion of calcitonin (CT) by the thyroid gland. CT normally acts to decrease the resorption of calcium from bone. The net effect of these actions of 1,25$(OH)_2$D, PTH, and CT on intestine and bone is to maintain serum calcium levels within tight limits.

In this complex homeostatic mechanism, many steps could contribute to the decline in intestinal absorption with age. Key steps in this mechanism (Fig. 5-1) include the sensitivity of the intestine to 1,25$(OH)_2$D (step 1), the serum levels of 1,25$(OH)_2$D itself (step 2), renal production of 1,25$(OH)_2$D from 25(OH)D (step 3), serum levels of PTH (step 4), the stimulation of renal 1,25$(OH)_2$D production by PTH (step 5), and serum levels of CT (step 6). Age-related changes in any or all of these steps could account for the observed age-related changes in intestinal absorption and adaptation.

Age-Related Changes in Intestinal Absorption of Calcium

To study changes in calcium absorption and homeostasis with age, we have developed the rat as an animal model. In a typical experiment, male rats of each age group were divided into two dietary groups. One group was fed a high calcium (1.2% calcium) diet, and the second group was fed a low calcium (0.02% calcium) diet. The low calcium diet tested the capacity of the animals to adapt to a calcium-poor diet. Both diets contained adequate amounts of vitamin D and phosphorus. After 4 weeks on the diets, the rats were sacrificed, and their adaption to dietary calcium restriction was studied as a function of age.

In initial studies, the capacity of the intestine to absorb calcium actively from a test solution was measured using the everted gut sac technique (10–12). Calcium absorption by the intestine declined with age regardless of diet (Fig. 5-2). At 1.5 months of age, the intestines of rats fed the low calcium diet demonstrated a significantly greater capacity to absorb calcium actively than intestines from rats fed the high calcium diet. However, this intestinal adaption to a low calcium diet declined with age. By 12 months of age there was no significant difference in intestinal absorption between the two groups. No further changes in absorption were seen between 12 and 24 months of age. This pattern in age and diet is very similar to that seen in humans (7).

One possible reason for the age-related decline in intestinal absorption of calcium is that there is an age-related decline in intestinal responsiveness to 1,25$(OH)_2$D (Fig. 5-1, step 1). This possibility has been explored by administering 1,25$(OH)_2$D to young and old rats (12,13). In general, 1,25$(OH)_2D_3$ administration results in a significant stimulation of calcium absorption in both young and old animals. However, the level of calcium

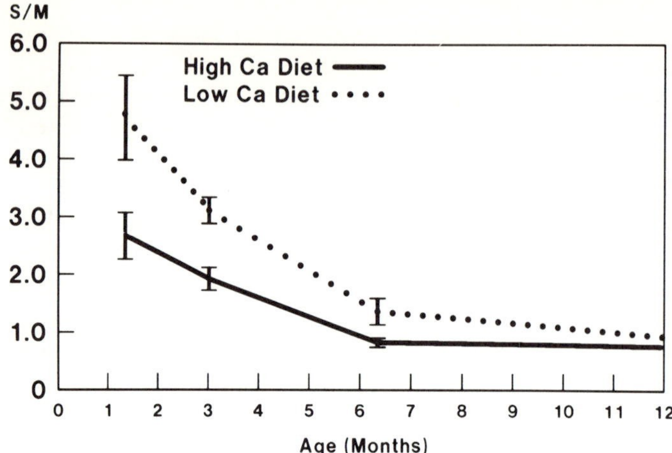

Figure 5-2. Change in intestinal calcium absorption with age and diet. Active transport of calcium was measured using the everted gut sac. S/M is the ratio of serosal (S) to mucosal (M) concentration of calcium after a 1.5-hour incubation of the everted gut sac. Each data point is the mean ± SE of four to eight animals. Modified from Armbrecht HJ et al (10).

absorption in the old rat after $1,25(OH)_2D_3$ stimulation is less than in the young. In clinical studies, $1,25(OH)_2D_3$ has been shown to be effective in stimulating calcium absorption in elderly patients (3).

Age-Related Changes in Vitamin D Metabolism

Since the adult intestine does respond to $1,25(OH)_2D_3$, another possibility is that the serum $1,25(OH)_2D$ level itself declines with age (Fig. 5-1, step 2). Therefore, serum $1,25(OH)_2D$ levels were measured in the rat as a function of age and diet (9). In animals fed the low calcium diet, serum $1,25(OH)_2D$ levels declined markedly with age (Fig. 5-3). Feeding 3-month-old animals the low calcium diet markedly stimulated serum $1,25(OH)_2D$ levels. However, the low calcium diet produced only a slight elevation of serum $1,25(OH)_2D$ in 13-month-old animals and no significant elevation in 25-month-old animals. In animals fed the high calcium diet, serum $1,25(OH)_2D$ declined slightly but significantly with age, as it had in a previous study (14). An age-related decline in serum $1,25(OH)_2D$ levels has also been reported in humans (3). This change in serum $1,25(OH)_2D$ is very similar to the observed change in calcium absorption with age and diet (Fig. 5-2). Another study found that the decline in calcium absorption with age was positively correlated with decreased levels of $1,25(OH)_2D$ in serum and intestinal mucosa (12). Therefore, age-

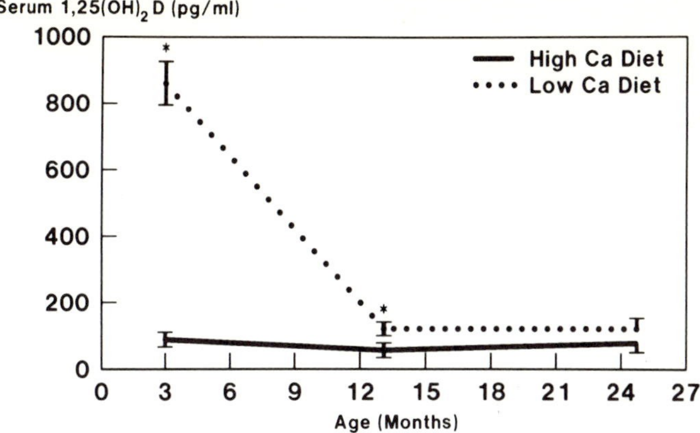

Figure 5-3. Effect of age and dietary calcium on serum $1,25(OH)_2D$ levels. Each data point is the mean ± SE of six to seven animals. The lower limit of detection was 4 pg/mL. The asterisk indicates a value significantly different than the high calcium diet group of the same age ($P < .05$, *t*-test). Modified from Armbrecht HJ et al (9).

related changes in serum $1,25(OH)_2D$ could account for the age-related changes in calcium absorption.

One explanation for the age-related decline in serum $1,25(OH)_2D$ levels is that there is an age-related decline in the conversion of 25(OH)D to $1,25(OH)_2D$ by the kidney (Fig. 5-1, step 3). This is a likely possibility since $1,25(OH)_2D$ production by the kidney accounts for virtually all of the serum $1,25(OH)_2D$ (15). We have used the renal slice technique to examine changes in renal $1,25(OH)_2D$ production with age and diet (9,16). Briefly, renal cortical slices are incubated in Krebs-Ringer buffer containing tritiated $25(OH)D_3$. After 1 hour, the slices are extracted, and the extract is chromatographed to separate out the tritiated vitamin D_3 metabolites produced by the renal slices. A typical hexane/methanol/methylene chloride HPLC chromatographic separation of a renal extract is shown in Figure 5-4. Slices from 3-month-old animals contain large amounts of radioactivity migrating with the authentic $1,25(OH)_2D_3$ standard. Slices from 25-month-old rats contain very little radioactivity migrating with authentic $1,25(OH)_2D_3$, but they do contain large amounts of radioactivity migrating with authentic $24,25(OH)_2D_3$, another metabolite of vitamin D_3 produced by the kidney.

Using the renal slice technique, renal conversion of $25(OH)D_3$ to $1,25(OH)_2D_3$ and $24,25(OH)_2D_3$ was measured as a function of age and diet. In rats fed a low calcium diet, renal $1,25(OH)_2D_3$ production declined markedly with age (Fig. 5-5). The low calcium diet produced a significant increase in $1,25(OH)_2D_3$ production in 3-month-old, but not in

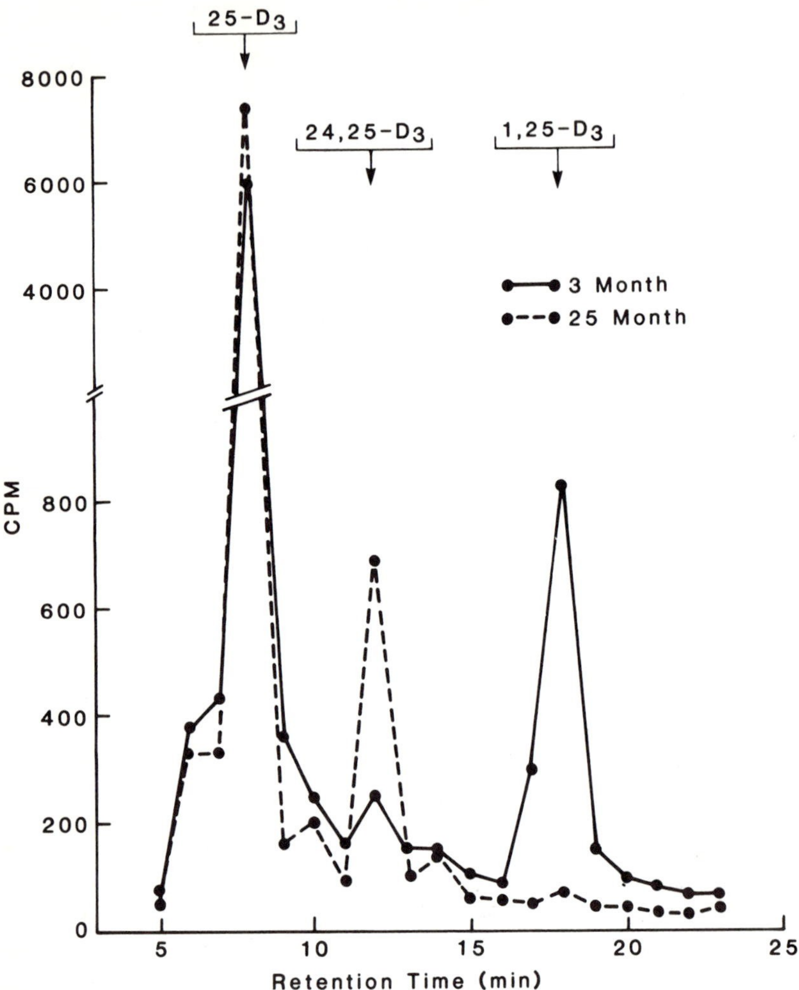

Figure 5-4. Effect of age on high pressure liquid chromatographic elution pattern of tritiated vitamin D metabolites extracted from renal cortical slices. Renal slices were from a 3-month and 25-month-old rat fed a low calcium diet for 4 weeks. Slices were incubated with tritiated $25(OH)D_3$ for one hour, and organic extracts of the slices were chromatographed on a Zorbax-SIL column (0.6 × 25 cm) equilibrated with hexane/methanol/methylene chloride (8:1:1). One-minute fractions were collected at a flow rate of 2 mL/min, and the fractions were analyzed for radioactivity. Retention times of vitamin D standards are indicated at top of figure. Total counts per minute (CPM) were normalized to 10,000 in each case.

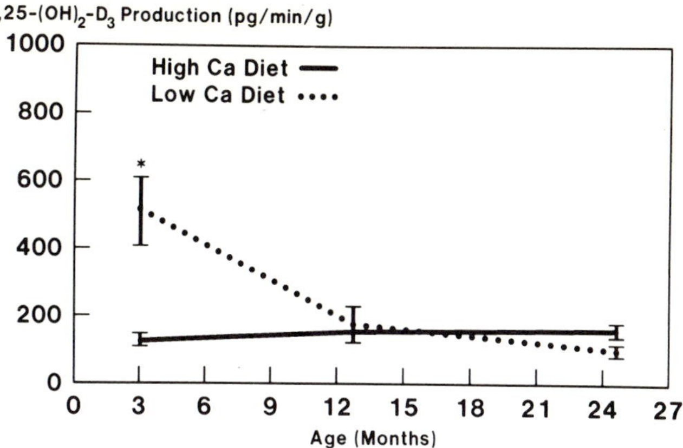

Figure 5-5. Effect of age and dietary calcium on renal $1{,}25(OH)_2D_3$ production. Each data point is the mean ± SE of eight renal slice incubations. The asterisk indicates a value significantly different from the high calcium diet group of the same age ($P < .05$, *t*-test). Modified from Armbrecht HJ et al (9).

13- and 25-month-old rats. This pattern is very similar to the changes in serum $1{,}25(OH)_2D$ seen with age and diet (Fig. 5-3). Therefore, age-related changes in renal $1{,}25(OH)_2D$ production may account for the age-related changes in serum $1{,}25(OH)_2D$.

Interestingly, in the same experiments renal $24{,}25(OH)_2D_3$ production increased with age regardless of diet (Fig. 5-6). Feeding a low calcium diet resulted in a significant decrease in renal $24{,}25(OH)_2D_3$ production in 3-month but not in 13- and 25-month-old animals. Therefore, the kidney does not lose its capacity to hydroxylate $25(OH)D_3$ with age. Rather, it preferentially produces $24{,}25(OH)_2D_3$ rather than $1{,}25(OH)_2D_3$. The biologic role of $24{,}25(OH)_2D_3$ is still controversial: it may play a role in bone metabolism (17), or it may simply be a catabolic pathway for $25(OH)D_3$ (18).

Age-Related Changes in PTH

Since PTH is a potent stimulator of renal $1{,}25(OH)_2D_3$ production, one possible reason for the age-related decline in renal $1{,}25(OH)_2D_3$ production is that there is an age-related decline in serum PTH levels (Fig. 5-1, step 4). Therefore, serum immunoactive PTH (iPTH) levels were measured as a function of age and diet (9) and and were found to increase with age regardless of diet (Fig. 5-7). In the 3-month-old animals, a low calcium diet resulted in a significant increase in serum iPTH, but this ad-

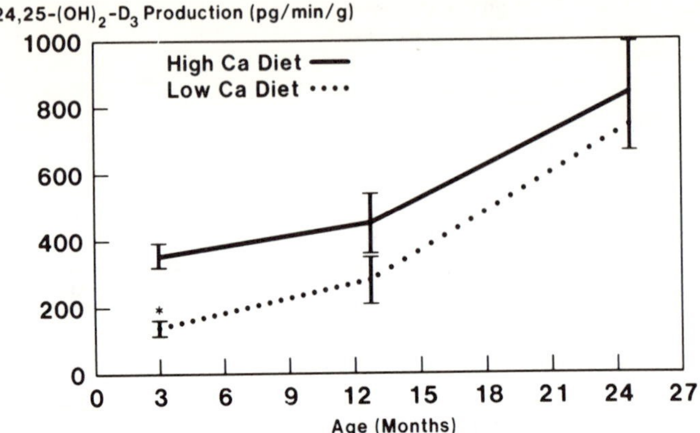

Figure 5-6. Effect of age and dietary calcium on renal 24,25$(OH)_2D_3$ production. Each data point is the mean ± SE of eight renal slice incubations. The asterisk indicates a value significantly different from the high calcium diet group of the same age ($P < .05$, t-test). Modified from Armbrecht HJ, et al (9).

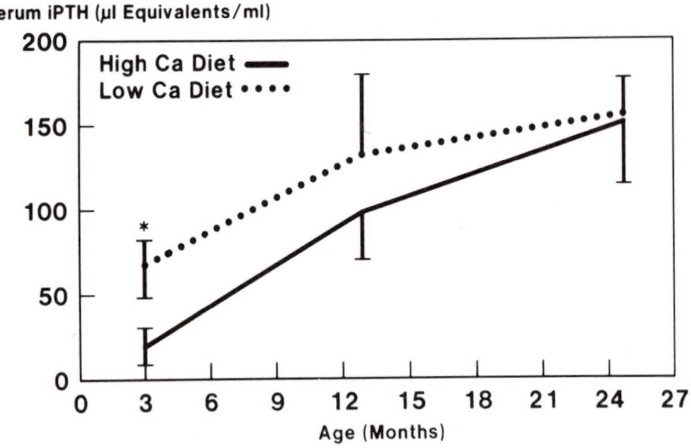

Figure 5-7. Effect of age and dietary calcium on serum iPTH levels. Each data point is the mean ± SE of six to seven animals. The lower limit of detection was 1.4 μL equivalents/mL. The asterisk indicates a value significantly different from the high calcium diet group of the same age ($P < .05$, t-test). Modified from Armbrecht HJ, et al (9).

aptation was lost in 13- and 25-month-old animals. Similar age-related increases in iPTH levels have been reported in humans (8,19).

The fact that renal $1,25(OH)_2D_3$ production declines with age despite an age-related increase in serum iPTH suggests that the adult kidney may be refractory to PTH (Fig. 5-1, step 5). Therefore, we used the renal slice technique to study the in vitro responsiveness of the kidney to PTH with age (20). In addition, the responsiveness of the kidney to forskolin, a compound that mimics the action of PTH by stimulating directly the catalytic unit of adenylate cyclase, was also examined (21). When renal slices from young rats were incubated for four hours with PTH or forskolin in vitro, renal $1,25(OH)_2D_3$ production was significantly increased (Fig. 5-8). However, these compounds did not increase $1,25(OH)_2D_3$ production when incubated with renal slices from adult rats. These results demonstrate that the adult kidney is refractory to PTH and forskolin in terms of renal $1,25(OH)_2D_3$ production. The lack of forskolin stimulation indicates that the refractoriness is not caused by down-regulation of PTH receptors. This refractoriness to PTH may partly explain the age-related decline in renal $1,25(OH)_2D_3$ production.

The mechanism responsible for the diminished PTH responsiveness of the adult kidney is still under investigation. There is evidence that PTH stimulates renal $1,25(OH)_2D_3$ production by increasing intracellular cAMP levels, stimulating cAMP-dependent protein kinase activity, and

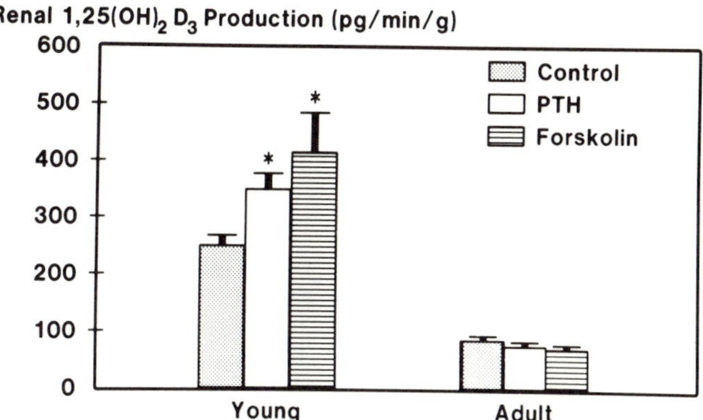

Figure 5-8. Effect of PTH and forskolin on renal $1,25(OH)_2D_3$ production. Renal slices were prepared from young (3-month) and adult (12-month) rats fed a vitamin D-deficient, low calcium diet and then thyroparathyroidectomized 18 hours prior to sacrifice. Renal slices were preincubated for 3 hours in the presence or absence of PTH (5 units/mL) or forskolin (3 μM). $1,25(OH)_2D_3$ production was then measured by transferring slices to identical media containing tritiated $25(OH)D_3$ for 1 hour. Control slices received vehicle only. Bars represent the mean ± SE of 9 to 21 individual slice incubations. The asterisk indicates a value significantly different from control of the same age group ($P < .05$, *t*-test).

phosphorylating key intracellular proteins (22–25). Several studies have reported that PTH-dependent adenylate cyclase decreases with age (20,26). However, it is not known if this moderate decrease in intracellular cAMP can account for the striking decline in renal $1,25(OH)_2D_3$ production with age. It is possible that age-related changes in cAMP-dependent protein kinase activity or protein phosphorylation may account for the age-related decline in renal $1,25(OH)_2D_3$ production.

Age-Related Changes in CT

CT may play a role in maintaining constant serum calcium levels by preventing hypercalcemia (27). Therefore, we measured serum immunoreactive CT (iCT) (Fig. 5-1, step 6) with age and diet (28). Serum iCT increased markedly with age in animals fed a low calcium diet (Fig. 5-9). A similar increase was seen in rats fed the high calcium diet, except that there was no further increase in serum iCT between 13 and 25 months of age. This age-related rise in serum iCT has been observed in both male (29) and female (30) rats of different strains.

The increase in serum iCT with age was significantly correlated with the increase in serum iPTH in this study (Fig. 5-10). This suggests that these two hormones may work together to regulate calcium resorption from bone throughout the life span. A concurrent rise in both serum iPTH and iCT with age has been observed in male (29) but not female rats (30) of different strains. A role for CT in preventing hypercalcemia

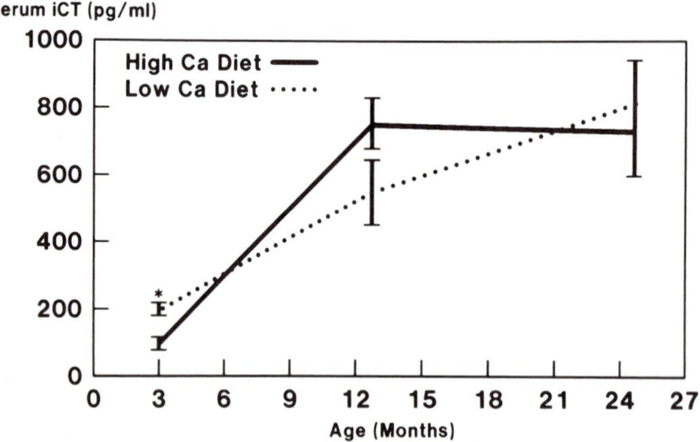

Figure 5-9. Effect of age and dietary calcium on serum iCT levels. Each data point is the mean ± SE of six to seven animals. The lower limit of detection was 100 pg/mL. The asterisk indicates a value significantly different from the high calcium diet group of the same age ($P < .05$, *t*-test).

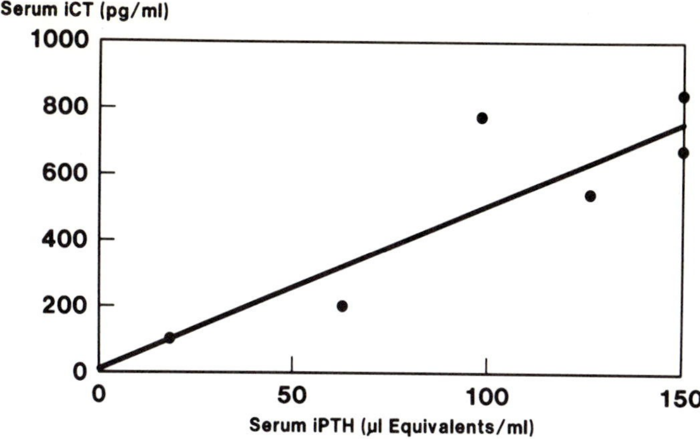

Figure 5-10. Correlation of serum iPTH with serum iCT. Serum iCT (Fig. 5-9) was plotted versus serum iPTH (Fig. 5-7) for each age and dietary calcium group. The line ($y = 5.0x + 15.8$) was determined by least squares analysis. There was a significant correlation ($r = .87$, $P < .05$) between the two parameters.

in the adult rat is suggested by the fact that removal of the thyroparathyroid complex results in a slower fall in serum calcium in adult rats than in young rats (20,29). Although serum iCT increases with age in the rat, its physiologic effects may be less in the adult. It has been reported that CT has less of a hypocalcemic effect in adult animals compared to young animals (31). The relevance of these studies to the human is not known, since serum iCT has been reported to decline with age in man (32–34).

Effect of Dietary Restriction on Calcium Homeostasis

These data clearly demonstrate that there are age-related changes in many of the parameters associated with calcium homeostasis. The question of how these age-related changes are related to longevity itself then arises. One of the most reproducible ways of increasing maximal life span is dietary restriction (see Chapters 6 to 8). Recently, the effect of dietary restriction on several parameters associated with calcium homeostasis has been explored (35,36). In these studies, total calories were restricted but calcium, phosphorus, and vitamin D were not. Lifelong dietary restriction had little effect on serum calcium levels, which remained constant from 1.5 to 24 months and rose slightly at 27 months of age. However, lifelong dietary restriction almost completely inhibited the age-related increase in serum iPTH (36), and it blunted the age-related increase in serum iCT (35).

Lifelong dietary restriction also had an effect on bone parameters. In the nonrestricted animals, bone length, weight, density, and calcium content plateaued at about 12 months of age, and the sealing off of the epiphyseal growth plate by bone occurred at 18 months (36). In the lifelong restricted group, plateauing of bone parameters and sealing off of the epiphyseal growth plate did not occur until 24 months of age.

The mechanism by which lifelong dietary restriction delays these age-related changes in calcium homeostasis is not known. However, these effects on calcium homeostasis are similar to the effects of dietary restriction on other physiologic and pathologic processes (see Chapter 6). By varying feeding schedules and diet composition, it was found that the effects of lifelong food restriction on calcium homeostasis did not result specifically from restriction of protein or food intake during the period of rapid growth (35,36). Since the changes in calcium homeostasis with age and food restriction are so dramatic, further studies of food restriction and calcium homeostasis may give new insight into both the mechanism by which food restriction exerts its effects and the mechanisms responsible for the age-related changes in calcium homeostasis.

Summary and Conclusions

In summary, the rat model shows changes in the intestinal absorption of calcium with age and diet that are similar to those seen in humans. This age-related decline in calcium absorption can be explained in terms of an age-related decline in serum $1,25(OH)_2D$ levels (Fig. 5-1, step 2). The decreased serum $1,25(OH)_2D$ levels, in turn, can be said to result from an age-related decline in renal $1,25(OH)_2D_3$ production (Fig. 5-1, step 3). The decrease in renal $1,25(OH)_2D_3$ production is not caused by an age-related decline in serum iPTH, but rather may result from an age-related decrease in sensitivity to PTH (Fig. 5-1, step 5).

The net result of these biochemical changes is that the intestine makes less of a contribution to the maintenance of serum calcium with increasing age (Fig. 5-1). Instead, the adult animal relies on bone resorption to maintain serum calcium, and this may result in negative calcium balance. This lack of dietary calcium intake, in conjunction with other factors such as loss of estrogen and lack of exercise, can lead to or aggravate bone diseases such as osteoporosis in the elderly (see Chapter 11).

These findings bring us to the question of what can be done to improve dietary calcium intake in the elderly. One way is to increase the amount of calcium in the diet, which will result in a greater absolute amount of calcium being absorbed. Using balance studies, it has been demonstrated that feeding old rats a diet high in calcium can alter calcium balance from negative to positive (37). In humans, a high calcium diet has been shown to decrease bone resorption in adult women (2). Additionally, administration of $1,25(OH)_2D_3$ has been demonstrated to enhance intestinal calcium absorption in rats (12,13) and in man (3,38), and to alter calcium balance in osteoporotic women from negative to positive (18). Care must be taken with 1,25$(OH)_2D_3$ administration to avoid hypercalcemia and excessive bone resorption (38). Finally, certain nutrients such as the milk sugar lactose and some amino acids have been shown to enhance calcium absorption in both rat (39) and man (40). This suggests that certain foods such as milk, which contain high amounts of both calcium and lactose, may be especially beneficial in maintaining calcium homeostasis in the elderly. It is hoped that further research will suggest new ways of improving calcium metabolism and maintaining bone integrity in the elderly.

Acknowledgments

The author gratefully acknowledges the excellent secretarial assistance of Mrs. Cheryl Duff. Serum iPTH and iCT measurements were made by Dr. Leonard R. Forte, Veterans Administration Medical Center, Columbia, Missouri. This research was supported in part by the Veterans Administration.

References

1. Avioli LV: Osteoporosis: Pathogenesis and therapy, in Avioli LV and Krane SM (eds): *Metabolic Bone Disease,* vol 1. New York, Academic Press, 1977, pp 307–370.
2. Nordin BEC, Horsman A, Gallagher JC: Effect of various therapies on bone loss in women, in Kuhlencordt F, Kruse H (eds): *Calcium Metabolism, Bone and Metabolic Bone Diseases.* Berlin, Springer-Verlag, 1975, pp 233–242.
3. Gallagher JC, Riggs BL, Eisman J, et al: Intestinal calcium absorption and serum vitamin D metabolites in normal subjects and osteoporotic patients. *J Clin Invest* 1979; 64:729–736.
4. Abraham S: Dietary intake findings, United States, 1971–1974, in *National Health Survey, Vital and Health Statistics,* Series II, No. 202, publication (HRA) 77-1647. US Dept. of Health, Education, and Welfare, Public Health Service, 1977.
5. Avioli LV, McDonald JE, Lee SW: Influence of aging on the intestinal absorption of ^{47}Ca in women and its relation to ^{47}Ca absorption in postmenopausal osteoporosis. *J Clin Invest* 1965; 44:1960–1967.
6. Bullamore JR, Gallagher JC, Wilkinson R, Nordin BEC: Effect of age on calcium absorption. *Lancet* 1970; II:535–537.
7. Ireland P, Fordtran JS: Effect of dietary calcium and age on jejunal calcium absorption in humans studied by intestinal perfusion. *J Clin Invest* 1973; 52:2672–2681.
8. Wiske PS, Epstein S, Bell NH, et al: Increases in immunoreactive parathyroid hormone with age. *N Engl J Med* 1979; 300:1419–1421.

9. Armbrecht HJ, Forte LR, Halloran BP: Effect of age and dietary calcium on renal 25-OH-D metabolism, serum 1,25$(OH)_2$D, and PTH. *Am J Physiol* 1984; 246:E266–E270.
10. Armbrecht HJ, Zenser TV, Bruns MEH, Davis BB: Effect of age on intestinal calcium absorption and adaptation to dietary calcium. *Am J Physiol* 1979; 236:E769–E774.
11. Armbrecht HJ, Zenser TV, Gross CJ, Davis BB: Adaptation to dietary calcium and phosphorus restriction changes with age. *Am J Physiol* 1980; 239:E322–E327.
12. Horst RL, DeLuca HF, Jorgenson NA: The effect of age on calcium absorption and accumulation of 1,25-dihydroxyvitamin D_3 in intestinal mucosa of rats. *Metab Bone Dis Relat Res* 1978; 1:29–33.
13. Armbrecht HJ, Zenser TV, Davis BB: Effects of vitamin D metabolites on intestinal calcium absorption and calcium binding protein in young and adult rats. *Endocrinology* 1980; 106:469–475.
14. Gray RW, Gambert SR: Effect of age on plasma 1,25-$(OH)_2$ vitamin D in the rat. *Age* 1982; 5:54–56.
15. Reeve L, Tanaka Y, DeLuca HF: Studies on the site of 1,25-dihydroxyvitamin D_3 synthesis *in vivo*. *J Biol Chem* 1983; 258:3615–3617.
16. Armbrecht HJ, Zenser TV, Davis BB: Effect of age on the conversion of 25-hydroxyvitamin D_3 to 1,25-dihydroxyvitamin D_3 by the kidney of the rat. *J Clin Invest* 66:1118–1123.
17. Pavlovitch JH, Cournot-Witmer G, Bourdeau A, et al: Suppressive effects of 24,25-dihydroxycholecalciferol on bone resorption induced by acute bilateral nephrectomy in rats. *J Clin Invest* 1981; 68:803–810.
18. DeLuca HF: The vitamin D system in the regulation of calcium and phosphorus metabolism. *Nutr Rev* 1979; 37:161–193.
19. Gallagher JC, Riggs BL, Jerpbak CM, Arnaud CD: The effect of age on serum immunoreactive parathyroid hormone in normal and osteoporotic women. *J Lab Clin Med* 1980; 95:373–385.
20. Armbrecht HJ, Wongsurawat N, Zenser TV, Davis BB: Differential effects of parathyroid hormone on the renal 1,25-dihydroxyvitamin D_3 and 24,25-dihydroxyvitamin D_3 production of young and adult rats. *Endocrinology* 1982; 111:1339–1344.
21. Armbrecht HJ, Forte LR, Wongsurawat N, et al: Forskolin increases 1,25-dihydroxyvitamin D_3 production by rat renal slices *in vitro*. *Endocrinology* 1984; 114:644–649.
22. Rost CR, Bikle DD, Kaplan RA: In vitro stimulation of 25-hydroxycholecalciferol 1α-hydroxylation by parathyroid hormone in chick kidney slices: Evidence for a role for adenosine 3′, 5′-monophosphate. *Endocrinology* 1981; 108:1002–1005.
23. Henry HL: Insulin permits parathyroid hormone stimulation of 1,25-dihydroxyvitamin D_3 production in cultured kidney cells. *Endocrinology* 1981; 108:733–735.
24. Noland TA, Henry HL: Protein phosphorylation in chick kidney. Response to parathyroid hormone, cyclic AMP, calcium, and phosphatidylserine. *J Biol Chem* 1983; 258:538–546.
25. Armbrecht HJ, Wongsurawat N, Zenser TV, Davis BB: Effect of PTH and

$1,25(OH)_2D_3$ on renal $25(OH)D_3$ metabolism, adenylate cyclase and protein kinase. *Am J Physiol* 1984; 246:E102–E107.

26. Marcus R, Gonzales D: Age-related changes in parathyroid hormone-dependent cyclic AMP formation in rat kidney. *Mech Ageing Dev* 1982; 20:353–360.
27. Talmage RV, Cooper CW: Physiology and mode of action of calcitonin, in DeGroot LJ, Cahill GF, Martini L, et al (eds): *Endocrinology,* vol 2. New York, Grune & Stratton, 1979, pp 647–651.
28. Anast CS, David L, Winnacker J, et al: Serum calcitonin-lowering effect of magnesium in patients with medullary carcinoma of the thyroid. *J Clin Invest* 1975; 56:1615–1621.
29. Queener SF, Bell NH, Larson SM, et al: Comparison of the regulation of calcitonin in serum of old and young buffalo rats. *J Endocrinol* 1980; 87:73–80.
30. Thomas ML, Armbrecht HJ, Forte LR: Effects of long-term vitamin D deficiency and response to D-repletion in the mature and aging male and female rat. *Mech Ageing Dev* 1984; 25:161–175.
31. Copp DH, Kuczerpa AV: A new bioassay for calcitonin and effect of age and dietary Ca on the response, in Taylor S (ed): Calcitonin. New York, Springer-Verlag, 1968, pp 18–24.
32. Heath H, Sizemore GW: Plasma calcitonin in normal man. Differences between men and women. *J Clin Invest* 1977; 60:1135–1140.
33. Hillgard CJ, Stevenson JC, MacIntyre I: Relative deficiency of plasma calcitonin in normal women. *Lancet* 1978; I:961–962.
34. Shamonki IM, Fumar AM, Tataryn IV, et al: Age-related changes of calcitonin secretion in females. *J Clin Endocrinol Metab* 1980; 50:437–439.
35. Kalu, DN, Cockerham R, Yu BP, Roos BA: Lifelong dietary modulation of calcitonin levels in rats. *Endocrinology* 1983; 113:2010–2016.
36. Kalu DN, Hardin RH, Cockerham R, Yu BP: Aging and dietary modulation of rat skeleton and parathyroid hormone. *Endocrinology* 1984; (in press).
37. Armbrecht, HJ, Gross CJ, Zenser TV. Effect of dietary calcium and phosphorus restriction on calcium and phosphorus balance in young and old rats. *Arch Biochem Biophys* 1981; 210:179–185.
38. Peacock M, Gallagher JC, Nordin BEC: Action of 1α-hydroxyvitamin D_3 on calcium absorption and bone resorption in man. *Lancet* 1974; I:385–389.
39. Armbrecht HJ, Wasserman RH: Enhancement of Ca^{++} uptake by lactose in the rat small intestine. *J Nutr* 1976; 106:1265–1271.
40. Condon JR, Nassim JR, Millard FJC, Stainthorpe EM: Calcium and phosphorus metabolism in relation to lactose intolerance. *Lancet* 1970; I:1027–1029.

Part II

Effect of Nutrition on Aging—Length of Life

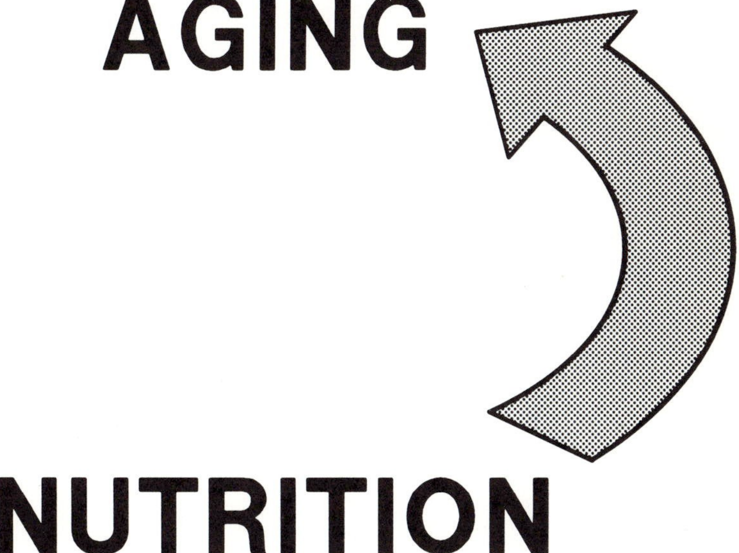

6

Dietary Restriction and Metabolism and Disease

Edward J. Masoro

In 1935, McCay and his colleagues (1) reported that severe food restriction started in rats at weaning resulted in many early deaths but also in a remarkably long life for those rats that survived past the first year of life. This finding has become a cornerstone of experimental gerontology. It has been repeated many times in several rodent species and has been found to be effective even when the food restriction is not severe enough to retard maturation markedly (2).

Of course the fact that an intervention increases the length of life does not necessarily mean that it acts by slowing the aging process (3). However, food restriction does much more than influence longevity. Its action on the aging of rodents can be summarized as follows:

1. extension of life span
2. retardation of age-related physiologic deterioration
3. retardation of age-related disease processes

Because food restriction provides a potentially powerful approach for the exploration of the aging process and because of the possible practical significance of modulating aging by nutritional means, our laboratory, for the past 8 years, has intensively explored in two successive studies many aspects of the action of food restriction on aging in rats. This chapter focuses on our findings.

Male Fischer 344 rats (specific pathogen-free) were maintained in a barrier facility throughout the course of these studies. In the first study, there were two dietary groups: Group A was fed ad libitum throughout life a standard semisynthetic diet (caloric composition of 21% protein, 57% carbohydrate, and 22% fat) and Group R was provided the same diet but was restricted to 60% of the mean food intake of the ad libitum-fed Group A rats starting at 6 weeks of age. In the second study, there were five dietary groups: Groups 1 and 2 were a repeat of Groups A and R, respectively; Group 3 was restricted to 60% of the food intake of Group 1 from 6 weeks to 6 months and thereafter fed ad libitum; Group 4 was restricted to 60% of the food intake of Group 1 starting at 6 months of age; Group 5 was fed ad libitum throughout life, but the diet (caloric composition of 12.6% protein, 65.4% carbohydrate, and 22% fat) was different in composition from that of Group 1. Thus, the second study expands the first study by examining a group that is food restricted during early life only, a group in which food restriction was not initiated until adult life and a group in which protein, but not calories, was restricted.

Longevity

The longevity findings of our first study (4) are presented in Figure 6-1 in the form of survival curves. The survival curve of the Group A rats is quite rectangular, as would be expected for highly protected barrier-maintained rats. The survival curve for Group R is much less rectangular, which is somewhat surprising because the effects of technology and medicine on human survival curves have been to make them increasingly rectangular. What food restriction does is to shift the survival curve to the right, thereby increasing not only the median length of life but also the life span (ie, the maximum length of life of the rat population). In con-

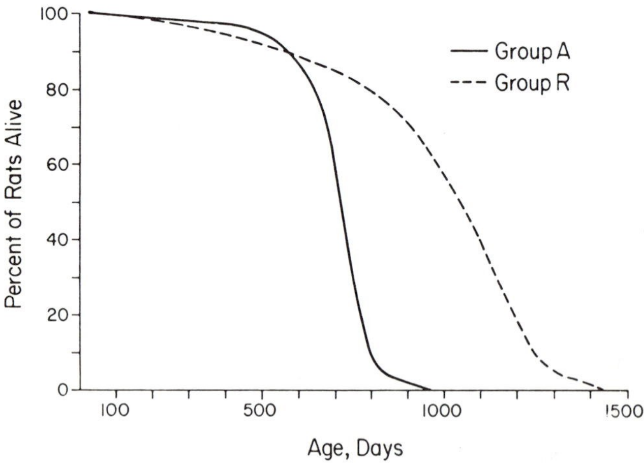

Figure 6-1. Survival curves of ad libitum fed (Group A) and restricted (Group R) rats of the first study. From Yu et al (4).

trast, technology and medicine have increased the median length of life of humans, but have had little or no effect on the human life span.

The survival curves for Group A and R rats were generated from a population of 115 rats for each group. This number of rats made the longevity study costly to execute. Thus, in the second study, only 40 rats per dietary group were used for the longevity study. The survival curve of Group 1 almost perfectly replicated that of Group A and the survival curve of Group 2 was similar to that of Group R. Thus, in barrier-maintained rats and highly controlled environmental and nutritional conditions, longevity findings are highly reproducible and can be reliably measured with an *n* of 40 rats per dietary group.

Food restriction limited to the period of from 6 weeks to 6 months of age caused a small but significant increase in the median length of life (808 days for Group 3 rats compared with 701 days for Group 1 rats) and in the maximum length of life (1,040 days for Group 3 rats compared with 941 days for Group 1 rats). In contrast, restriction of rats starting at adult life markedly increased median length of life (941 days for Group 4 rats) and increased the maximum length of life as effectively as food restriction started at 6 weeks of age (1,299 days for Group 4 rats compared with 1,296 days for Group 2 rats).

Protein restriction in the absence of caloric restriction significantly increased the median length of life (810 days for Group 5 rats compared with 701 days for Group 1 rats), but did not appreciably influence the maximum length of life (969 days for Group 5 rats compared with 941 days for Group 1 rats). Not only was the caloric intake of Group 1 rats and Group 5 rats the same, but the rates of growth of the rats in each of these dietary groups were also the same.

Physiological Deterioration

Most physiologic processes undergo age-related change (5) of such a nature that it seems reasonable to conclude that there is physiologic deterioration with advancing age. Food restriction has been found to retard these age-related physiologic changes (6). Typical of this are our findings (7) on serum cholesterol concentrations shown in Figure 6-2. At 6 months and 12 months of age, the serum cholesterol concentration was similar in Group 1 and Group 2 rats. However, with increasing age, serum cholesterol increased markedly in Group 1 rats while in Group 2 rats this increase was less marked and was delayed. The serum cholesterol concentration changes with age in Group 4 rats were identical to those seen in Group 2 rats while the changes in Group 3 rats were similar to those seen in Group 1 rats. Thus, food restriction started in early life or in adult life and continued throughout the rest of life delayed and blunted this age-related physiologic change, while food restriction limited to early life had little effect.

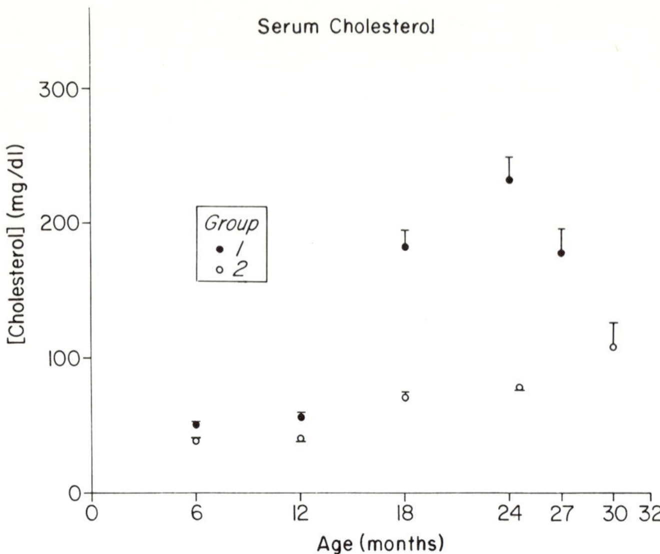

Figure 6-2. Age changes in serum cholesterol concentrations in ad libitum fed (Group 1) and restricted (Group 2) rats of the second study. Modified from Masoro et al (7).

Most other physiologic activities that have been studied are influenced by food restriction in a similar way. For instance, in our laboratory (6) the loss in response of fat cells to hormones, the increase in serum calcitonin and parathyroid hormone levels, the loss of skeletal muscle mass, the deterioration in the mechanical response of skeletal muscle, the loss of bone mass were all delayed and partially or totally prevented by food restriction (see also Chapter 5). Levin et al (8) found the age-related loss of dopamine receptors in the rat corpus striatum to be retarded by food restriction. Also, the age-related deterioration of the immune system in mice has been found to be delayed by food restriction (9, 10).

Age-Related Disease

A major age-related disease process in the male Fischer 344 rat is chronic nephropathy. This lesion is in many ways similar to atherosclerosis in humans. It starts early and progresses throughout life. The severity varies from individual to individual and clinical expression of the disease is seen only with the most severe lesions (ie, Grade E lesions). Many, but by no means all of the population, eventually develop Grade E lesions during adult life. Food restriction (both in Groups 2 and 4) markedly curtailed the progression of this disease process. At death, 51% of the Group 1 rats had Grade E lesions; in contrast, only 4% of the Group 4 rats and 2% of Group 2 rats exhibited Grade E lesions at death. Food restriction limited to early life was not very effective in retarding the progression of chronic nephropathy; 32% of the Group 3 rats had Grade E lesions at death. However, restricting dietary protein, but not calories, was quite effective in slowing the progression of chronic nephropathy. Only 10% of the Group 5 rats had Grade E lesions at death. It is surprising that restricting protein had such a marked effect on chronic nephropathy and yet exerted such a small effect on longevity. Clearly, the marked prolongation of life by food restriction is not primarily related to its ability to retard the development of chronic nephropathy.

Food restriction retarded the development of cardiomyopathy in a fashion similar to that just described for chronic nephropathy. Grade 3 cardiomyopathy involves a marked degeneration of myocardial cells and thus almost certainly indicates the existence of clinically expressed heart disease. At death, 21% of the Group 1 rats, 0% of the Group 2 rats, 13% of the Group 3 rats, 2% of the Group 4 rats, and 7% of the Group 5 rats exhibited Grade 3 lesions. Again, food restriction through most of adult life was very effective in retarding the development of the disease process. Protein restriction without caloric restriction was also quite effective.

Rats sacrificed in cross-sectional studies showed that food restriction during adult life (Groups 2 and 4) delayed the occurrence of neoplastic disease. However, at death, it was a significant clinical problem in rats of all groups. Thus, 68% of both the Group 2 and 4 rats had neoplastic disease at death, but of course death in these rats occurred at very old ages.

Mechanisms by Which Food Restriction Influences Aging

During the past 50 years, four major hypotheses have dominated thought about the mechanism by which food restriction retards aging. The first of these was the view that food restriction slows the aging process by retarding maturation. Indeed, this hypothesis was the basis for the initial studies of McCay and his colleagues. They postulated that aging is a postmaturational event and that if maturation could be prevented, aging would not occur. They interpreted their findings as supporting this view; ie, food restriction prolonged life and retarded aging by slowing maturation. Our finding that food restriction started in adult life (Group 4 rats) is about as effective as food restriction started early in life (Group 2 rats) in increasing the life span and in retarding physiologic deterioration and age-related disease is not in accord with this view.

A hypothesis closely related to that of McCay is the view that food restriction retards aging by slowing the rate of growth and prolonging its duration. Indeed, there are considerable data indicating that the length of life of rats and mice correlates inversely with rate of growth and directly with duration of growth (11). However, again, our finding that adult onset food restriction is as effective as food restriction started early in life makes this hypothesis about mechanism an unlikely one.

For many years now, it has been generally believed that in humans greater adiposity than the so-called ideal level results in decreased longevity. This widely held view has recently been reviewed and challenged by Andres (12). Nevertheless, many nutritionists seem to assume that food restriction influences longevity and the aging process by reducing body fat. Data obtained in our laboratory do not support this concept (13). In the case of the Group A rats of our first study (body fat ranged from 12% to 25% of body weight), there was no correlation between body fat and length of life. Moreover, in the case of the Group R rats (body fat ranged from 7% to 14% of body weight), there was a positive correlation; ie, the fatter the rat, the longer it lived.

In 1977, Sacher (3) proposed that food restriction increased the length of life by reducing the metabolic rate per gram of body mass. He based this conclusion on his analysis of data published by Ross (14). From those data, he calculated that the average lifetime caloric expenditure for ad libitum-fed rats and rats fed various life-prolonging restricted diets was the same for all groups, specifically 102 kcal, with no group varying from this value by more than 4.5%. This view is in line with the "rate of living theory of aging" proposed in 1928 by Pearl (15). Indeed, Rubner (16) stated at the turn of the century that there was an inverse correlation between the life span of domestic animals and their metabolic rate per unit body weight.

This hypothesis was thoroughly studied in our laboratory (17) and we conclude that food restriction does not influence the aging process by lowering the metabolic rate per unit body mass. Group R rats of our first study consumed more calories per day per gram body weight than Group A rats. If calculated on the basis of lean body mass, Group A and R rats consumed the same number of calories per day. During their lifetime, the average caloric intake per gram body mass of Group R rats was 134 kcal per gram body weight compared to 92 kcal per gram body weight for ad-libitum-fed rats. Thus, the food-restricted rats consumed more calories per gram body weight per lifetime and lived longer than the ad libitum fed rats. A likely reason for the discrepancy between our results and those of Sacher is the fact that Sacher's calculation was based on the limited amount of data available in a published paper of Ross, and thus required assumptions, while our calculations were made directly from the raw data, requiring no assumptions to be made. Indeed, if Sacher had chosen different assumptions, his calculations from Ross's data would have led him to a conclusion similar to ours.

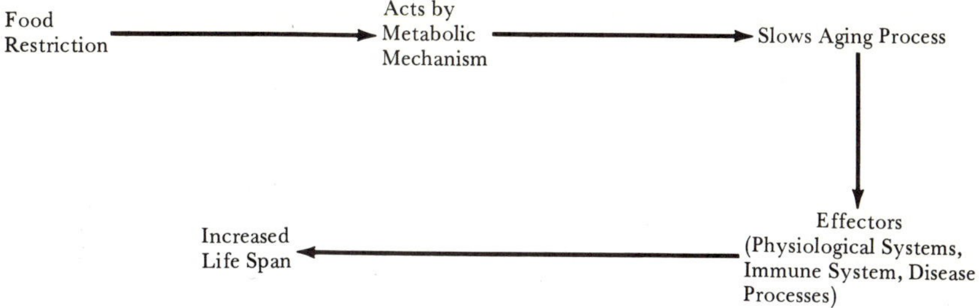

Figure 6-3. A general metabolic hypothesis. From Masoro (18).

Conclusion

If all hypotheses about the mechanism of food restriction so far proposed appear not to be correct, how, then should this subject area be further explored? My colleague, Dr. Byung P. Yu, and I feel that the framework shown in Figure 6-3, which we call a general metabolic hypothesis, can serve as a useful guide for further studies (18). This hypothesis proposes that food restriction slows the aging process by one or more specific metabolic action(s). By slowing the aging process, food restriction retards age-related physiologic deterioration, including that of the immune system and the development of age-related disease. A sequela of these actions is the increase in longevity. Future research on food restriction should focus on the specific metabolic event(s) coupling food restriction with the slowing of the aging process.

References

1. McCay CM, Crowell MF, Maynard LA: The effect of retarded growth upon the length of life span and upon the ultimate body size. *J Nutr* 1935; 10:63–79.
2. Berg BN, Simms HS: Nutrition and longevity. II. Longevity and onset of disease with different levels of food intake. *J Nutr* 1960; 71:251–263.
3. Sacher GA: Life table modification and life prolongation, in Finch C, Hayflick L (eds): *Handbook of Biology of Aging*. New York, Van Nostrand Reinhold, 1977, pp 582–638.
4. Yu BP, Masoro EJ, Murata I, et al: Life span study of SPF Fischer 344 male rats fed ad libitum or restricted diets: Longevity, growth, lean body mass and disease. *J Geront.* 1982; 37:130–141.
5. Masoro EJ: Physiologic changes with aging, in Winick M (ed): *Nutrition and Aging*, New York, Wiley, 1976, pp 61–76.
6. Masoro EJ, Yu BP, Bertrand HA, Lynd FT: Nutritional probe of the aging process. *Fed Proc* 1980; 39:3178–3182.
7. Masoro EJ, Compton C, Yu BP, Bertrand H: Temporal and compositional

dietary restrictions modulate age-related changes in serum lipids. *J Nutr* 1983; 113:880–892.

8. Levin P, Janda JK, Joseph JA, et al. Dietary restriction retards the age-associated loss of rat striatal dopaminergic receptors. *Science* 1981; 214:561–562.
9. Weindruch R, Kristie JA, Cheney KE, Walford RL: Influence of controlled dietary restriction on immunologic function and aging. *Fed Proc* 1979; 38:2007–2016.
10. Fernandes G, Friend P, Yunis EJ, Good RA: Influence of dietary restriction on immunologic function and renal disease in (NZB × NZW)F_1 mice. *Proc Natl Acad Sci USA* 1978; 75:1500–1504.
11. Goodrick CL: Effects of long-term voluntary wheel exercise on male and female Wistar rats. I. Longevity. *Gerontology* 1980; 26:22–33.
12. Andres R: Influence of obesity on longevity in the aged, in Borek C, Ferraglio C, King D (eds): *Aging, Cancer and Cell Membranes.* New York, Thieme S. Stuttgart 1980, pp 238–246.
13. Bertrand HA, Lynd FT, Masoro EJ, Yu BP: Changes in adipose mass and cellularity through the adult life of rats fed ad libitum or a life-prolonging restricted diet. *J Geront* 1980; 35:827–835.
14. Ross MH: Aging, nutrition and hepatic enzyme activity patterns in the rat. *J Nutr* 1969; 97 (suppl 1; part II):563–602.
15. Pearl R: *The Rate of Living.* New York, Knopf, 1928.
16. Rubner M: Das Problem der Lebensdauer und Seine Beziehungen Zun Wachstum und Ernährung. München, Oldenborerg, 1908.
17. Masoro EJ, Yu BP, Bertrand HA: Action of food restriction in delaying the aging process. *Proc Natl Acad Sci* USA 1982; 79:4239–4241.
18. Masoro EJ: Food restriction and the aging process. *J Am Geriatr Soc* 1984; 32:296–300.

7

Dietary Restriction and Biologic Variables

Charles H. Barrows, Jr. and Gertrude C. Kokkonen

Dietary restriction has been shown to increase the life span of a variety of young growing laboratory animals (1). For example, this phenomenon has been reported in the following model systems: *Tokophrya, Campanularia flexuosa, Daphnia* sp., rotifers, *Drosophila* sp., and fish. In addition, a number of laboratory experiments have been carried out on rodents. It has been generally believed that nutritional manipulations that increase life span had to be imposed during early growth. This concept originated from the early work of Minot, who postulated that senescence follows the cessation of growth (2,3). Furthermore, Lansing indicated that aging in the rotifer involved the appearance of a cytoplasmic factor that coincided with the cessation of growth (4). However, recent studies have indicated that dietary restriction imposed in adult life was effective in increasing the life span of rotifers, *Daphnia* sp., rats, hamsters, and mice (11). In studies using both young growing and adult animals, dietary restriction has been brought about by: (a) reducing the daily dietary intake of a nutritionally adequate diet (one that supports maximal growth); (b) intermittently feeding a nutritionally adequate diet (eg, feeding every second, third, or fourth day); and (c) feeding ad libitum a diet containing insufficient amounts of protein to support maximal growth.

Mechanisms of Dietary Restriction

Thus far there have been few attempts to explain the mechanism involved in the extension of life span associated with dietary restriction. Part of the difficulty lies in the small amount of data presently available on which to base a testable hypothesis. In the past, studies on the effects of dietary restriction on biochemical variables have produced two generally compatible pieces of information. Leto et al (5) showed that the life span of C57BL/6J female mice could be increased from 685 ± 23 to 852 ± 27 days by feeding low dietary protein (4%) from weaning. A variety of enzymatic activities were determined in liver, kidney, and heart. The only meaningful data concerning intracellular proteins such as enzymes are those based on some index of cell number. The study by Leto et al (6) estimated cell number based on the DNA per wet weight of the tissue; its validity was based on our finding of the constancy of nuclear DNA in the livers of rats of different ages (7). Similar data in the brains of mice have been described by Franks (8). Enzymatic activities of the tissues of normal and dietarily restricted mice are shown in Figures 7-1, 7-2, and 7-3 (6). In general these data indicate a reduced enzymatic activity per unit DNA in these three tissues. It would seem that this manipulation affects liver the most, kidney intermediately, and heart the least. Similar findings have been described by Ross (9), who determined the activity of catalase, alkaline phosphatase, histidase, and adenosine triphosphatase in normal and dietarily restricted Sprague-Dawley rats. In these studies Ross's enzymatic activity is expressed per hepatocyte, based on counts in histologic sections. The data obtained on catalase are shown in Figure 7-4. The data of Leto and Ross thus indicate a reduced cellular enzymatic activity in most, but not all systems tested. These data led to the proposal that an increase in life span due to dietary restriction was caused by a reduced enzymatic synthesis.

Effect of Dietary Restriction on Biochemical Variables

In an effort to establish whether the various dietary manipulations that increase life span do so by a common biologic mechanism, a recent study measured biochemical variables in mice fed two dietary regimens reported to increase life span, namely, low protein and intermittent feeding.

Methods

Twenty-one day-old C57BL/6J female mice were obtained from Jackson Laboratories, Bar Harbor, Maine. All animals when received were individually housed in a room maintained at 24°C on a 12-hour light–dark

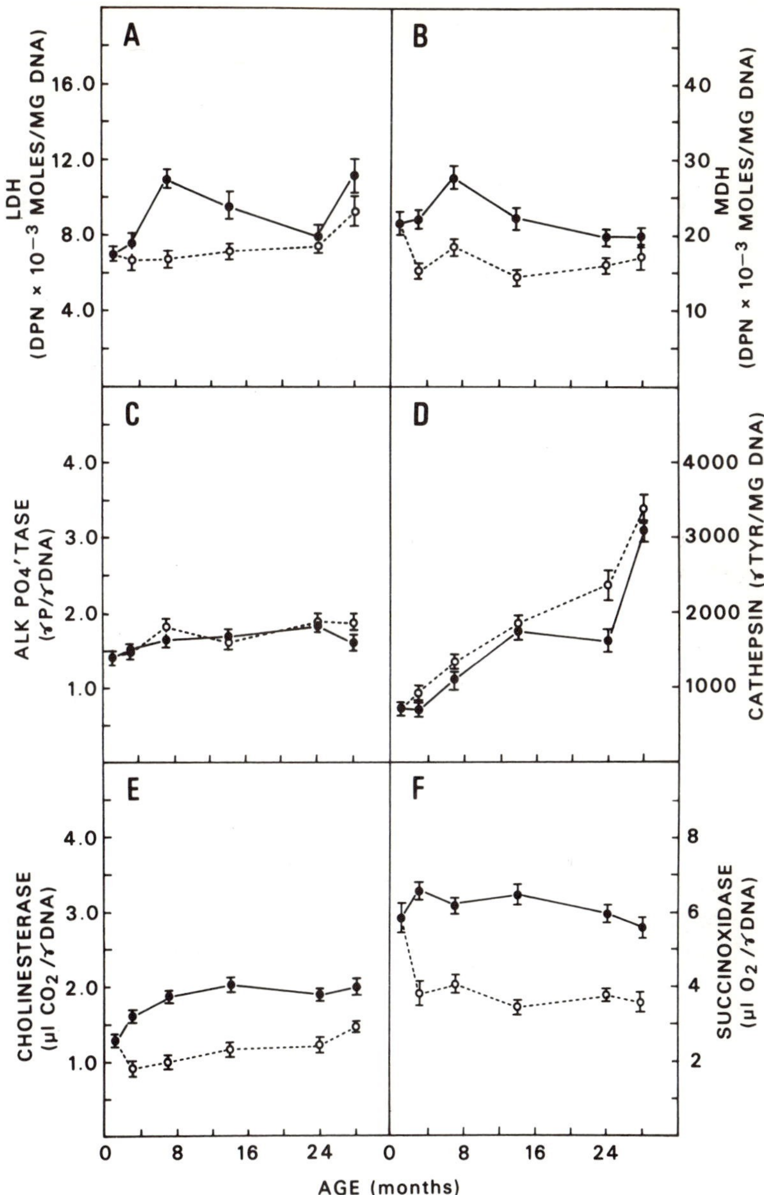

Figure 7-1. Effect of age and diet on the enzymatic activities of liver of female C57BL/6J mice fed (●) 26% casein diet or (○) 4% casein diet. Vertical bars represent SEM. The mean life span and SEM of the animals fed either the low-protein or control diet was 852 ± 27.4 days and 685 ± 22.8 days, respectively.

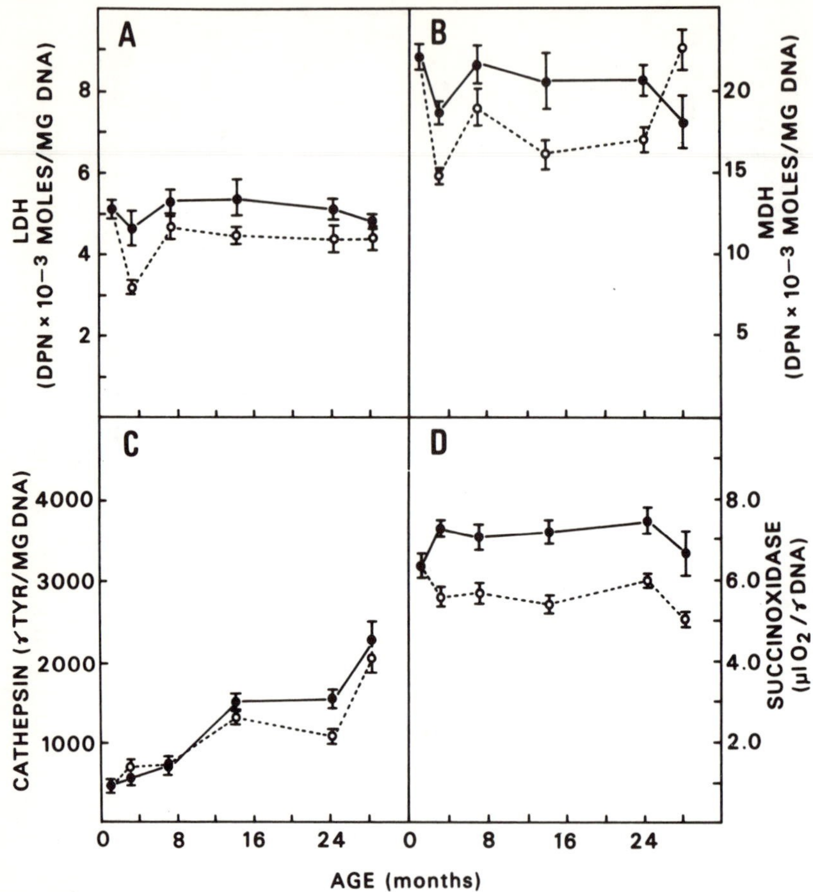

Figure 7-2. Effect of age and diet on the enzymatic activities of kidneys of female C57BL/6J mice fed (●) 26% casein diet or (○) 4% casein diet. Vertical bars represent SEM. The mean life span and SEM of the animals fed either the low-protein or control diet was 852 ± 27.4 days and 685 ± 22.8 days, respectively.

cycle and randomly distributed among three dietary manipulations. Two diets prepared and pelleted by Tekland Mills, Madison, Wisconsin, were used in the experiment: 28% casein (24% protein) and 4.6% casein (4% protein). All diets contained 4% hydrogenated vegetable oil, 15% cornstarch, 4% USP XIV salt mixture, adequate amounts of all known vitamins and 47% to 70% sucrose to compensate for the protein content in order to keep the diets isocaloric. The protein source was crude casein. Water was offered ad libitum. The dietary manipulations were (a) 24% protein ad libitum, (b) 4% protein ad libitum, or (c) 24% protein intermittently fed (diet offered for 24 hours on Monday and Wednesday, and

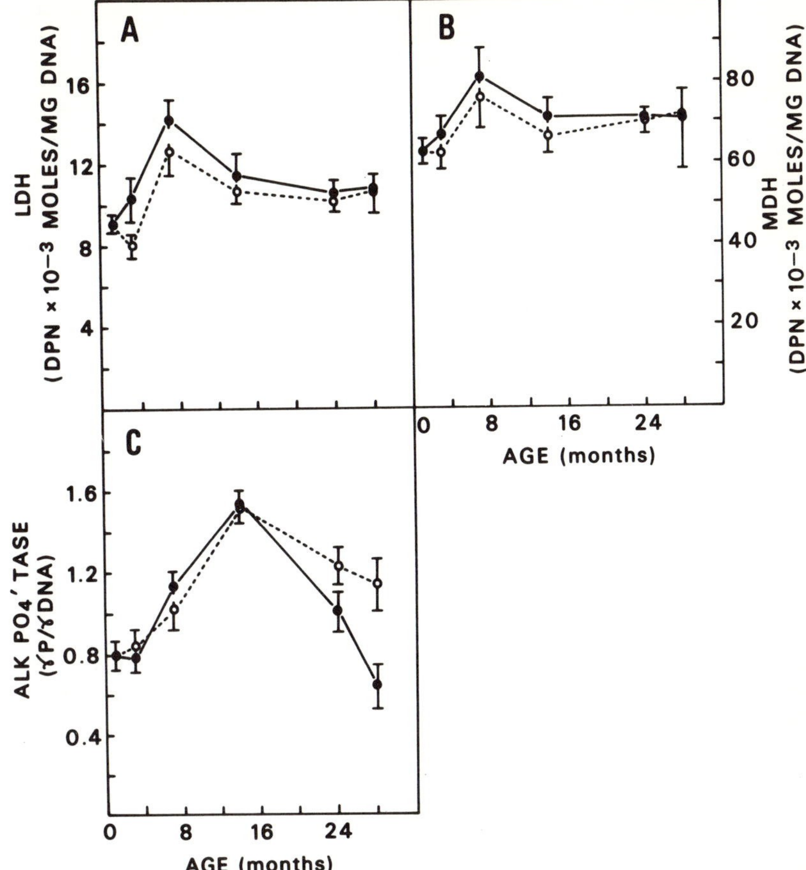

Figure 7-3. Effect of age and diet on the enzymatic activities of hearts of female C57BL/6J mice fed (●) 26% casein diet or (○) 4% casein diet. Vertical bars represent SEM. The mean life span and SEM of the animals fed either the low-protein or control diet was 852 ± 27.4 days and 685 ± 22.8 days, respectively.

for 8 hours on Friday). Those animals referred to as intermittent-fed were sacrificed either on Tuesdays or Thursdays, ie, following a 24-hour feeding period. Those referred to as intermittent-fasted were sacrificed either on Wednesdays or Fridays, ie, following a 24-hour fasting period. The animals were sacrificed at 2 and 7 months of age by cervical dislocation and their livers and kidneys rapidly excised, iced, and weighed. Distilled water homogenates were prepared for assays.

The methods used for the measurements of succinoxidase and cholinesterase have been reported (10). Malic dehydrogenase activity was measured by following the decrease in absorption at 340 nm caused by the

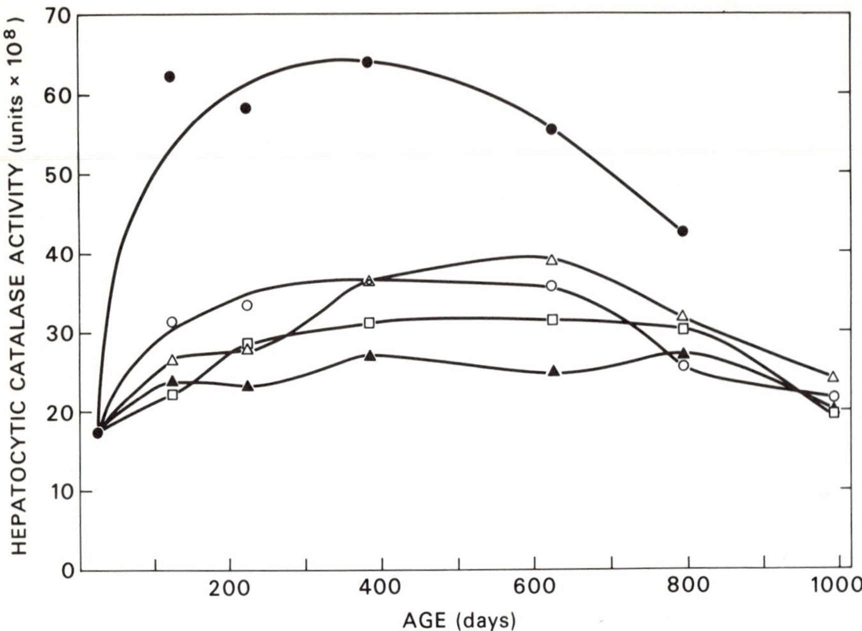

Figure 7-4. Effect of diet and age on the activity of hepatic catalase in male Sprague-Dawley rats. Rats maintained on commercial diet ad libitum (●); rats whose daily food allotment was restricted: (○) Diet A; (△) Diet B; (□) Diet C; (▲) Diet D. From Ross MH (9).

oxidation of DPNH (reduced diphosphopyridine nucleotide). Tissue DNA was isolated by the Munro and Fleck modification of the Schmidt-Tannhauser method (11). DNA concentrations of the samples were measured by the method of Ceriotti (12). Protein assay of the trichloroacetic acid (7%) precipitates of the tissues was performed according to Miller's modification of the Lowry procedure (13).

Results

The DNA per milligram of tissue in the livers of young growing mice fed the 4% protein diet was significantly higher than that of the control animals (Table 7-1). Although the values for the intermittent-fasted animals were higher than the controls and those of the intermittent-fed lower, the mean values were approximately the same as the animals fed the 24% protein diet ad libitum. If an increase in the DNA per unit wet weight represents a decrease in the size of hepatic cells, then these data suggest small cells in the livers of animals fed 4% protein diet. Further-

Table 7-1. Concentration of Protein and DNA in the Livers and Kidneys of Female C57BL/6J Mice Fed Different Dietary Regimes from Weaning

	No.	*24% Protein*	*4% Protein*	*Intermittent Fed*	*Intermittent Fasted*
			DNA (γ/mg tissue)		
Liver					
2-mo old	10	3.52 ± 0.08	4.04 ± 0.07	3.19 ± 0.09	4.16 ± 0.19
7-mo old	10	4.13 ± 0.19	4.55 ± 0.17	3.49 ± 0.11	5.24 ± 0.18
Kidney					
2-mo old	10	6.46 ± 0.33	8.08 ± 0.13	5.89 ± 0.11	6.45 ± 0.15
7-mo old	10	6.63 ± 0.18	8.82 ± 0.18	6.00 ± 0.11	7.36 ± 0.18
			Protein (mg/mg DNA)		
Liver					
2-mo old	10	54.7 ± 1.7	41.1 ± 0.8	63.8 ± 0.6	51.6 ± 1.6
7-mo old	10	46.7 ± 0.9	34.8 ± 1.1	54.8 ± 1.8	39.6 ± 1.9
Kidney					
2-mo old	10	27.4 ± 1.7	22.1 ± 0.5	33.0 ± 1.0	26.8 ± 0.6
7-mo old	10	26.2 ± 0.8	20.4 ± 0.6	27.3 ± 0.5	23.4 ± 0.9

more, they suggest that hepatic cells decrease in size during a period of fasting and return to the original size during a period of refeeding. Essentially the same results were obtained when kidneys were examined. There was a significant decrease in the protein per milligram of DNA in the livers and kidneys of young growing animals fed the diet containing 4% protein. The mean values of protein per milligram of DNA in animals fed either of the intermittent regimes were essentially the same as those of the controls. Similar results were obtained when specific enzymes such as malic dehydrogenase, succinoxidase, and cholinesterase were examined (Table 7-2).

It was of interest to determine whether a relationship existed between cell size and cellular protein among the different dietary groups. Therefore, in liver, the cellular protein (mg protein/mg DNA) was plotted against cell size (mg DNA/mg wet wt) for each dietary group. The results shown in Figure 7-5 indicate that, among animals fed the 24% diet ad libitum, the larger the cell (low mg DNA/wet wt) the higher the cellular protein. This relationship was maintained in the animals fed the low protein diet. In addition to small cells, as indicated by a shift of the values to higher concentrations of DNA per wet weight, there was a decrease in the cellular protein content of the same sized cells as indicated by the values lying outside of the distribution of the control animals (Fig 7-5B). A 24-hour fasting period also resulted in small cells, but the cellular protein content of the same sized cell was higher than in control animals (Fig. 7-5D). A 24-hour period of ad libitum feeding increased cellular size, and the cellular protein content seemed to be returning to the control level (Fig. 7-5C). Similar data were obtained when the activities of the specific enzymes malic dehydrogenase (Fig. 7-6) and succinoxidase (Fig. 7-7) were examined. On the other hand, the cellular activity of acetylcholinesterase was independent of cellular size (Fig. 7-8A). Nevertheless, the effect of low dietary protein was the same as in the other enzymes (Fig. 7-8B). Although starvation resulted in small cells, the enzymatic activity of the same cellular size was the same as the control animals (Fig. 7-8D), and refeeding resulted in high enzymatic activities (Fig 7-8C). This latter finding is different from that observed in enzymes whose activities are related to cell size. Although the same relationship existed for cell size and protein content, dietary restriction had very little effect in the kidney (Fig. 7-9).

Discussion

These data do not indicate the existence of a common biochemical alteration to explain the increase in life span brought on by dietary restriction, nor do they support the concept that the benefits of dietary restriction are exclusively associated with low protein synthesis. The data

Table 7-2. The Effect of Various Dietary Regimens on Enzymatic Activities in Livers of Female Mice

	24% Protein	*4% Protein*	*Intermittent Fed*	*Intermittent Fasted*
		Malic dehydrogenase (mmol DPNH/hr/mg DNA)		
2-mo-old	10.211 ± 0.293	7.344 ± 0.148	11.578 ± 0.178	10.371 ± 0.506
7-mo-old	7.998 ± 0.343	5.543 ± 0.383	9.714 ± 0.409	7.009 ± 0.218
		Succinoxidase (μ 10_2/hr/γDNA)		
2-mo-old	6.71 ± 0.37	4.00 ± 0.12	7.53 ± 0.20	6.73 ± 0.21
7-mo-old	5.96 ± 0.26	3.21 ± 0.16	6.99 ± 0.22	5.87 ± 0.20
		Cholinesterase (μ lCO_2/hr/λDNA)		
2-mo-old	7.34 ± 0.31	5.02 ± 0.30	9.79 ± 0.49	6.36 ± 0.32
7-mo-old	6.82 ± 0.44	3.95 ± 0.32	8.47 ± 0.27	6.06 ± 0.31

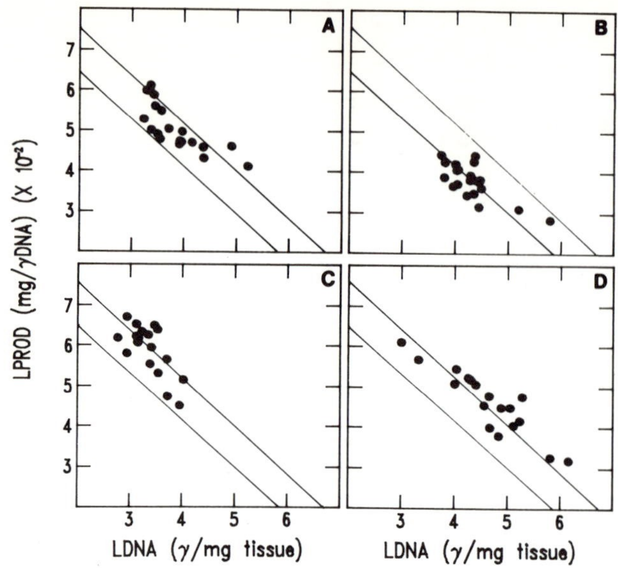

Figure 7-5. Effect of dietary regimen on the relationship between cellular protein and DNA in the livers of C57BL/6J female mice.

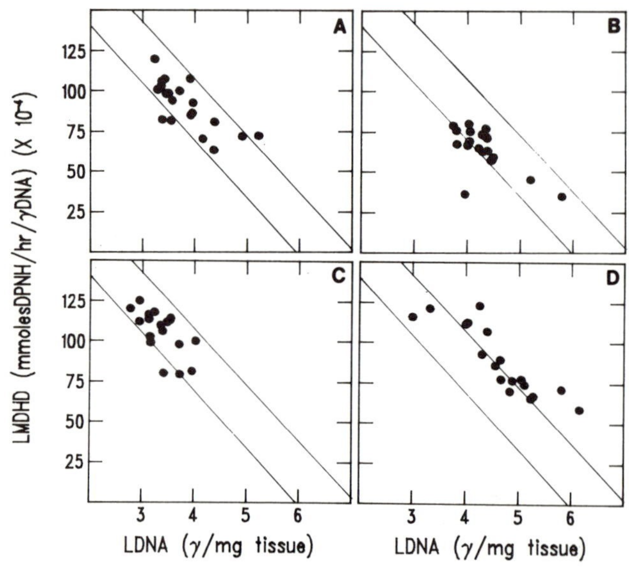

Figure 7-6. Effect of dietary regimen on the relationship between malic dehydrogenase and DNA in the livers of C57BL/6J female mice.

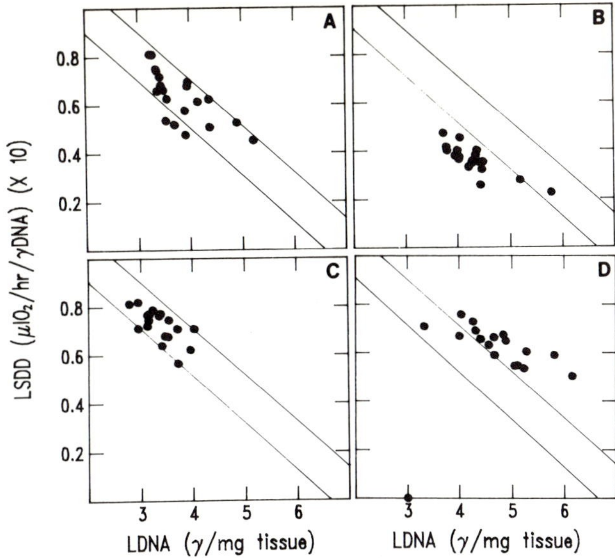

Figure 7-7. Effect of dietary regimen on the relationship between succinic oxidase and DNA in the livers of C57BL/6J female mice.

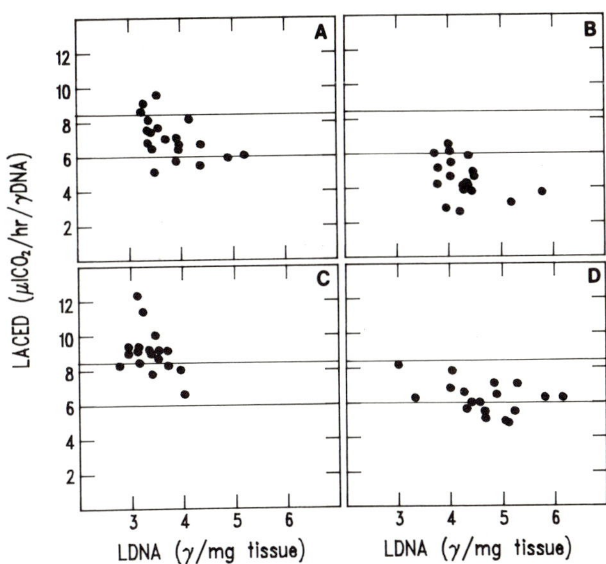

Figure 7-8. Effect of dietary regimen on the relationship between acetylcholinesterase and DNA in the livers of C57BL/6J female mice.

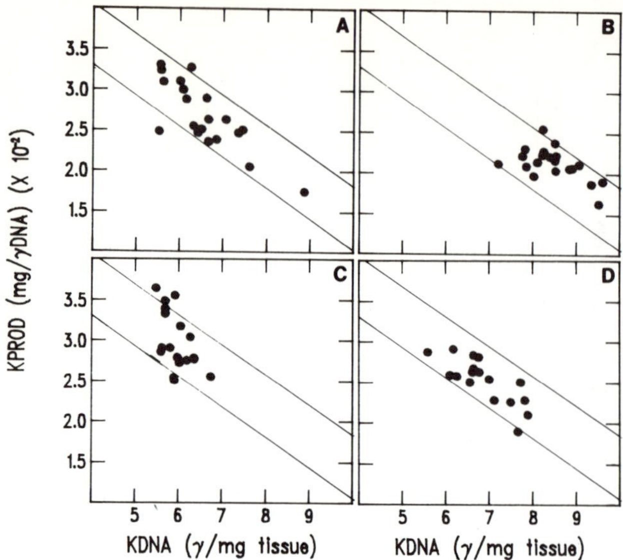

Figure 7-9. Effect of dietary regimen on the relationship between cellular protein and DNA in the kidneys of C57BL/6J female mice.

may suggest that various dietary regimens that increase life span do so by independent mechanisms, which produce different effects on such variables as age-associated disease, physiologic changes, and biochemical alterations.

Effect of Dietary Restriction on Disease

In order to investigate this possibility, previous studies of the effect of dietary restriction on disease were examined. In studies of the effect of dietary restriction on the immune system, the most frequently studied immune function was the mitogenic responses of lymphocytes. Available data indicate that the effect of low protein feeding or intake restrictions on this function is an initial suppression during the first months of life (14,15). As the animals mature and age, the effect of low protein feeding diminishes (16). On the other hand, the cells of animals with restricted intake exhibit markedly higher responses than controls to a variety of mitogens (15). Indeed, the data of Mann (14) obtained on the animals in the present report clearly indicate that in mature animals (7 months) the mitogenic responses of intermittently fed animals are markedly higher than those of controls, which suggests that cells containing high concentrations of enzymes are more responsive and may be more efficient.

Bras (17) studied the effect of dietary restriction on renal diseases in rats. The restricted animals were fed synthetic diets that contained high or low levels of calories or dietary proteins. Progressive glomerulonephrosis was diagnosed in the control animals, who were fed a commercial diet and assigned a disease index of 100. Thus, a value less than 100 indicated the beneficial effects of the experimental diet. Animals whose dietary intake was restricted and who were fed the high calorie–high protein diet had a disease index of 24.7. In animals fed a high calorie–low protein diet, the disease index was 10.5, indicating the beneficial effects of low dietary protein. However, when the caloric intake was reduced to a greater degree, the disease index was reduced to approximately 1.5. Thus there is a differential effect on renal disease depending upon the type of dietary restriction imposed.

Ross and Bras (18,19) have also extensively studied the relationship among spontaneous tumors, age, protein, and caloric restriction. Because of the high degree of specificity about the effectiveness of given diets on particular tumors, the investigations are difficult to summarize. Nevertheless, data similar to those reported for renal disease were observed when the incidence of malignant lymphomas was examined.

Time of Initiation of Dietary Restriction

The characteristics of young growing animals subjected to dietary restriction leave doubt about the applicability of this phenomenon to young growing human populations. For example, during early life, dietarily restricted animals are growth retarded, exhibit suppressed immunologic function and cellular enzymatic activity, and have low body temperature and increased basal metabolic rate (1). Data obtained on invertebrates suggest that fertility may be adversely affected (20,21). Therefore, it seems that if dietary restriction has any practical role in human populations it must be initiated during middle life. During the past 15 to 20 years a number of studies have shown that life span can be increased when dietary restriction is initiated during the middle life of the rat (12 to 16 months) (1). When the dietary protein is reduced from 24% to 12% in 16-month-old female rats, the increased life span is accompanied by little if any change in the body weight of the animals (22). Beauchene (23) and McCay (24) have also indicated that increases in life span may be brought about when body weights are reduced only approximately 10%. Thus there are dietary manipulations that seem beneficial and that do not involve radical changes in physiologic state as evidenced by body weight.

There are a number of studies indicating beneficial effects on physiologic function when dietary restriction is initiated in middle life. For example, both the data of Tucker et al (25) and Everitt et al (26) indicated improvement in renal function associated with adult dietary restriction. Bertrand (27) reported that the loss of responsiveness of adipocytes to glucagon could be totally reversed in adult animals subjected to dietary restriction. Weindruch et al (28) showed improved mitogenic response of splenic lymphocytes to phytohemagglutinin (PHA) and concanavalin A (Con A) stimulation in animals dietarily restricted at 12, 17, and 22 months of age. Similarly, Barrows and Roeder (29) showed that the biochemical characteristics associated with dietary restriction was the same in 12-month-old animals as in weanling animals. Saxton (30) reported that dietary restriction imposed in middle life reduced the frequency of a degenerative disease of the kidneys of rats. Dietary restriction imposed in 12- to 13-month-old mice by Weindruch and Walford (31) reduced the overall incidence of cancer and lymphoma to levels of borderline significance ($P < .07$). These authors also indicated that dietary restriction imposed at the age of 12 months showed a reduced tumor incidence in animals killed between 19 and 25 months of age. They conclude that apparently restriction of the diet, even when started in middle-aged mice, can inhibit cancer. Thus, data exist showing that relatively moderate dietary restriction imposed in middle life can increase life span, reduce diseases, and apparently reverse age-associated physiologic and biochemical age changes.

Conclusion

There is a relationship among cellular protein, enzymatic activity, and size. That is, small cells have low protein and low activity of some but not all enzymes. This relationship holds for both liver and kidney. Low protein feeding produces smaller cells with less protein and less enzyme per cell size than normal animals. Animals fed intermittently also have smaller cells than controls. In the fed state the cells have a protein content and enzymatic activities comparable to controls or higher. However, in the fasted state these cellular variables are always high. Kidney is less responsive than liver to diet. Thus, the biochemical characteristics of the two types of dietarily restricted animals are indeed markedly different. At present, there is no biochemical evidence for a common mechanism to explain the increased life span brought about by dietary restriction.

References

1. Barrows CH, Kokkonen, GC: Relationship between nutrition and aging, in Draper HH, (ed): *Advances in Nutritional Research* vol 1. New York, Plenum Press, 1972, pp 253–298.
2. Minot, CS: The problem of age, growth, and death; a study of cytomorphis. Based on lectures at the Lovell Institute, March 1907. London, Lovell Institute, 1908.

3. Minot CS: *Moderne Probleme der Biologie.* Jena, 1913.
4. Lansing A: Evidence of aging as a consequence of growth cessation. *Proc Natl Acad Sci* 1948; 34:304.
5. Leto S, Kokkonen GC, Barrows CH: Dietary protein, lifespan, and physiological variables in female mice. *J Gerontol* 1976; 31:149–154.
6. Leto S, Kokkonen GC, Barrows CH: Dietary protein, lifespan, and biochemical variables in female mice. *J Gerontol* 1976; 31:144–148.
7. Falzone JA, Barrows CH, Shock NW: Age and polyploidy of rat liver nuclei as measured by volume and DNA content. *J Gerontol* 1959; 14:2–8.
8. Franks L, Wilson P, Whelan R: The effects of age on total DNA and cell number in the mouse brain. *Gerontologia* 1974; 20:21–26.
9. Ross MH: Aging, nutrition, and hepatic enzyme activity patterns in the rat. *J Nutr* 1969; 97:565–602.
10. Barrows CH, Roeder LM: Effect of age on protein synthesis in rats. *J Geront* 1961; 16:321–325.
11. Munro HN, Fleck A: Determination of nucleic acids, in Glick D (ed): *Methods of Biochemical Analysis,* vol 14. New York, Interscience, pp 113–176.
12. Ceriotti GJ: A microchemical determination of desoxyribonucleic acid. *J Biol Chem* 1952; 198:297–303.
13. Miller GL: Protein determination for large numbers of samples. *Anal Chem* 1959; 31:964.
14. Mann PL: The effect of various dietary restricted regimes on some immunological parameters of mice. *Growth* 1978; 42:87–103.
15. Gerbase-DeLima M, Lui RK, Cheney KE, et al: Immune function and survival in a long-lived mouse strain subjected to undernutrition. *Gerontologia* 1975; 21:184–202.
16. Stoltzner G: Effects of life-long dietary protein restriction on mortality, growth, organ weights, blood counts, liver aldolase, and kidney catalase in BALB/C mice. *Growth* 1977; 42:337–348.
17. Bras G: Age-associated kidney lesions in the rat. *J Infect Dis* 1969; 120:131–135.
18. Ross MH, Bras G: Lasting influence of early caloric restriction on prevalence of neoplasms in the rat. *J Natl Cancer Inst* 1971; 47:1095.
19. Ross MH, Bras G: Tumor incidence patterns and nutrition in the rat. *J Nutr* 1965; 87:245–260.
20. Fanestil DD, Barrows CH: Aging in the rotifer *J Gerontol* 1965; 20:462–469.
21. Ingle E, Wood TR, Banta AM: A study of longevity, growth, reproduction, and heart rate in Daphnia longispina as influenced by limitations in quantity of food. *J Exp Zool* 1937; 76:325–352.
22. Barrows CH, Kokkonen GC: Protein synthesis, development, growth, and life span. *Growth* 1975; 39:525–533.
23. Beauchene RE, Bales CW, Smith CA, et al: The effect of food restriction on body composition and longevity of rats. *Physiologist* 1979; 22:4.
24. McCay C, Maynard LA, Sperling G, Osgood H: Nutritional requirements during the latter half of life. *J Nutr* 1941; 21:45–60.
25. Tucker SM, Mason RL, Beauchene RE: Influence of diet and feed restriction on kidney function of aging male rats. *J Gerontol* 1976; 31:264–270.
26. Everitt AV, Seedsman NJ, Jones F: The effect of hypophysectomy and continuous food restriction, begun at ages 70 and 400 days, on collagen aging,

proteinura incidence of pathology and longevity in the male rat. *Mech Ageing Dev* 1980; 12:161–172.

27. Bertrand HA, Masoro EJ, Yu BP: Nutritional reversal of an age-related deficit, abstracted. *Fed Proc* 1982; 41:1674.
28. Weindruch R, Gottesman SRS, Walford RL: Modification of age-related immune decline in mice dietarily restricted from or after midadulthood. *Proc Natl Acad Sci USA* 1982; 79:898–902.
29. Barrows CH, Roeder LM, Fanestil DC: The effects of restriction of total dietary intake and protein intake, and of fasting interval on the biochemical composition of rat tissues. *J Gerontol* 1965; 20:374–378.
30. Saxton JA: Pathology of senescent animals, in Shock NW (ed): *Conference on Problems of Aging,* vol 135. New York, Josiah Macy, Jr. Foundation, 1950.
31. Weindruch R, Walford RL: Dietary restriction in mice beginning at 1 year of age: Effect on life-span and spontaneous cancer incidence. *Science* 1982; 215:1415–1418.

8

Aging in the Food-restricted Rat: Body Temperature, Receptor Function, and Morphologic Changes in the Brain

Christopher D. West, Ladislav Volicer, and Deborah W. Vaughan

This investigation examined three different aspects of aging rats maintained on a food-restricted diet that prolonged life: body temperature in young and old adults, receptor sensitivity in young and old adults, and neuromorphologic changes in extreme old age. We were interested to see 1) whether lower body temperature was a factor in the longevity of food-restricted rats, 2) whether receptor function was one of the age-sensitive variables affected by food restriction, and 3) whether certain morphologic changes found in the brains of old humans and certain very old monkeys and dogs would be found in the brains of the oldest food-restricted rats.

Food Restriction and Longevity

Restricting food intake without restricting dietary components essential to life has been shown to increase both the average life span and the maximum life span in several species of animals. It has been reported in certain protozoa, rotifers, in certain arthropods, and in species of fish, mice, rats, and cattle (1–7).

In man, Henschen (8) suggested that food restriction imposed on the population during World War II was responsible for the reduced mortality rates of people in Nordic countries during that time. He cited records from Sweden and from Stockholm that showed reduced mortality and incidence of arteriosclerosis and chronic myocarditis in 1942 and 1943. Records from Finland showed reduced incidence of arteriosclerosis mortality and less mortality in general in 1943 and 1944.

In laboratory investigations, not all experimental studies of mice, (9,10) or rats (11) have demonstrated increased longevity with restricted diets. However, the mammal in which this phenomenon has been most consistently documented is the laboratory rat.

Early studies of McCay et al (12) indicated that restricting food intake not only prolonged life, but also retarded skeletal growth and sexual maturation. However, Carlson and Hoelzel (13), with intermittent fasting, and Berg and Simms (14), with 46% reduced diet, were able to produce enhanced longevity without affecting early development. Their animals showed no significant delay in sexual maturity or skeletal growth. Nolan (15) allowed rats 3 months ad libitum feeding through the period of early growth to young adulthood before restricting their diet to 60% or 80% of control and also produced enhanced longevity without affecting maturation.

Food restriction instituted as late as the second half of life was shown to be effective in prolonging life. Rats raised ad libitum for over 1 year by McCay et al (16) had mildly enhanced longevity with diets reduced by only 10% of control. Ross (17) found that reduced ad libitum food intake of rats at 300 days by 40% led to a 20% increase in life expectancy. From correlations of weight changes with longevity, he concluded that for every 10% weight loss following food restriction, there was a 13.5% gain in life expectancy. If, instead of being restricted, animals were switched to diets on which they gained weight, the opposite was true. Ross (18) delineated the limits beyond which reducing food intake ceased to increase life expectancy and began to shorten it. Rats raised ad libitum on a 21% casein diet to 300 days of age and then restricted to 8 g of food per day lived longer than controls; those restricted to 6 g per day died prematurely.

Food Restriction and Longevity—Body Weight, Adiposity, and Metabolism

In an experiment approximating the dietary conditions of humans in developed countries where people, fat and thin, select their own diets and eat ad libitum, Ross et al (19) allowed rats to select ad libitum among three diets differing in protein–carbohydrate composition. The life span of these rats was not strongly correlated with the kind of diet they selected, but it was strongly correlated with the rate at which they gained weight on the diets, particularly in early adult life. The number of days to double body weight from 200 to 300 g to 400 to 600 g was the best predictor of a rat's longevity. The maximum weight attained by a rat, however, was unrelated to its longevity.

Bertrand et al (20) and Masoro et al (21) examined the interaction of adiposity and longevity in the Fischer 344 rat, a strain of rat that does not show the extreme obesity of the Sprague-Dawley rat when housed in single cages and fed ad libitum. These investigators found no relationship between the amount of body fat measured in middle or late adult life and the longevity of the ad-libitum-fed rat. Food-restricted rats, limited to 60% of ad libitum intake, had a mean life span 40% greater than controls. Although they were smaller and had less absolute amounts of fat than controls, there was some overlap with the control population in the amount of fat per gram of body weight. Thus, the fattest food-restricted rats had a greater percentage of body fat than the leanest controls. In contrast to the ad-libitum-fed controls, food-restricted rats, which were better able to build up fat, particularly in middle life, had greater life expectancy.

In a study of metabolism and the mechanisms of longevity enhancement in food-restricted rats, Masoro et al (22) found that the amount of food ingested by food-restricted animals each week was the same per gram lean body mass as the amount ingested by controls. They concluded that food restriction did not prolong life by decreasing the overall metabolic rate. However, they did not rule out that changes in certain metabolic rates and processes might be involved.

Food Restriction and Body Temperature

Since Weindruch et al (23) had reported that mice exposed to food restriction early in life had lower body temperature than controls, and that this might be one of the mechanisms by which food restriction extended life, we decided to measure body temperature in our food-restricted rats. The means, highs, lows, and pattern of daily temperature variation were similar in our food-restricted and control rats as were body temperature responses to stress, feeding, and fasting. There were age-associated differences in the body temperature and the magnitude of stress responses between young and old adult rats, but these were independent of the diet (24).

The rats used in our studies, like those used by Ross in studies of dietary restriction and in several neuromorphologic studies of aging in ad-libitum-fed rats, were Charles River, Sprague-Dawley-derived, barrier-sustained, cesarean-delivered, male albino rats. They were housed three per cage (25⅜ in × 9½ in × 7 in wire mesh cages) to avoid the excessive obesity of singly caged rats (25) and to avoid any behavioral or neuromorphologic changes associated with restricted movement, sensory deprivation, or social isolation (26,27). All rats were fed ad libitum for 2 months to avoid changes affecting the development of the brain and other organs prior to sexual maturity (28). At 2 months of age, the rats were placed on limited rations to hold their body weights at 280 to 300 g for the first year and approximately 300 g thereafter (Fig. 8-1). This was achieved by giving them two 1-in, 4.5 g pellets of chow per animal per day. Food-restricted rats were switched to powdered chow in three 3-in spillproof cups placed in three corners of the cage for 15 minutes per day, after fighting was observed that resulted in weight variation, injuries, and cannibalism. When rats were 11 months old, fighting was observed to diminish and body weight limits could be maintained on the

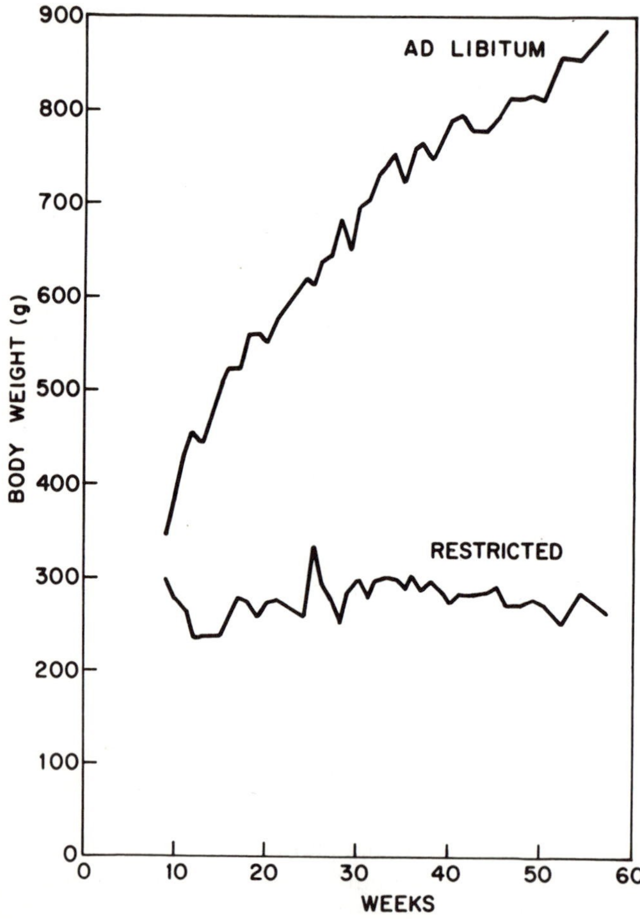

Figure 8-1. Body weights of ad-libitum-fed rats and rats on restricted diet.

two-pellet daily ration once again. Control rats were supplied at all times with an overabundance of chow pellets on which they fed ad libitum. Water was constantly available to all groups. The housing facility was kept on a 12-hour light–dark cycle (light 6 AM to 6 PM) at 27°C. The rat colony was started by placing 120 rats in each of the two groups. Since several animals were sacrificed from each group every 6 months, the life spans of all animals could not be determined. The last four surviving rats from the ad-libitum-fed group were sacrificed at 34 months of age when their death appeared imminent, but before they were moribund or in the terminal stage of an illness. By contrast, the last four surviving food-restricted rats were similarly sacrificed between 46 and 48 months of age. Since the same number of rats was sacrificed in each group, this indicates that the food restriction prolonged life span in our rats. Figure 8-2 shows population mortality from a group of the same breeding population raised, multiply housed, and maintained with ad libitum feeding at Charles River Laboratories in Wilmington, Massachusetts. The arrows in Figure 8-2 indicate the dates of sacrifice of the last four surviving food-restricted rats from our colony at the Research Service of the Veterans Administration Hospital in Bedford, Massachusetts.

To measure the body temperature in rats, the tail was secured outside a wire mesh cage and a Yellow Spring rectal probe was inserted to a depth of 6 cm. Temperature was recorded continuously on a Narco-Bio physiograph or monitored with a Yellow Spring Instrument Telethermometer. Room temperature was held at 27 ± 1.5°C. Food-restricted rats were fed between 8:30 and 9:00 AM, 30 minutes before the experiments. During the 24 hours that temperature was continuously recorded, ad-libitum-fed rats had continuous access to food and water while food-restricted rats had access to water only but no food. One hour before termination of the recording, food-restricted rats were given two chow pellets each.

When the circadian variations in body temperature in 24-month-old restricted and ad libitum fed rats were compared, no differences were found in mean temperature, temperature extremes, or the time of day at which the temperature extremes occurred (Table 8-1). However, we did observe that the initial temperature reading was higher in restricted rats than in controls. And the temperature of ad-libitum-fed controls increased at the beginning of the experiment after the tail was secured and the rectal probe inserted; in the food-restricted rat it remained nearly constant. We also observed that feeding the restricted rats at the end of the 24-hour temperature recording session resulted in an initial small decrease followed by an increase in body temperature that averaged 0.78 ± 0.09°C. and peaked 43.0 ± 7.5 minutes after feeding. The initial small decline probably resulted from the rapid ingestion of room-temperature material, which cooled the abdominal area. The subsequent increase was most likely caused by the calorigenic effect of the food and motor activity of feeding. A feeding-induced increase of body temperature also ex-

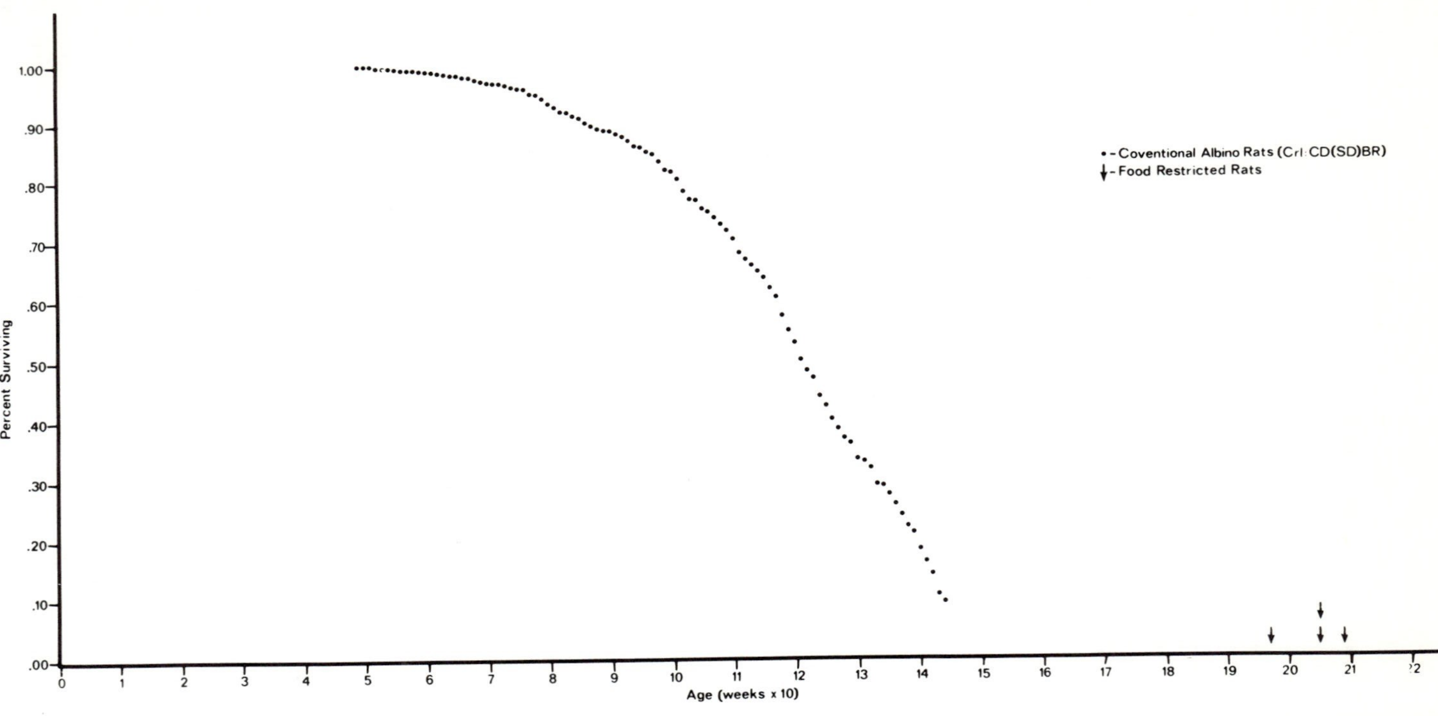

Figure 8-2. Survival distribution of male Sprague-Dawley-derived rats maintained on ad libitum diet at Charles River Laboratories. The four arrows indicate the age at sacrifice of the last four surviving rats maintained on a food-restricted diet at the Research Service of the Bedford Veteran's Administration Hospital.

plains the difference in the initial temperatures of restricted and control rats, as the experiments were started 30 minutes after the daily feeding period of the restricted rats, when such an increase would be near its peak.

In order to control for the food intake of the restricted rats just prior to the beginning of the experiment, we added two more groups of ad-libitum-fed rats. Both groups were fasted for 24 hours, and one of them was fed 30 minutes prior to the experiment, like the restricted rats. When this was done, a similar increase in initial body temperature was observed in the rats that were fasted for 24 hours and fed 30 minutes prior to the experiment, but not in the rats that were simply fasted.

Four groups of six-month-old rats were also studied: an ad libitum group with continuous access to food, an ad libitum group fasted for 24 hours, an ad libitum group fasted 24 hours and fed 30 minutes prior to the experiment, and a restricted group fed its daily ration 30 minutes prior to the experiment (Fig. 8-3).

Body temperature observed immediately after probe insertion was affected both by age ($f = 6.11, P < .02$), and by dietary status ($f = 8.72, P < .001$) (Table 8-2). The interaction between age and dietary status was not statistically significant ($f = 2.24, P < .05$). This indicates that six-month-old rats had a higher initial body temperature than two-year-old rats. An orthogonal contrast showed that the individual body temperature in ad-libitum-fed rats that had continuous access to food was similar to the temperature in ad-libitum-fed rats that were fasted for 24 hours ($f = 0.57, P < .05$). Body temperature was also similar in rats on restricted diets fed prior to measurement and in ad-libitum-fed rats that were fasted for 24 hours and fed prior to measurement ($f = 0.05, P < .05$). There was a significant difference of initial body temperature between rats fed prior to measurement and ad libitum rats either kept with continuous access to food or fasted 24 hours without feeding prior to measurement. This indicated that feeding before measurement significantly

Table 8-1. Twenty-four-hour Body Temperatures of Ad-Libitum-Fed Rats and Rats on a Restricted Diet*

		Temperature			
	Body Weight	Peak		Trough	
Diet	(g)	C°	Time	°C	Time
Ad libitum	519	38.75	21:39	36.60	8:18
	±77	±0.32	± 3:02	±0.40	± 49
Restricted	338	38.72	20:18	37.01	6:36
	±22	±0.18	± 50	±0.10	±1:57

*The numbers are means ± SEM. The time is expressed in hours and minutes. Four 24-month-old rats were used in each group.

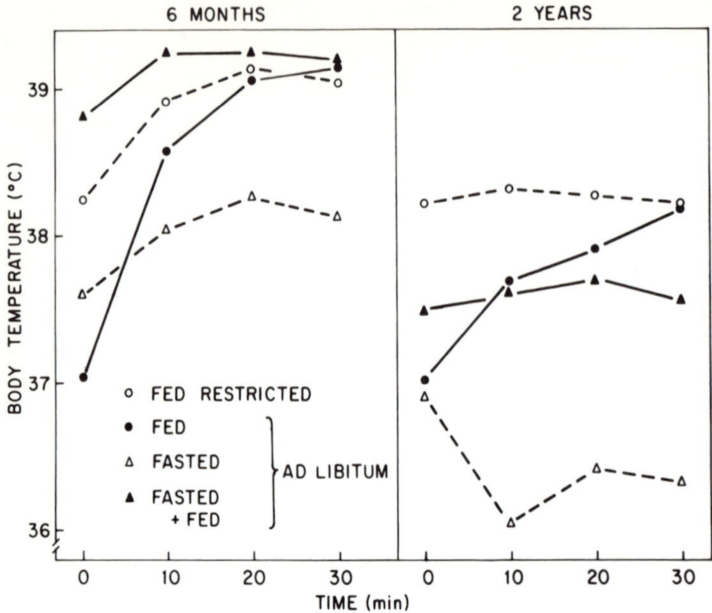

Figure 8-3. The effect of feeding and stress on body temperature of ad-libitum-fed rats and rats on restricted diet. Five six-month-old rats were used for each group except for the fasted and fed ad libitum rats where four were used. Ten ad-libitum-fed two-year-old rats with continuous access to food, three fasted, three fasted and fed, and nine restricted two-year-old rats were used. See text for statistical analysis.

increased body temperature in all rats. The interaction between feeding and age was not significant ($f = 0.05, P < .05$) indicating that the feeding effect occurred both in young and old rats.

In most groups of rats, body temperature increased in the beginning of the observation period. This increase was most likely the result of the

Table 8-2. Stress-induced Temperature Change*

Diet	Nutritional State	Age: 6 Mo	Age: 2 Yr
Restricted	fed	0.80 ± 0.23 (5)†	0.00 ± 0.12 (9)
Ad libitum	fed	2.10 ± 0.19 (5)	0.97 ± 0.14 (10)
Ad libitum	fasted	0.54 ± 0.30 (5)	−0.57 ± 0.06 (3)
Ad libitum	fasted & fed	0.37 ± 0.20 (4)	0.07 ± 0.55 (3)

*The stress was induced by insertion of the thermometer probe and by fixation of the animal's tail outside the cage.

†Numbers represent means ± SEM and numbers of observations are in parentheses. For statistical analysis see text.

stress to which the animals were exposed when their tails were secured and the probe inserted. Stress-induced increase of body temperature has been observed previously both in rats (29) and in man (30).

The effect of stress resulting from fixation of the tail and insertion of the probe was evaluated by analyzing the change in body temperature during a 30-minute observation period (Table 8-2). The temperature changes were affected by age ($f = 25.64, P < .001$) and dietary status ($f = 17.32, P < .001$). The interaction of these two factors was not significant ($f = 1.34, P < .05$), indicating that the stress increased body temperature more in six-month-old rats than in two-year-old rats without regard to dietary status (Fig. 8-3).

Our data showed a smaller stress response in restricted rats than in ad-libitum rats with continuous access to food. This difference might have resulted from the fact that food-restricted rats were fed prior to measurement, causing the food-induced temperature increase somehow to mask or to limit the degree of stress-induced hyperthermia. However, the stress-induced temperature increase was also diminished by fasting the ad libitum rats for 24 hours, which had no effect on their initial body temperature. We concluded that the decreased stress-induced hyperthermic response in the food-restricted rat was caused by short-term fasting and was not the result of chronic food restriction.

The 24-hour temperature means were similar in food-restricted rats and in controls. This contrasts with the observations of decreased body temperature in food-restricted mice (7,23). The effect of food restriction or the means of producing it by intermittent fasting (23) or by a low protein diet (7) could affect body temperature differently in rats and mice. For example, Webb et al (31) reported a marked decrease in body temperature following fasts of 24 to 48 hours, and in the study of Weindruch et al (23), food-restricted mice were fed on Fridays and their temperatures measured after a prolonged fast on Sundays.

In the rat, however, our study indicated that a 24-hour fast had no effect on mean body temperature in ad-libitum-fed rats or in food-restricted rats given limited amounts of food once a day. The feeding of our restricted rats induced a brief increase in body temperature, which occurred at a time of day when body temperature of ad libitum rats was low. Because for the rest of the day the circadian variation of body temperatures was similar in restricted and control rats, the increased longevity of restricted rats in our colony cannot be explained by a decrease of body temperature.

Food Restriction and Aging

In addition to prolonging life, food-restricted diets retard the rates of certain aging changes. It is equally significant that the rates of other aging changes are unaffected. Thus aging is not affected as a unitary process by food restriction. McCay et al (32) reported that the texture of hair of food-restricted rats was similar to ad-libitum-fed controls of a younger age. X-ray examination showed that food-restricted rats had less extensive calcification than age-matched controls of the intercostal cartilage, but more extensive calcification of the aorta and kidneys. The calcium content of the eye was unaffected. Tail collagen from food-restricted rats studied by Chvapil and Hruza (33) had elastic properties similar to that of younger controls, and liver and muscle cells from food-restricted rats prepared by tissue culture by Holeckova et al (34) had a shorter latency period than those from age-matched control. Recently, a study of age age-related decrease in receptor sites by Levin et al (35) indicated that the number of dopamine receptors in two-year-old dietarily restricted rats were comparable to younger three- to six-month-old controls.

Food Restriction and Aging in β-Adrenergic Receptors

Decreased responsiveness with age of β-adrenergic receptors has been described in heart (36), liver (37), tracheal smooth muscle (38), erythrocytes (39–40), fat cells (41–43), and in the cerebellum (44). We decided to look at β-adrenergic receptor sensitivity in cultures of aortic smooth muscle cells from rats of different ages and found a decreased response with age to epinephrine stimulation. The magnitude of this decrease was clearly reduced by food restriction although cell growth was only minimally affected (45).

Rats anesthetized with chloral hydrate solution were clamped just below the arch of the descending aorta. Before aldehyde perfusion, a portion of the thoracic aorta was removed and prepared for explant in a sterile manner. The aorta was cut longitudinally and the intimal-medial layer was removed under a microscope. Cell cultures were prepared as described earlier (45). Before the drug incubation, cell count and viability of representative dishes were determined by the dye exclusion method in a hemocytometer. Only if the cell count was higher than 200,000 cells per dish and the viability was at least 75% were the cells used for drug incubation. The entire contents of the culture dish were transferred to a test tube for isolation of cAMP and determination of cellular DNA content. The samples were centrifuged at 1,600 g and 5°C for 30 minutes. cAMP was isolated from the supernatant by column chromatography and measured by radioimmunoassay. The DNA content was determined in the cell pellet using the method of Burton. Each drug incubation was usually done in triplicate and the means of the triplicates used was calculated by statistical analysis (45).

Cells from 24-month-old and 34-month-old rats started to grow from explants after the same latency period regardless of diet and age. However, cells from 34-month-old animals grew slower in the explant and first and second passage stages than cells from 24-month-old animals, and they achieved lower final densities in first and second passage. Differences between food-restricted animals and age-matched controls were greatest in the 34-month-old age group where the final density of cells in second passage was significantly less for controls ($f = 3.95, P < .05$) (Fig. 8-4).

The elevation of the cAMP level in response to epinephrine was decreased with age. cAMP levels in second-passage cells (Table 8-3) show that epinephrine at 10^{-6} mol/L concentration increased the cAMP levels significantly in cells from 3-month-old and 18-month-old rats. The magnitude of cAMP response to epinephrine declined with age until there was no increase in 34-month-old, ad-libitum-fed rats at this concentration.

Figure 8-5 shows that cAMP levels grow with increasing concentration to a maximum at 10^{-5} mol/L epinephrine concentration in all groups except the 30- to 34-month-old ad libitum group where the peak may not have been reached. Cells from food-restricted animals responded more

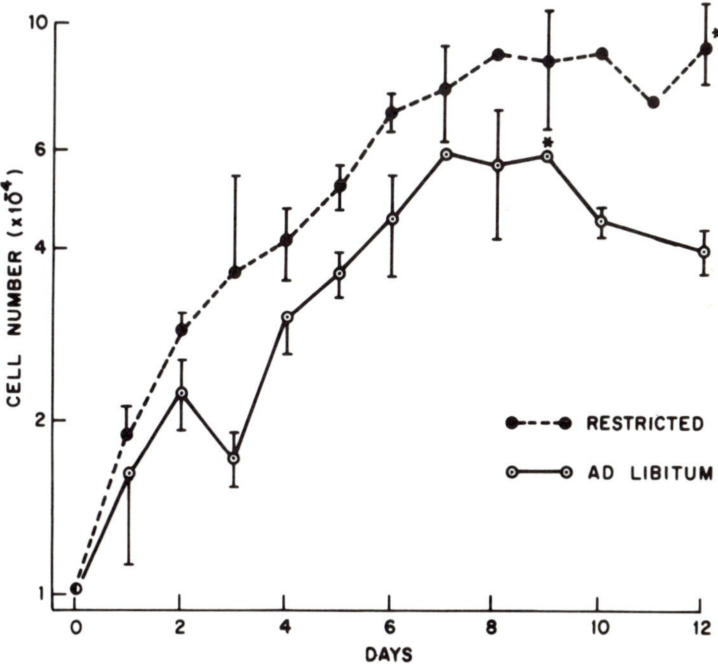

Figure 8-4. Growth curves of vascular smooth muscle cells from 34-month-old rats in the second passage. The points are means and bars indicate SEM. Cultures from four animals were used for ad libitum group and from three animals for the restricted group. $^*P < .05$ compared to ad libitum group.

Table 8-3. Age-Related Changes of Basal and Epinephrine-induced cAMP Levels in Vascular Smooth Muscle*

Diet	Treatment	Age (months)				
		3	18	24	30	34
Ad libitum	Basal	0.25 ± 0.06	0.85 ± 0.15	0.24, 0.36	0.12	0.33 ± 0.14
	Epinephrine	49.24 ± 9.08†	5.94 ± 1.18†	3.25, 3.30	0.35	0.28 ± 0.08
		(5)	(3)	(2)	(1)	(3)
Restricted	Basal	—	0.81 ± 0.04	0.67	1.26, 0.33	0.19, 0.09
	Epinephrine	—	10.76 ± 2.83*	4.67	3.53, 1.39	0.32, 0.17
			(3)	(1)	(2)	(2)

*Smooth muscle cells were incubated with epinephrine (10^{-6}mol/L) for 2 min and the results are expressed as pmol cAMP/μg DNA.
†$P < .02$ compared to the basal levels

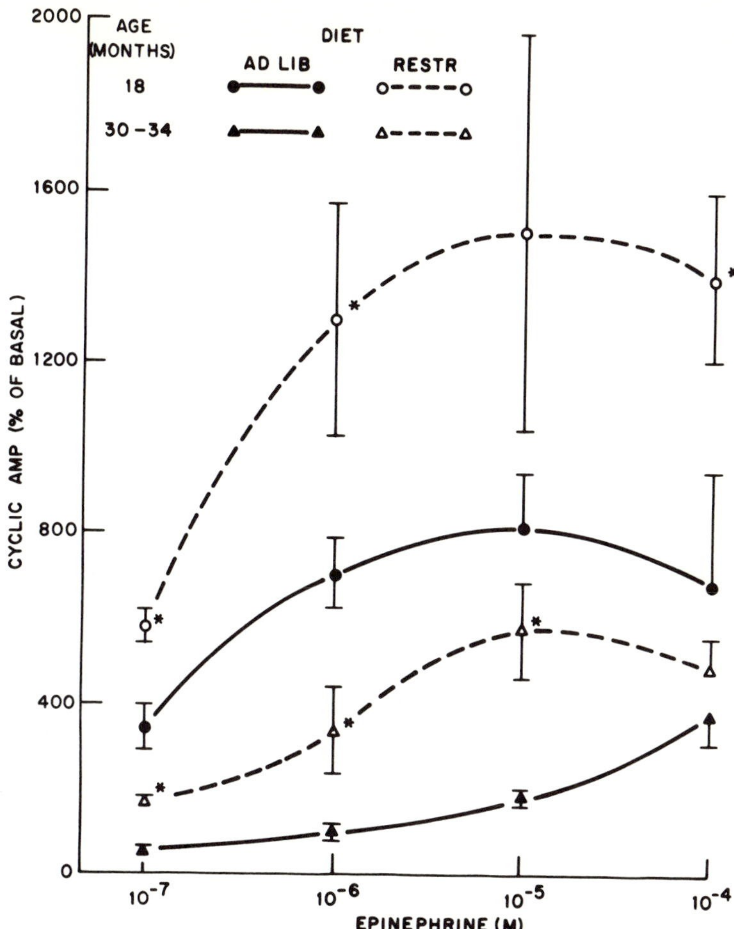

Figure 8-5. Increase of cAMP response to various epinephrine concentrations in cultured smooth muscle cells. The points are means of three to five rats and the bars indicate SEM. *$P < 0.05$ compared to ad-libitum-fed controls of the same age.

to epinephrine than did cells from age-matched animals fed ad libitum. An analysis of variance indicated that the cAMP response to epinephrine was concentration dependent ($f = 10.33$, $P < .001$), was larger in younger rats than in older ones ($f = 83.32$, $P < .001$), and was larger in restricted rats than in rats on ad libitum diet ($f = 31.38$, $P < .001$). There was a significant interaction of age with diet ($f = 6.35$, $P < .015$), indicating that food restriction maintained the epinephrine responsiveness of receptors better at younger than at older ages.

Food restriction did not change the growth of cultured smooth muscle cells very much in our experiments. Specifically we did not observe a decrease in the length of the latency period at the explant stage, as was reported by Holeckova et al (34) in explants of muscle and liver. The only difference observed between the cells grown from our food-restricted and ad-libitum-fed rats was at 34 months of age when cells of food-restricted animals achieved higher final densities.

Our results showed an age-induced decrease in the β-adrenergic responsiveness of smooth muscle cells grown in culture. This age-induced decrease was attenuated by food restriction. Since cell growth was only minimally affected, the preservation of epinephrine responsiveness in β-adrenergic receptors could be considered a selective effect of the restricted diet.

Food Restriction and Disease

One of the factors apparently contributing to the longevity of food-restricted rats is the delayed onset of several age-associated diseases. Ross and Bras (46,47) found that food-restricted diets reduced the incidence of certain tumors, particularly if control rats not only ate ad libitum but also selected among different ad libitum diets. Berg and Simms (14) and Berg et al (48) concluded from their studies of several nonneoplastic (48), age-associated diseases that the incidence of renal, cardiac, arterial, and degenerative muscle disease was shifted to a later date in food-restricted rats. Only the incidence of radiculoneuropathy, the one nervous system disease evaluated, was unaffected.

Food Restriction and Morphologic Aging Changes in the Brain

Our observations of the brains of ad-libitum-fed rats at several ages and of food-restricted rats at extreme old age indicated that the incidence of many morphologic aging changes in neurons, glia, and cerebral blood vessels are also unaffected by food-restricted diets.

Rats for the investigations of the nervous system came from our colony and from a colony of rats (male, retired breeders) multiply housed, and fed ad libitum at Charles River Breeding Laboratories in Wilmington, Massachusetts. Animals were anesthetized with chloral hydrate and respirated through a tracheotomy prior to perfusion through the ascending aorta with aldehyde fixative warmed to 40°C. In a two-stage perfusion (49) a solution of 1% paraformaldehyde and 1.25% glutaraldehyde in .08 mol/L cacodylate buffer with $CaCl_2$ at pH 7.2 was followed without interruption by a more concentrated mixture containing 4% paraformaldehyde and 5% glutaraldehyde in the same buffer. Each mixture was delivered for 10 to 15 minutes. Perfused animals were left intact and refrigerated in sealed polyethylene bags overnight before dissection of the brain. Blocks of cerebral cortex were taken from Kreig's area 41. Following postfixation in cacodylate-buffered 2% osmium, tissue was dehydrated in ethanol and embedded in Araldite. Prior to thin sectioning, 1-μm/sections were taken and stained with toluidine blue. Thin sections were then made and stained with uranyl acetate and lead citrate.

Morphologic changes in neurons of the auditory cortex, such as abnormal myelinated axons, intradentritic membranous bodies (49), and lipofuscin, increase with age (50,51). These changes were found with greater frequency and in greater amounts in the oldest surviving food-

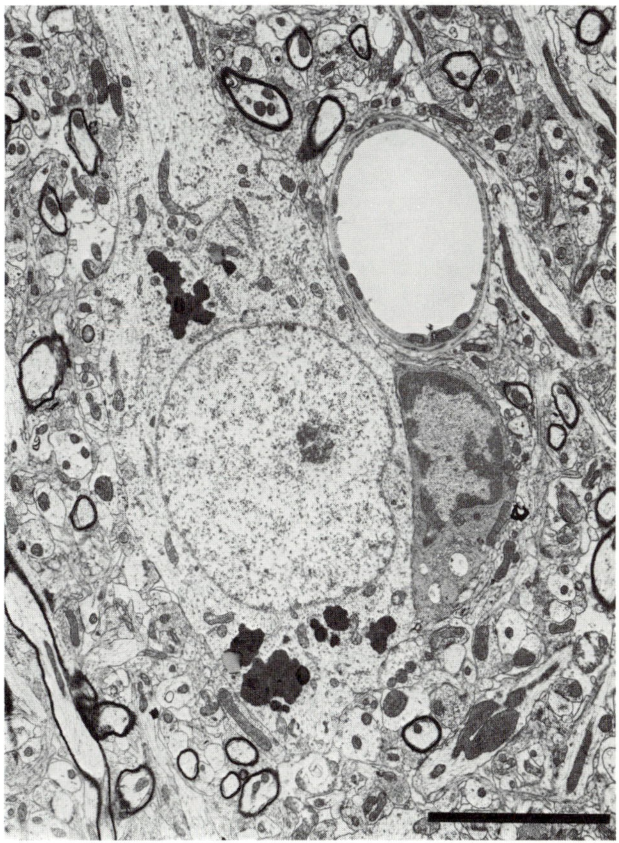

Figure 8-6. *Neurons.* Most neurons have one or more satellite neuroglial cells. Neurons often contain large amounts of lipofuscin and show other signs of advanced age. Food-restricted four-year-old rat. Bar = 5 μm.

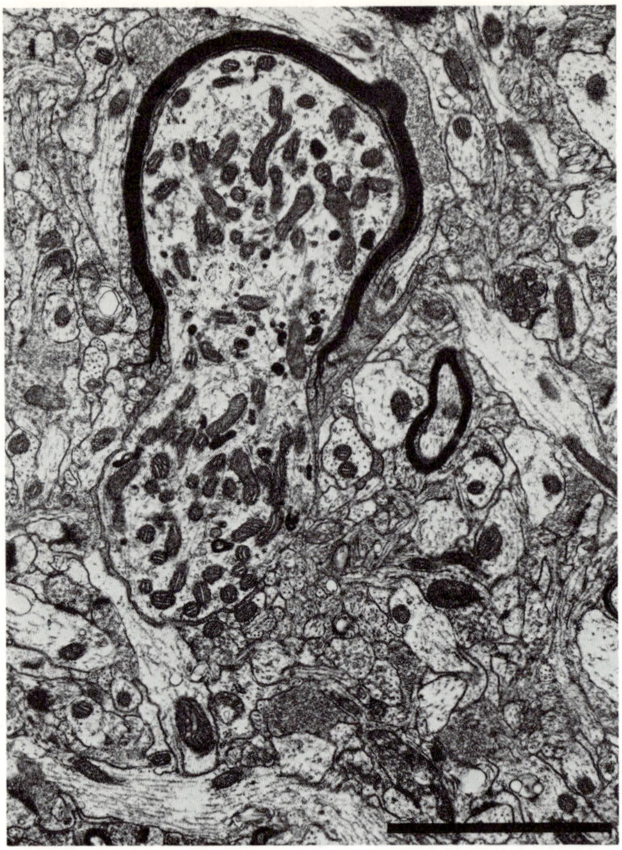

Figure 8-7. *Axons:* Abnormal myelinated axons are prevalent. Both the myelin sheath and the axon develop degenerative changes. Food-restricted four-year-old rat. Bar = 5 μm.

restricted rats (four years old) when compared with the oldest surviving ad-libitum-fed rats (three years old) (Figs. 8-6, 8-7, and 8-8). Although three-year-old, food-restricted rats were not available for comparison with three-year-old controls, no significant differences were seen when two-year-old, food-restricted rats were compared with two-year-old controls. Neuroglia of the auditory cortex also showed aging changes of greater magnitude in four-year-old, food-restricted rats than in three-year-old controls. Microglia, astroglia, and oligodendroglia showed increased proliferation and increased accumulation of dense debris (Figs. 8-9 and 8-10).

Certain changes seen rarely or not at all as a result of aging in the auditory cortex of the oldest rats on ad libitum diets at three years of age

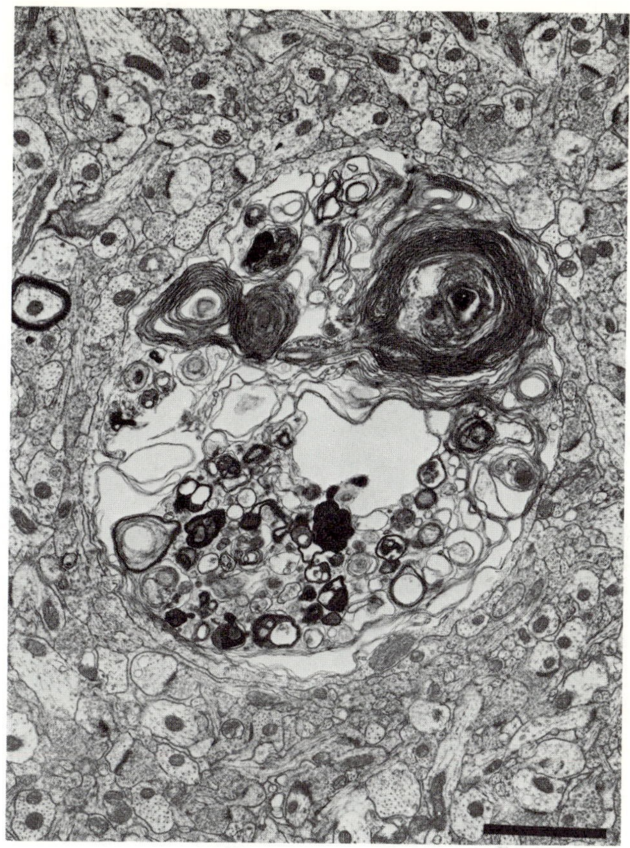

Figure 8-8. *Dendrites:* Dendrites greatly enlarged by abnormal membranous bodies are common. Food-restricted four-year-old rat. Bar = 5 μm.

were common in the brains of the four-year-old, food-restricted rats. One of these, a thickening of the basal lamina in blood vessels, was rarely seen at younger ages except in vessels of the olfactory bulb (52). Another change, foci of neuropil vacuolarization, had been seen in cortex before, but not necessarily as an aging change (53,54).

Vaughan and Peters (54) had described three rats, 38 to 30 months old, that had neuritic plaques with amyloid filamentous cores, degenerating neurites, reactive microglia, and vacuolarized neuropil. The amyloid filaments appeared to be extracellular and were birefringent when stained with Congo red and examined with polarized light. They were always accompanied by vacuolarized neuropil. With the birefringent amyloid core as a definitive criterion, Vaughan and Peters described the constellation of changes as neuritic plaques. Neuritic plaques are encountered in the

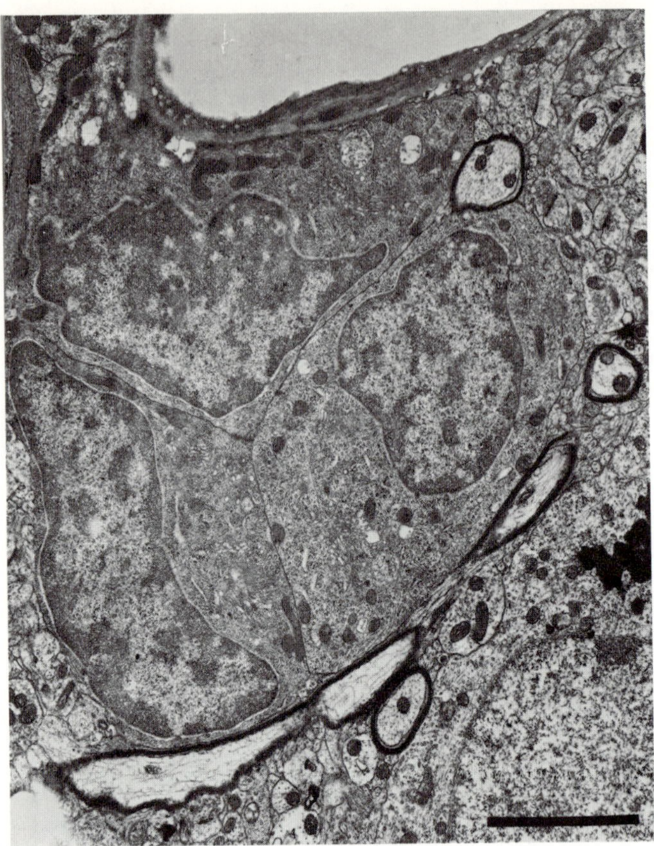

Figure 8-9. *Neuroglia:* All three types of neuroglia greatly increase in numbers. Oligodendroglia frequently occur in groups of two or more. Food-restricted four-year old rat. Bar = 5 μm.

brains of normal, nondemented, elderly humans and have been described in the brains of very old dogs (55) and monkeys (56). They are found with greater frequency in middle-aged, Down's syndrome individuals, in Alzheimer's disease and senile dementia of the Alzheimer's type, and in certain other diseases (51,57–60).

The etiology of the neuritic plaques described by Vaughan and Peters was unknown, and normal aging processes per se were not implicated as only a small number of animals studied in that age group showed the lesions. Instead, an infectious agent of some unknown etiology was suggested (54). Such an agent might have been similar to viral agents implicated in neuritic plaque-forming disorders of Creutzfeldt-Jakob

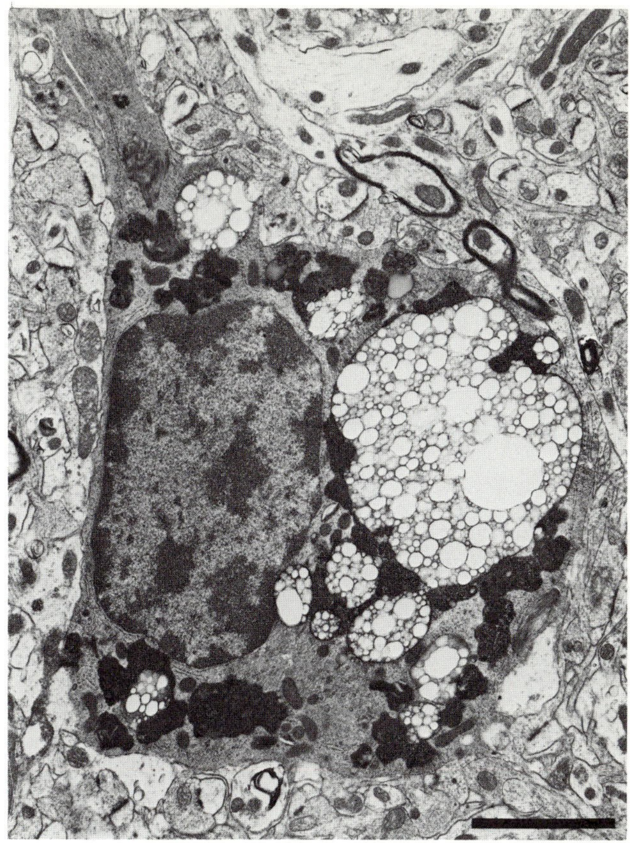

Figure 8-10. *Neuroglia:* Microglia, oligodendroglia, and astrocytes accumulate dense debris characteristic of each cell type. Microglial cells accumulate the greatest volume of debris. Food-restricted four-year-old rat. Bar = 5 μm.

disease and Kuru, or to the scrapievirus used to induce neuritic plaque formation in experimentally infected mice.

Focal neuropil vacuolarization does not appear as an obvious component of the neuritic plaques illustrated in studies of aging man or monkey (56–58). However, it is evident near an amyloid deposit in an illustration from the brain of an aged dog in Figure 19 of the study by Wisniewski et al (55). Since thickening of blood vessel walls and other changes have been associated with neuritic plaques in the brains of other old animals (55,56), it is possible that the changes in the four-year-old, diet-restricted rats—all of which had both thickening of the basal lamina and foci of neuropil vacuolarization—were the beginnings of age-associated neuritic plaques.

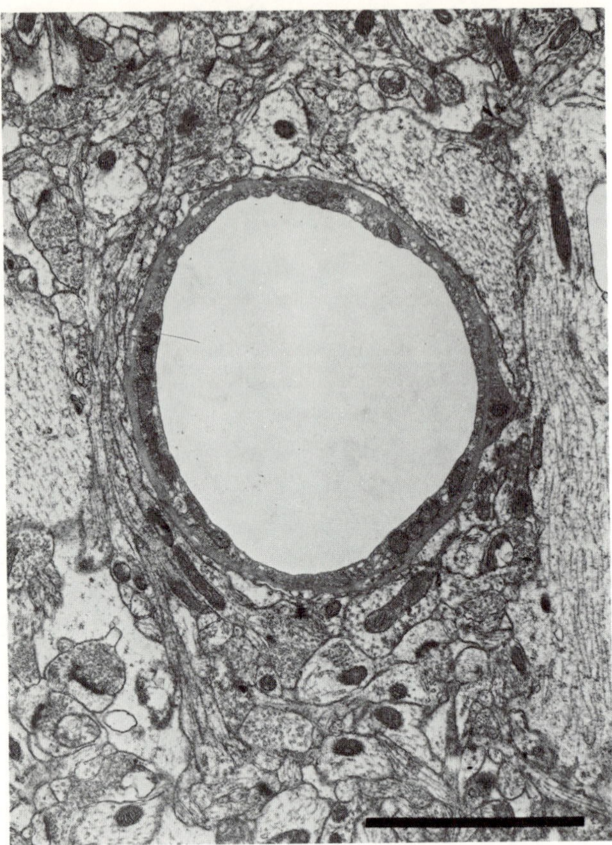

Figure 8-11. *Capillaries:* Endothelial cells are often thin and contain vesicles. The basal lamina is obviously thickened and often has basal spurs and cavitations. Food-restricted four-year-old rat. Bar = 5 μm.

An age-associated process would not preclude the participation of infectious, autoimmune, or toxic agents in neuritic plaque formation, because an age-associated breakdown of the blood–brain barrier at the basal lamina could be the mechanism by which a plaque-producing agent gained access to the brain parenchyma. The demonstration of amyloid formation by Wisniewski et al (61) along a viral-infected needle track, and neuritic plaque formation adjacent to an experimental stab wound in the mouse brain supports a relationship between blood–brain barrier integrity and plaque formation (57,58,62). The fact that foci of neuropil vacuoles and basal lamina thickening appear for the first time simultaneously in the cortex of the four-year-old, food-restricted rat may be further evidence of such a relationship.

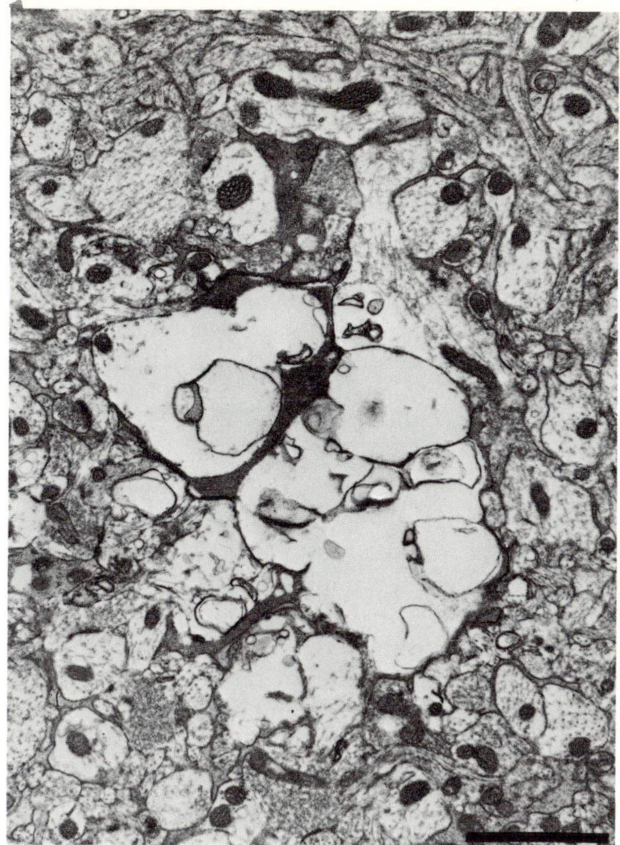

Figure 8-12. *Vacuoles:* Patches of vacuoles, similar to those associated with the neuritic plaques we found in three younger ad-libitum-fed rats, may have reactive microglia associated, but in the four-year-old diet-restricted rat extracellular amyloid filaments have not been observed. Food-restricted four-year-old rat. Bar = 5 μm.

Conclusions

The food-restricted rat provides an attractive animal model for studying aging changes in the brain in general and for the experimental production of neuritic plaques in particular. If the changes seen in the four-year-old, food-restricted rat brain are precursors of neuritic plaques, then two of the four morphologic components of neuritic plaques in rats are already present: the foci of vacuolarized neuropil and the reactive microglia. Any experimental manipulation that could add the other two components, degenerating neurites and amyloid filaments, would certainly be of relevance for research in the pathogenesis of Alzheimer's disease and senile dementia of the Alzheimer's type.

The last portion of this study was designed to utilize the longevity-producing properties of the restricted diet to study those age-associated changes that specifically were not retarded by food restriction as opposed to those that were retarded. By allowing rats to survive to near the maximum age achieved in previous studies of food restriction and longevity, we were able to examine aging changes that did not appear to be affected in their time course by food restriction. These restrictions had progressed to extremes not present in the oldest living ad-libitum-fed rats. Some of these changes, such as lipofuscin accumulation, glial proliferation, myelin abnormalities, and intradendritic membranous bodies, were present in three-year-old rats and were simply more advanced in the food-restricted four-year-olds. Others, such as thickening of the basal lamina of blood vessels in cortex, had only been seen with age in other parts of the brain. Still others, such as the focal neuropil vacuolarization, appeared as age-associated changes for the first time.

Since populations of wild rats exist in areas of food abundance as well as in areas of food scarcity, it is impossible to say what normal old age in the rat really is. However, the data from our four-year-old rats suggest that morphologic studies of the brains of the oldest rats produced on ad libitum diets may have been studies of rat brains that were in some respects more similar to human brains in middle age than in old age. For example, most of the morphologic aging changes seen in the three-year-old rat brain were extensions of changes seen in lesser amounts at two years. Similarly, changes in the middle-aged human brain such as lipofuscin accumulation are also seen in lesser amounts at younger ages (51). At four years, however, the brain of the food-restricted rat showed changes that may be precursors of neuritic plaques. If so, this is an aging change that is not characteristic of the normal human brain in middle age, but limited primarily to the normal human brain in old age (37,58).

The significance of the food-restricted rat is expanding in aging research. In addition to the study of mechanisms of longevity, it is being used more frequently in research on functional changes with age and on age-associated diseases. The food-restricted rat is coming to be recognized as a normal laboratory animal, and it is as appropriate an animal in which to study aging as the ad-libitum-fed rat. The food-restricted rat grows and ages in a nutritional environment that is every bit as normal as the nutritional environment of the ad-libitum-fed rat and probably as common. In the wild, limited food supply is as often the rule as the exception. Truncating the life span that is normal in times of food scarcity may be a mechanism by which this species maximizes a breeding population's potential for adaptive genetic change in areas of food abundance (63). This may or may not be partly true for human populations as well. In any event, both dietary regimes are appropriate models for the study of aging, because human populations exist both in areas of food scarcity and in areas where food is abundant and ad-libitum-feeding is a common practice.

The principles by which food-restricted diets function to prolong life may eventually be revealed as laboratory investigations continue. In applying these principles to extend the life of human beings, it becomes important to consider just which portions of human life will be extended: the learning period in youth, the productive period in adulthood, and the period of wisdom in old age, or possibly the period of terminal dependency, incapacity, and senility.

Our studies of food restriction in rats and aging in the nervous system suggest that the rates of several morphologic aging changes in neurons and other cell types in the brain may continue unabated. And, although senile dementia may not be an inevitable result of age, at present the probability of its occurring increases with age. On the other hand, our studies and those of others (35) indicate that receptors, which are critical elements in the proper functioning of the nervous system and other systems throughout the body, are partially insulated from deterioration with age by a life-prolonging, food-restricted diet. If disease processes are implicated in the development of senile dementia and controlled at some future date, then principles developed in laboratory experiments on food-restricted diets may someday provide man with a longer, fuller life.

Summary

A food-restricted diet that prolonged life in rats reduced the rate of certain aging changes but left others apparently unaffected. Mean body temperature, the highs and lows and time at which they occurred, were unaffected by the food-restricted diet as was body temperature response to feeding, fasting, and stress. Cell growth of vascular smooth muscle in culture was mildly affected. Response of β-adrenergic receptors to epinephrine stimulation decreased less with age in rats maintained on the restricted diet than in ad-libitum-fed rats. The progress of morphologic aging changes in neuronal, glial, and vascular components of the brain did not appear to be affected by the food-restricted diet.

Acknowledgments

We thank Arlene Chase, Louise Greene, Christopher Cahill and Anthony Carboni for their contributions to this project. This research was supported in part by MIRS Grant No. 9313-01, renewal no. 476468001, from the Veterans Administration and USPHS Grant No. 1 R23 AG00607-01 from Harvard Medical School.

References

1. McCay CM, Dilley WE, Crowell MF: Growth rates of brook trout reared upon purified rations, upon dry skim milk diets, and upon feed combinations of cereal grains. *J Nutr* 1929; 1:233–244.
2. McCay CM, Crowell MF, Maynard LA: The effect of retarded growth upon the length of lifespan and upon the ultimate body size. *J Nutr* 1935; 10:63–74.
3. Sinclair HM: Nutrition and aging, in Yapp WB, Bourne GH (eds): *The Biology of Ageing.* New York, Hafner 1959, pp 101–109.
4. Hansen K, Steensber V: Forsekelligt op draettede Koers holdbarked og ydelse, no 246. Kovenhavn, Udgivet af Statens Hysdrybrugsudvalg, 1950.
5. Comfort A: Effect of delayed and resumed growth on the longevity of fish (*Lebistes reticulatus,* Peters) in captivity. *Gerontologia* 1963; 8:150–155.
6. Fanestil DD, Barrows CH, Jr: Aging in the rotifer. *J Gerontol* 1965; 20:452–469.
7. Leto S, Kokkonen GC, Barrows CH, Jr: Dietary protein, lifespan and biochemical variables in female mice. *J Gerontol* 1976; 31:144–148.
8. Henschen F: Geographic and historical pathology of arteriosclerosis. *J Gerontol* 1953; 8:1–5.
9. Silberberg R, Jarrett SR, Silberberg H: Lifespan of mice fed enriched or restricted diets during growth. *Am J Physiol* 1961; 200:332–334.
10. Silberberg R, Silberberg J, Jarrett S: Effects of diet during growth: Studies in male mice of various strains. *Pathol Microbiol* 1962; 25:56–66.
11. Nakagawa I, Sasaki A, Kajimoto M, et al: Effect of protein nutrition on growth, longevity and incidence of lesions in the rat. *J Nutr* 1974; 104:1576–1583.
12. McCay CM, Maynard LA, Sperling G, Barnes LL: Retarded growth, lifespan, ultimate body size and age changes in the albino rat after feeding diets restricted in calories. *J Nutr* 1939; 18:1–13.
13. Carlson AJ, Hoelzel F: Apparent prolongation of the lifespan of rats by intermittent fasting. *J Nutr* 1946; 31:363–375.
14. Berg BN, Simms HS: Nutrition and longevity in the rat. II. Longevity and onset of disease with different levels of food intake. *J Nutr* 1960; 71:255–263.
15. Nolan GA: Effect of various restricted dietary regimens on the growth, health and longevity of albino rats. *J Nutr* 1972; 102:1477–1493.
16. McCay CM, Maynard L, Sperling G, Osgood H: Nutrition requirements in the latter half of life. *J Nutr* 1941; 21:45–60.
17. Ross MH: Life expectancy modification by change in dietary regimen of the mature rat. Kuhnau J (ed): *Proc 7th Internat Cong Nutr.* vol 5. New York, Pergamon Press, 1966, pp 35–38.
18. Ross MH: Length of life and caloric intake. *Am J Clin Nutr* 1972; 25:834–838.
19. Ross MH, Lustbader E, Bras G: Dietary practices and growth responses as predictors of longevity. *Nature* 1976; 262:548–553.
20. Bertrand HA, Lynd FT, Masoro EJ, Yu RP: Change in adipose mass and cellularity through the adult life of rats fed ad libitum on life prolonging restricted diet. *J Gerontol* 1980; 35:827–835.

21. Masoro EJ, Yu BP, Bertrand HA, Lynd FT: Nutritional probe of the aging process. *Fed Proc* 1980; 39:3178–3182.
22. Masoro EJ, Yu BP, Bertrand HA: Action of food restriction in delaying the aging process. *Proc Natl Acad Sci* 1982; 79:4239–4241.
23. Weindruch RH, Kristie, JA, Cheney KE, Walford RL: Influence of controlled dietary restriction on immunologic function and aging. *Fed Proc* 1979; 38:2007–2016.
24. Volicer L, West CD, Greene L: Effect of dietary restriction and stress on body temperature in rats. *J Gerontol* 1984; 39:178–182.
25. Ingle DJ: A simple means of producing obesity in the rat. *Proc Soc Exp Biol Med* 1934; 72:604–605.
26. Diamond MC, Krech D, Rosenzweig MR: The effects of an enriched environment on the histology of the rat cerebral cortex. *J Comp Neurol* 1964; 123:111–120.
27. Holloway RL, Jr: Dendritic branching: Some preliminary results of training and complexity in rat visual cortex. *Brain Res* 1966; 2:393–396.
28. West CD, Kemper TL: The effect of a low protein diet on the developing rat brain. *Brain Res* 1976; 107:221–237.
29. Briese E, Dequijada MG: Colonic temperature of rats during handling. *Acta Physiol Lat Am* 1970; 20:97–102.
30. Renbourn ET: Body temperature and pulse rate in body and young men prior to sporting contests. A study of emotional hyperthermia: With a review of the literature. *J Psychosom Res* 1960; 4:149–175.
31. Webb GP, Jaget YA, Rogers PD, Jackson ME: The effect of fasting on thermoregulation in normal and obese mice. *IRCS Med Sci* 1980; 8:163–164.
32. McCay CM, Ellis GJ, Barnes LL, et al: Chemical and pathological changes in aging after retarded growth. *J Nutr* 1939; 18:15–25.
33. Chvapil M, Hruza Z: The influence of aging and undernutrition on chemical contractility and relaxation of collagen fibers in rats. *Gerontologia* 1959; 3:241–252.
34. Holeckova E, Fabry P, Poupa A: Studies in the adaptation of metabolism. VIII: The latent period of explanted tissues of rats adapted to intermittent starvation. *Physiol Bohemoslov* 1959; 8:15–22.
35. Levin P, Janada J, Joseph JA: Dietary restriction retards the age-associated loss of rat striatal dopaminergic receptors. *Science* 1981; 214:561–562.
36. Lakatta EG: Age-related alterations in the cardiovascular response to adrenergic mediated stress. *Fed Proc* 1980; 39:3173–3177.
37. Bitinsky MW, Russell V, Blanco M: Independent variations of glucagon and epinephrine responsive components of hepatic adenyl cyclase as a function of age, sex and steroid hormones. *Endocrinology* 1970; 86:154–159.
38. Duncan PG, Brink C, Douglas JJ: Beta-receptors during aging in respiratory tissues. *Eur J Pharmacol* 1982; 78:45–52.
39. Sheppard H, Burghardt CR: Age-dependent changes in the adenylate cyclase and phosphodiesterase activity of rat erythrocytes. *Biochem Pharmacol* 1973; 22:427–429.
40. Bylund B, Tellex-Inon T, Hollenberg D: Age-related parallel decline in beta-adrenerginc receptors, adenylate cyclase and phosphodiesterase activity in rat erythrocyte membranes. *Life Sci* 1970; 21:403–410.

41. Forn J, Schonhoffer PS, Skidmore IF, Krishna G: Effect of aging on the adenyl cyclase and phosphodiesterase activity of isolated fat cells of rats. *Biochim Biophys Acta* 1970; 208:304–309.
42. Cooper B, Gregerman RI: Hormone-sensitive fat cell adenylate cyclase in the rat. Influences of growth, cell size and aging. *J Clin Invest* 1976; 57:161–168.
43. Giudicelli Y, Pequery R: Beta-adrenergic receptors and catecholamine sensitive adenylate cyclase in rat fat cell membranes. Influence of growth, cell size and aging. *Eur J Biochem* 1978, 413–419.
44. Schmidt MJ, Thornberry JF: Cyclic AMP and cyclic GMP accumulation *in vitro* in brain regions of young, old and aged rats. *Brain Res* 1978; 139:169–177.
45. Volicer L, West CD, Chase AR, Greene L: Beta-adrenergic receptor sensitivity in cultured vascular smooth muscle cells: Effect of age and dietary restriction. *Mech Ageing Dev* 1983; 21:283–293.
46. Ross MH, Bras G: Influence of protein under- and overnutrition on spontaneous tumor prevalence in the rat. *J Nutr* 1973; 103:944–963.
47. Ross MH, Bras G: Dietary preference and diseases of age. *Nature* 1974; 250:263–265.
48. Berg BN, Wolf A, Simms HS: Nutrition and longevity in the rat. IV. Food restriction and the radiculoneuropathy of aging rats. *J Nutr* 1962; 77:439–442.
49. Vaughan DW: Membranous bodies in the cerebral cortex of aging rats: An electron microscope study. *J Neuropathol Exp Neurol* 1976; 35:152–166.
50. Vaughan DW, Vincent JM: Ultrastructure of neurons in the auditory cortex of aging rats: a morphometric study. *J Neurocytol* 1979; 8:215–228.
51. West CD: A quantitative study of lipofuscin accumulation with age in normals and individuals with Down's syndrome, phenylketonuria, Progeria and transneuronal atrophy. *J Comp Neurol* 1979; 186:109–116.
52. Hinds JW, McNelly NA: Capillaries in aging rat olfactory bulb: A quantitative light and electronmicroscopic study. *Neurobiol Aging* 1982; 3:197–207.
53. Vaughan DW, West CD: Deteriorative changes in the neocortex of aging rats on restricted diets. *Anat Rec* 1983; 205:206.
54. Vaughan DW, Peters A: The structure of neuritic plaques in the cerebral cortex of aged rats. *J Neuropathol Exp Neurol* 1981; 40:471–487.
55. Wisniewski HM, Johnson AB, Rain CS, et al: Senile plaques and cerebral amyloidosis in aged dogs. *Lab Invest* 1970; 23:287–296.
56. Wisniewski HM, Ghetti B, Terry RD: Neuritic (senile) plaques and filamentous changes in aged Rhesus monkeys. *J Neuropathol Exp Neurol* 1973; 32:566–584.
57. Wisniewski HM, Terry RD: Morphology of the aging brain, human and animal, in Ford DH (ed): *Progress in Brain Research,* vol 40. Amsterdam, Elsevier Press, 1973.
58. Terry RD: Some biological aspects of the aging brain. *Mech Ageing Dev* 1980; 14:191–201.
59. Klatzo I, Gajdusek DC, Zigas V: Pathology of Kuru. *Lab Invest* 1959; 8:799–847.
60. Chou SM, Martin JD: Kuru-plaques in a case of Creutzfeldt-Jakob disease. *Acta Neuropathol* 1971; 17:150–155.
61. Wisniewski HM, Bruce ME, Fraser H: Infectious aetiology of neurotic (senile) plaques in mice. *Science* 1975; 190:1108–1110.

62. Wisniewski HM, Moretz RC, Lossinsky AS: Evidence for induction of localized amyloid deposits and neuritic plaques by an infectious agent. *Ann Neurol* 1981; 10:517–522.
63. Stunkard AJ: Nutrition, aging and obesity, in Rockstein M, Sussman ML (eds): *Nutrition, Longevity, and Aging.* New York, Academic Press, 1976, pp 253–284.

9

Dietary Antioxidants, Membrane Lipids, and Aging

Grace Y. Sun and Albert Y. Sun

The continuous generation and propagation of free radical-containing compounds are damaging to body organs and subcellular organelles. One consequence is the peroxidative attack of the oxygen-containing radicals on membrane lipids. In fact, free radical-induced lipid peroxidation has become an important basis for explaining the biochemical phenomenon of cellular aging. Many types of organ damage can be directly or indirectly traced to an increase in lipid peroxidation. This chapter briefly describes the types of oxygen-containing free radical reactions and the biochemical interaction between the radicals and membrane lipids. Some examples of the effects of dietary antioxidants on membrane lipids and age-related changes in cellular functions will be described. The important role played by antioxidants in protecting the cells and organs from the lipid peroxidative processes and in alleviating the deleterious effects imposed by the free radicals on aging cells will be discussed. Recent research has focused on attempts to identify the types of biochemical changes occurring in the body systems that are caused by antioxidant deficiency and to assess the level of dietary antioxidants needed to insure proper protection.

Active Forms of Oxygen and Free Radical Reactions

The abundance of oxygen in the atmosphere has had an overt effect on the oxidative mechanisms in biologic systems. Many biochemical reactions utilize molecular oxygen as substrate and subsequently incorporate the molecule into biologically active compounds. Oxygen can also become activated by nonenzymatic mechanisms such as radiation, air pollutants, toxic gases, and drugs to form superoxide radicals ($\cdot\bar{O}_2$) (1). This free radical can react spontaneously with another superoxide radical to give rise to hydrogen peroxide (H_2O_2) and singlet oxygen (reaction 1).

$$\cdot\bar{O}_2 + \cdot\bar{O}_2 \xrightarrow[\text{spontaneous dismutation}]{+ 2H^+} H_2O_2 + {}^1O_2 \qquad (1)$$

In the cellular system, superoxide radicals are metabolized by superoxide dismutase to form H_2O_2 and triplet oxygen, as shown in reaction 2:

$$\cdot\bar{O}_2 + \cdot\bar{O}_2 \xrightarrow[\text{superoxide dismutase}]{+ 2H^+} H_2O_2 + {}^3O_2 \qquad (2)$$

The H_2O_2 generated by enzymatic or nonenzymatic means is unstable and can be reduced by catalase or glutathione peroxidase to H_2O (reaction 3). On the other hand, it can be further oxidized to form hydroxy radicals ($\cdot OH$) (reaction 4). A significant proportion of the oxygen consumed by biologic systems results in production of the superoxide radicals (2). Among the various forms of activated oxygen, hydroxy radicals are most reactive and therefore most destructive to the cells and tissue organs in biologic systems. Formation of hydroxy radicals from H_2O_2 and O_2 is greatly facilitated by Fe^{2+}. This reaction is known as the Haber-Weiss reaction (reaction 4).

$$2H_2O_2 \xrightarrow{\text{catalase}} 2H_2O + O_2 \qquad (3)$$

$$H_2O_2 + O_2 \xrightarrow[\text{Haber-Weiss reaction}]{Fe^{2+}} O_2 + OH^- + \dot{O}H \qquad (4)$$

Because of these reactive mechanisms, Leibovitz and Siegel (3) concluded that removal of superoxide radicals by superoxide dismutase not only can terminate the chain reactions involving propagation of free radicals, but can also inhibit other reactions leading to production of the hydroxy radicals. Superoxide radicals are produced in measurable amounts in both prokaryotes and eukaryotes (4) and in subcellular organelles such as mitochondria and peroxisomes (5,6). Enzymes such as xanthine oxidase, aldehyde oxidase, flavin dehydrogenases, and indolamine dioxygenase also produce superoxide radicals during the course of the catalysis (4). Examples of biologically active compounds that can undergo auto-oxidation and result in free radical formation are hydroquinones, flavins, catacholamines, thiols, ferridoxin, and hemoglobin (3). Therefore, in the absence of a proper control mechanism, free radicals formed during activation of oxygen are liable to be propagated rapidly and to cause damage to other biomolecules in the cellular system. The free radical hypothesis has become an important basis for explaining the biochemical phenomenon of cellular aging (7,8), and there is increasing evidence of free radical involvement in tissue pathology and various disease states (9–11).

Lipid Peroxidation and Membrane Function

Among the primary targets for free radical attack are the double bonds of polyunsaturated fatty acids (PUFA). These fatty acids are largely esterified to the phospholipids that form the primary structure of the lipid bilayer in membranes. Leibovitz and Siegel (3) have pointed out that the allylic hydrogens on the fatty acid chain are especially susceptible to free radical attack and, in the presence of oxygen, lipid peroxy radicals are formed easily, as shown by reaction 5. The lipid peroxy radical can further react with another double bond on the acyl chain to form a hydroperoxy ring structure. Rearrangement of the ring structure with bond splitting results in malondialdehyde (MDA) formation (12). This type of reaction mechanism is similar to the enzyme-mediated oxygenation of arachidonic acid for prostaglandin biosynthesis. Therefore, assay of MDA formation can be used as an indication of both enzymatic and nonenzymatic lipid peroxidation processes.

$$\underset{\text{PUFA}}{R-CH=CH-CH_2R} \xrightarrow{\text{electron and proton abstraction}} \underset{\text{allylic PUFA radical}}{R-CH=CH-\dot{C}H-R}$$

$$\xrightarrow{O_2} \underset{\text{lipid peroxy radical}}{R-CH=CH-CH(O-O^{\bullet})-R} \xrightarrow{LH \rightarrow L^{\bullet}} \underset{\text{lipid hydroperoxide}}{R-CH=CH-CH(O-OH)-R} \longrightarrow \text{MDA, ethane, pentane, etc.}$$

$$\underset{\text{lipid hydroperoxide}}{R-CH=CH-CH(O-OH)-R} \xrightarrow{2GSH \rightarrow GSSG} \underset{\text{hydroxy PUFA}}{R-CH=CH-CH(OH)-R} \qquad (5)$$

$$R = -CH=CH \text{------} \overset{O}{\overset{\|}{C}}OH$$

Lipid peroxidation is known to cause damaging effects to the biologic membranes. Insertion of peroxide molecules at the fatty acid double bonds could alter the acyl chain structure and impose additional restrictions to the freedom of motion of the chain (13). The physical changes include alteration of membrane fluidity, charges, proton conductivity, and permeability (14). In turn, these changes may be correlated to changes in membrane functions such as inhibition of membrane transport enzymes (15), loss of respiratory control, release of lysosomal enzymes, inhibition of thiol activity, and activation of phospholipases (14).

Recently, a number of biochemical studies have been initiated to correlate the effects of lipid peroxidation with membrane functions. Lee et al (16) found that lipid peroxidation induced by Fe^{2+} ion can cause both a specific hydrolysis of phosphatidylethanolamine in brain membranes and release of lysophospholipids. Some membrane proteins (eg, adenylate cyclase) were solubilized, probably by the detergent effects of the lysophospholipids. In another study, Libe et al (17) demonstrated that lipid peroxidation in brain cell membranes corresponded to changes in serotonin and diazepam binding. The effect was attributed to a change in the lipid environment for the interaction between the ligand and membrane receptor. Other types of environmental stress such as hyperoxia can also result in a decrease in serotonin-binding activity. On the other hand, membrane-protective agents such as Ionol were shown to give partial protection to the membrane oxidative activity and restore the receptor binding activity.

The effect of lipid peroxidation on mitochondrial swelling has been well demonstrated (14). The swelling process is always accompanied by uncoupling of oxidative phosphorylation, decrease in respiratory activity, and subsequently, breakdown of membrane phospholipids. Dudnik et al (18) observed a pronounced enhancement of lipid peroxidation in all subcellular fractions of liver homogenates upon ischemic treatment. The increase in lipid peroxidation activity was linked to a decrease in the readily oxidizable lipids such as cardiolipins with a concomitant increase in lysophospholipids. Chan and Fishman (19,20) showed that polyunsaturated fatty acids can induce brain edema, and this effect was attributed to the radical-mediated mechanism. Recently, Morel et al (21) showed that superoxide and/or hydrogen peroxide are involved in the formation of toxic low-density lipoprotein lipid species. Circulation of these oxidized lipid species could be the underlying cause for cell and organ injury in the body system.

Measurement of Lipid Peroxidation Products

Different laboratory procedures for measurement of the products resulting from lipid peroxidation have been described (12). The most common procedure is to measure the MDA generated from lipid peroxidation by complexing it with thiobarbituric acid (TBA). This complex exhibits an absorption maximum at 532 nm (equation 6). It is important to realize that in the biologic system MDA can also form a Schiff base with other amine-containing compounds (22). However, the TBA test is very sensitive and has been regarded as a useful procedure to indicate the extent of lipid peroxidation activity in cells and membranes.

$$\text{MDA} + 2\,\text{TBA} \xrightarrow[\text{heat}]{H^+} \text{MDA–TBA adduct} \qquad (6)$$

Another procedure is to measure exhaled gaseous hydrocarbons (23–25). The reaction mechanism for production of hydrocarbon gases from the lipid peroxides is shown in the equation below (reaction 7):

$$CH_3(CH_2)_4\,C(OOH)-R \xrightarrow{Fe^{2+} \to Fe^{3+}} CH_3(CH_2)_4\,C(\dot{O})-R + \dot{O}H$$

scission reaction

$$\longrightarrow CH_3(CH_2)_3\dot{C}H_2 + RC{=}O \xrightarrow{H^+} CH_3(CH_2)_3CH_3 \qquad (7)$$

In this mechanism, the hydrocarbon gases produced from peroxidative cleavage of the polyunsaturated fatty acid molecule are dependent on the position of the double bond attacked by the free radicals. For example, pentane is evolved from the $(n-6)$ fatty acids such as linoleic (18 : 2) and arachidonic (20 : 4), and ethane is evolved from the $(n-3)$ fatty acids such as docosahexaenoic acid (22 : 6).* Therefore, feeding rats diets supplemented with different types of fatty acids can result in production of different types of hydrocarbon gases (26).

A third method for determining lipid peroxides is to measure the intensity of chemiluminescence compounds produced (14). Under this condition, a linear relationship between the logarithm of lipid peroxide formed and the chemiluminescence intensity "quick flash" can be obtained. This procedure has been successfully used for studying lipid peroxidative mechanisms in mitochondria, as well as other systems (14).

*Nomenclature of fatty acids is $X : Y(n-Z)$, where X = number of carbon atoms, Y = number of double bonds, and Z = number of carbon atoms from the methyl group terminal of fatty acid chain to first double bond.

Other procedures include detection of fluorescence products such as the lipofuscin pigments that are accumulated during tissue aging (27). In some instances, it is also possible to detect the conjugated dienes that are formed and exhibit an absorption maximum at 233 nm. However, this latter method is not specific and lacks the sensitivity for practical application in biologic systems.

Protective Effects of Dietary Antioxidants on Cellular Function

Antioxidants are ubiquitous in cells and tissues and their role in protecting the radical-mediated peroxidative changes is well known. There is increasing emphasis on the nutritional requirement of antioxidants for combating the various chemical and environmental insults to the body. Dietary antioxidants have been shown to play an important role in modulation of the biologic aging processes (8,28), in protection against ischemic heart damage (13), and in inhibition of chemically induced carcinogenesis (10,11). Aside from the naturally occurring antioxidants, a number of chemically synthesized antioxidants such as butylated hydroxytoluene (BHT) and butylated hydroxyanisole (BHA) are commonly used in the food industry as preservatives. Dillard et al (29) showed that different types of antioxidants may exert different modes of action on the lipid peroxidative process. Therefore, when peroxidative activity was induced by treating rats with alloxan, the vitamin E-deficient animals were especially sensitive to the peroxidation insult. On the other hand, ascorbic acid was shown to prolong the effect of peroxidation instead of inhibiting the peroxidative changes. Dietary vitamin E and other antioxidants also exerted different effects on eicosanoid synthesis in young rabbits (30). Ames et al (9) described the role of uric acid as an antioxidant in the defense against oxidant and radical-caused aging and cancer (see Chapter 15). Since urate is a powerful scavenger for singlet oxygen, hydroxyl radicals, and other oxyheme oxidants, its presence in blood is important to protect the erythrocyte membrane from peroxidation and from lysis by lipid peroxides.

The role of vitamin E and selenium in terminating free radical reactions and in protection against lipid peroxidative processes in the body organs has been reviewed extensively (8,31,32). When the effects of dietary supplementation of *N,N'*-diphenyl-*p*-phenylenediamine or vitamin E on pentane production in vitamin E-deficient rats were compared, only vitamin E supplementation elicited a decrease in the production of pentane (23). In many instances, chemically synthesized antioxidants cannot effectively replace the action of the naturally occurring antioxidants. Microsomes (liver and lung) from vitamin E-deficient rats displayed an increase in lipid peroxidation as compared with those given vitamin E supplements (33). Furthermore, the vitamin E-deficient rats were more susceptible to lipid peroxidation induced by exposure to gaseous agents like NO_2. In vitamin E-deficient rabbits, the skeletal muscles showed extensive degeneration damages and morphologic changes such as appearance of streaming Z-lines, degenerated mitochondria, and fragmented sarcoplasmic reticulum (34). Vitamin E supplementation can result in significant improvement of the symptoms of the dystrophic muscle. In the ischemic myocardium, the increase in reactive Schiff products is correlated to a decrease in activities of superoxide dismutase, catalase, and glutathione peroxidase. One example is that pretreatment of animals with BHT resulted in improvement in their myocardial contractile function and suppression of lipid peroxidation activity. Drugs such as Inderal and Ionol were also effective to some extent. Dietary antioxidants have been shown to influence the incidence of mammary tumorogenesis induced by 7,12-DMBA (11,35,36). As a consequence of their peroxidative effect, polyunsaturated fatty acids are promoters of carcinogenesis (37,38); dietary BHT supplement is effective in reducing the incidence of tumors (10,38,39).

There is increasing interest in studying the effects of vitamin E on platelet functions and investigating whether antioxidants may exert an effect on platelet prostaglandin synthesis activity (40). Since α-tocopherol is incorporated into the platelet membrane, a modulation of the membrane microviscosity may result in a change in the platelet functions (41). Fong (42) observed that α-tocopherol added to human platelets could inhibit platelet aggregation induced by stimuli such as arachidonate, collagen, epinephrine, adenosine diphosphate, or thrombin. The in vitro addition of α-tocopherol to human platelets not only caused a change in the physical properties of the platelet membranes (43), but the platelet adhesiveness to collagen was also significantly reduced (44).

Agents that block membrane lipid peroxidation, including both the naturally occurring and synthetic antioxidants, were found to enhance the primary antigen response of mouse spleen cells simular to that elicited by 2-mercaptoethanol (45). Gavino et al (46) also showed that lipid peroxidation can influence the extent of proliferation of the cultured medial cells isolated from guinea pig aorta. Addition of PUFA to the culture resulted in an enhancement of lipid peroxidation as indicated by the amount of MDA formed. MDA formation can be inhibited by α-tocopherol, α-tocopherolquinone, and BHT, but not by 1,4-naphthoquinone. Recently, Fukuzawa et al (47) used liposomes to investigate the mechanistic aspects of the antioxidative action of vitamin E. Lipid peroxidation was induced by ascorbic acid and Fe^{2+}, and the peroxidative activity was correlated by measuring the amount of MDA produced. Using this system, it was found that the peroxidation reaction could be inhibited by α-tocopherol and 2,2,5,7,8-pentamethyl-6-hydroxy-chroman (TMC), but not by phytol, α-tocopherolquinone, or α-tocopherol acetate. Lipid peroxidation was accompanied by a decrease in membrane fluidity, and this change could be modified by α-tocopherol and TMC but not by cholesterol. Furthermore, the antioxidant effect of α-tocopherol could only be demonstrated after insertion of the molecule into the lipid bilayer. The conclusion is that the primary mode of action of vitamin E is to insert itself into the hydrophobic region of the membrane and thereby protect the fatty acyl chains from the peroxidative attack (48).

Dietary Antioxidants, Membrane Lipids, and Aging

Membrane Lipids and Aging

One effect of dietary antioxidants is to modulate membrane lipid changes during aging. The phospholipids in human brain myelin showed only a small decline in the PUFA content with age (49). Examination of myelin isolated from corpus callosum of Rhesus monkeys also indicated a similar change with age (50). On the other hand, the aging pattern for rodent brain myelin is different from that of the primates (51). Thus, aging in the human and primates is a gradual process, whereas in the rodents, acceleration of the aging process normally occurs after 24 months of age (52). Several comprehensive reviews of brain membrane lipid changes during aging are available (15,52–54).

Age-related changes in acyl group composition in the peripheral organs are different from those found in the brain membranes. Data in Tables 9-1 and 9-2 show the acyl group composition of phos-

Table 9-1. Phosphatidylcholine Acyl Group Composition in Rat Liver of Different Age Groups*

Fatty Acids	4 mo	14 mo	25 mo
		wt, %	
16 : 0	25.8 ± 1.1	17.0 ± 5.2	18.5 ± 2.6
18 : 0	17.6 ± 1.3	26.9 ± 2.6	21.7 ± 4.2
18 : 1	15.1 ± 0.8	11.8 ± 1.9	11.4 ± 2.7
18 : 2	15.9 ± 0.5	13.1 ± 1.7	16.3 ± 2.3
20 : 3	0.3 ± 0.1	0.4 ± 0.2	0.2 ± 0.0
20 : 3	1.8 ± 0.1	1.6 ± 0.4	1.9 ± 0.1
20 : 4	11.4 ± 1.8	13.5 ± 2.7	14.0 ± 1.6
20 : 5	2.4 ± 0.5	5.1 ± 1.6	1.9 ± 0.9
22 : 5	1.1 ± 0.2	1.4 ± 0.7	1.2 ± 0.4
22 : 6	8.7 ± 0.7	14.6 ± 3.8	13.6 ± 1.9
	(n = 4)	(n = 4)	(n = 4)

*Lipids in rat liver homogenate were extracted with chloroform-methanol, 2 : 1 (v/v), and the lipids were separated by one-dimensional thin-layer chromatography. Fatty acid methyl esters were obtained from phosphatidylcholines by base-methanolysis and were analyzed by gas–liquid chromatography. Results are mean ± SD from four samples.

Table 9-2. Phosphatidylethanolamine Acyl Group Composition in Rat Liver of Different Age Groups*

Fatty Acids	4 mo	14 mo	25 mo
		wt, %	
16 : 0	18.6 ± 2.0	15.6 ± 5.1	14.6 ± 2.4
18 : 0	22.2 ± 2.1	25.5 ± 2.7	22.3 ± 1.0
18 : 1	7.7 ± 0.6	5.5 ± 0.9	6.9 ± 2.0
18 : 2	7.7 ± 0.3	5.4 ± 0.7	7.6 ± 1.4
20 : 3	1.0 ± 0.1	0.4 ± 0.2	0.7 ± 0.3
20 : 4	16.2 ± 1.2	14.8 ± 2.4	15.5 ± 1.0
20 : 5	3.8 ± 0.4	4.8 ± 1.4	3.0 ± 0.7
22 : 5	2.9 ± 0.3	2.9 ± 1.3	2.4 ± 0.7
22 : 6	19.9 ± 1.2	28.2 ± 6.5	27.2 ± 3.4
	(n = 4)	(n = 4)	(n = 4)

*Experimental conditions were the same as in Table 9-1.

phatidylcholines (PC) and phosphatidylethanolamines (PE), respectively, in rat liver from three different age groups. Contrary to the brain membranes, there is an increase in the proportion of 22 : 6 ($n-3$) in both types of phospholipids and a concomitant decrease in 16 : 0 between the 4- and 14-month-old samples. Differences between the 14- and 25-month-old samples are not obvious.

Stege et al (55) compared the lipid peroxidation activity in hepatocytes isolated from Fischer-344 female rats aged 3, 12, and 25 months. All three groups of animals were fed an antioxidant-free diet for 21 days prior to the hepatocyte isolation. It was surprising to find that cells from young rats showed the highest level of lipid peroxidation. On the other hand, aged hepatocytes were more susceptible to the induced peroxidation process, and this was thought to result from a defective peroxidation defense mechanism in the aged group. Information regarding membrane peroxidative activity in various organs during aging is scarce, although this is certainly a pertinent subject for future investigation.

Effects of Dietary Antioxidant Deficiency on Membrane Lipids

Although it has been demonstrated that α-tocopherol exerts its primary effect by directly interacting with the cell membranes (48), little is known about its effect on the membrane lipids. Grinna (56) showed that aged rats are less susceptible to induction of dietary vitamin E deficiency, and therefore, the dietary tocopherol requirement also decreased with age. In this study, little change in membrane compositional and functional parameters was found in animals with vitamin E deficiency or with a supplement in the diet.

A study was carried out in our laboratory to examine the effects of dietary antioxidant deficiency on hepatic mitochondrial lipids (8). In this study, rats were given the following diets: (I) a basal diet supplemented by vitamin E and selenium; (II) a basal diet deficient in vitamin E and selenium; (III) a basal diet supplemented with vitamin E alone; (IV) a basal diet supplemented with selenium alone; and (V) a basal diet supplemented with BHT. These diets were initiated at weaning, and the various dietary regimes were maintained for 18 months. Obvious reduction in body weight was observed in rats fed the antioxidant-deficient diet (group II) and the deficient diet supplemented with BHT (group V) (Fig. 9-1). Besides, the life span of the antioxidant-deficient animals was greatly reduced (8). Among the body organs, the adrenal seemed to show a marked response to the dietary stress. Specifically, there was an increase in both adrenal cholesterol and cholesterylester levels in rats given the deficient (group II) and the BHT-supplemented diet (group V) (Fig. 9-2).

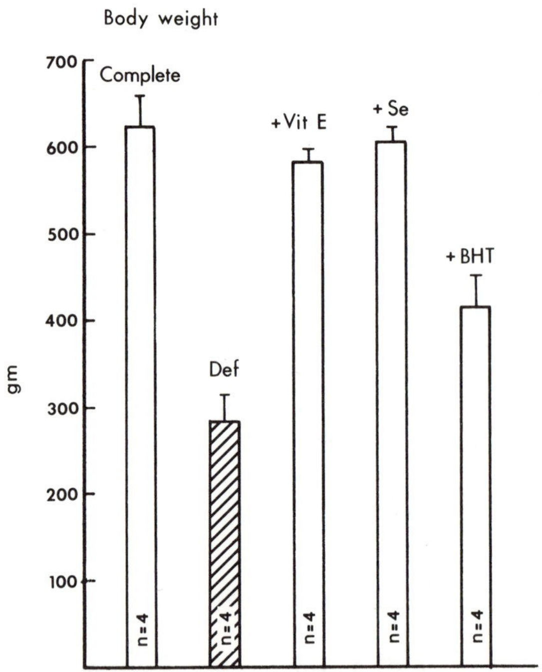

Figure 9-1. Body weight of rats given different antioxidant-deficient and -supplemented diets. Rats were given at weaning a formulated diet containing (as % of diet): Torula yeast, 30; sucrose, 57; vitamin E-free lard, 5; cod-liver oil, 3; salt mix, 5; vitamin mix, 1; and *dl*-methionine, 0.3. Group I was given the basal diet supplemented with 50 IU/kg of vitamin E and 0.5 ppm Na-selenite; Group II was given the basal antioxidant-deficient diet as control; Group III was supplemented with vitamin E; Group IV with selenium; and Group V with BHT (0.5%).

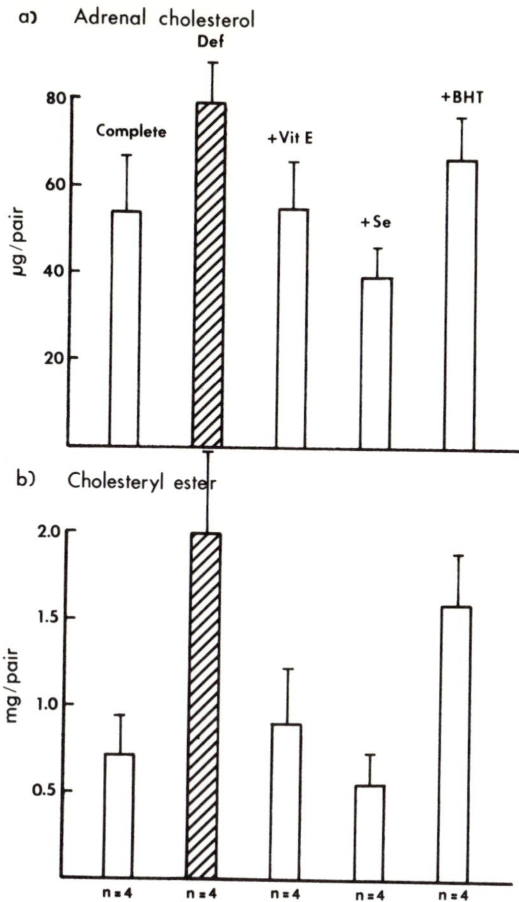

Figure 9-2. Adrenal cholesterol (a) and cholesteryl esters (b) levels in rats fed the various diets described in Figure 9-1.

A change in cholesterol level further suggests that some of the adrenal functions are altered by the dietary deficiency.

Analysis of the lipids from hepatic mitochondria indicated that the acyl groups of phospholipids in the antioxidant-deficient rats (group II) and rats fed the BHT diet (group V) were lower in PUFA of the $(n-3)$ series, such as 22 : $5(n-3)$ and 22 : $6(n-3)$, but not the $(n-6)$ series (Table 9-3). In fact, the proportion of 20 : $4(n-6)$ and 20 : $5(n-6)$ in phosphatidylethanolamine was higher in the deficient rats than in rats supplemented with vitamin E and selenium. The decrease in PUFA of the $(n-3)$ series was attributed to a decrease in the fatty acid desaturase activity specific for synthesis of the $(n-3)$ PUFA. A number of oxidative desaturases are present in the cell cytoplasm (57,58), and most of them are highly sus-

Table 9-3. Effect of Antioxidants on Major Polyunsaturated Fatty Acids from Phosphatidylcholines and Phosphatidylethanolamines in Rat Liver Mitochondria*

	Dietary Supplement				
Fatty Acids	(I) Complete	(II) Deficient	(III) + Vit E	(IV) + Selenium	(V) + BHT
			Phosphatidylcholine		
18 : 2	18.5	18.4	18.1	13.4	20.9
20 : 4	14.4	14.6	9.5	12.5	9.4
20 : 5	2.6	3.4	3.6	5.1	3.7
22 : 6	8.9	6.8	10.3	11.3	7.0
			Phosphatidylethanolamine		
18 : 2	8.6	9.7	8.2	6.0	10.3
20 : 4	16.9	23.2	12.6	14.6	14.3
20 : 5	3.2	5.3	3.7	5.7	3.7
22 : 6	19.4	13.8	21.7	20.4	15.4

*Analysis of the acyl group composition of mitochondrial phospholipids from rats fed various antioxidant diets. Results denote the percent distribution of the polyunsaturated fatty acids in the fraction.

ceptible to dietary and hormonal influences (59–61). It is not surprising that the PUFA desaturase activity is affected by lipid peroxidation, although this type of investigation has not been studied extensively. The resistance to change of PUFA of the $(n-6)$ series in the antioxidant-deficient group (group I) may be the result of an adaptive mechanism, probably because a critical level of arachidonic acid is needed for cellular metabolism and for conversion to the prostaglandins.

Free radical-induced lipid peroxidation can lead to phospholipid degradation and loss of membrane integrity (20,62). This effect, however, may be selective, depending on the types of lipids and their metabolic involvement in the membrane. Fatty acids of the retinal membranes (rod outer segments) comprise a high proportion of PUFA, such as $22:6(n-3)$ (63), and these membranes are highly susceptible to peroxidative insults (64). Recently, Wiegand et al (65) showed that prolonged exposure of the retina to light could result in a progressive loss of phospholipids, especially those containing the PUFA species. Therefore, peroxidation of long-chain PUFA in rod outer segments may be a determining factor in light-induced retinal degeneration.

Effects of a High Level of Dietary Vitamin E on Membrane Lipids

Not much is known about the consequences of an excess intake of vitamin E on membrane lipids. Large amounts of vitamin E can exert a protective effect on the membrane, since the hydrophobic portion of the molecule is expected to be inserted completely into the lipid bilayer (48). It is possible that upon excess intake of vitamin E, the membrane may adapt to the presence of the molecule by altering its lipid composition. In a recent experiment, weanling rats were given a dietary supplement with either 50 or 500 IU vitamin E/kg of diet and the rats with these two dietary vitamin E levels were maintained until 14 or 25 months of age. The phospholipids and acyl group composition of liver mitochondria were analyzed. At 14 months of age, animals given the higher level of vitamin E in the diet showed a lower level of cardiolipin (per mg protein) in the liver mitochondria, but the acyl groups of this phospholipid were higher in the proportion of $18:2$ (Table 9-4). Similar changes were observed in phosphatidylcholine, except that the increase in $18:2$ was marked by a decrease in $22:6(n-3)$, and the level of $20:4(n-6)$ was not changed (Table 9-5). From the results obtained, it is concluded that membrane lipids are altered by excess dietary vitamin E intake, probably to compensate for its presence. However, the physiologic significance of this type of membrane lipid change remains to be investigated.

The effects of a high dietary vitamin E (1,000 IU/kg) supplement were also evaluated in rabbits fed an atherogenic diet or a low-cholesterol diet (66). Aortic and coronary atherosclerosis were more frequent and exten-

Table 9-4. Effects of Vitamin E and Aging on the Acyl Group Composition of Phosphatidylcholines in Rat Liver Mitochondria*

Fatty Acids	14 mo		25 mo	
	Low E	High E	Low E	High E
Total μg/mg protein	19.2 ± 0.5	16.5 ± 2.4	20.2 ± 1.3	18.9 ± 2.1
		%, *wt*		
16 : 0	20.6 ± 0.7	21.4 ± 0.7	19.2 ± 1.6	16.0 ± 1.6
18 : 0	24.8 ± 0.8	24.1 ± 1.3	25.4 ± 2.2	28.0 ± 1.0
18 : 1	10.5 ± 0.3	9.7 ± 0.8	10.4 ± 0.9	9.3 ± 1.2
18 : 2	8.5 ± 0.4	12.9 ± 1.5	11.0 ± 1.1	13.6 ± 1.6
20 : 3	0.8 ± 0.1	0.7 ± 0.3	1.0 ± 0.3	1.2 ± 0.3
20 : 4	13.5 ± 0.2	13.9 ± 0.9	12.8 ± 1.7	13.3 ± 1.1
20 : 5	4.1 ± 0.3	4.5 ± 0.9	7.3 ± 1.6	6.4 ± 0.8
22 : 5	1.1 ± 0.1	0.6 ± 0.2	1.3 ± 0.2	1.1 ± 0.3
22 : 6	16.1 ± 0.2	12.1 ± 2.1	12.9 ± 0.9	10.7 ± 1.1
	(n = 4)	(n = 4)	(n = 7)	(n = 7)

*Rats at weaning were given the basal diet described in Figure 9-1 except that vitamin E-free lard was replaced by corn oil. The low-E and high-E groups were supplemented by 50 IU/kg diet and 500 IU/kg diet of vitamin E, respectively. Analysis of acyl group composition of phospholipids was the same as described in Table 9-1.

Table 9-5. Effects of Vitamin E and Aging on the Acyl Group Composition of Cardiolipin in Rat Liver Mitochondria*

Fatty Acids	14 mo		25 mo	
	Low E	High E	Low E	High E
Total μg/mg protein	17.9 ± 1.9	13.1 ± 0.4	14.4 ± 0.7	13.6 ± 2.4
		%, *wt*		
14 : 0	0.4 ± 0.3	0.4 ± 0.2	0.4 ± 0.2	—
16 : 0	4.9 ± 0.3	5.1 ± 1.0	4.1 ± 1.1	3.9 ± 1.0
16 : 1	8.8 ± 1.4	5.8 ± 1.2	6.5 ± 1.2	5.6 ± 0.7
18 : 0	5.9 ± 1.7	2.7 ± 1.3	3.2 ± 1.0	2.8 ± 0.5
18 : 1	26.8 ± 1.3	24.7 ± 1.2	25.8 ± 2.9	22.9 ± 2.3
18 : 2	53.4 ± 2.1	61.3 ± 5.9	60.1 ± 4.3	64.5 ± 3.4
	(n = 4)	(n = 3)	(n = 8)	(n = 5)

*Dietary regime and procedure for lipid analysis were same as in Table 9-4.

sive in rabbits fed either a basal diet or the basal diet supplemented with BHA and BHT than in rabbits fed the basal diet supplemented with vitamin E or the negative control diet (corn oil). In this study, a dramatic difference in serum lipid profile was observed among the various dietary groups. Animals given the diet supplemented with a high level of vitamin E showed a substantial decrease in serum cholesterol and phospholipids over those given a basal (butter) diet alone.

Some clinical trials have been initiated to investigate whether dietary supplement of a high level of vitamin E would influence human serum lipid components. However, most of the results are still highly controversial, and thus no clear-cut conclusions can be made at the present time (67,68).

Summary

Many biochemical reactions utilize molecular oxygen as substrate. Oxygen and oxygen-containing molecules can become activated by nonenzymatic and enzymatic mechanisms to form free radicals. Activated forms of oxygen (superoxide radicals and hydroxy radicals) are highly reactive molecules and can be propagated to give rise to other radical-containing compounds. One of the primary targets for free radical attack is the polyunsaturated fatty acids in membrane. The result is the formation of lipid peroxy radicals. Lipid peroxidation can give rise to changes in membrane physical properties and functions. An acceleration of this process has been correlated with cellular and subcellular mechanisms, including mitochondrial swelling, cell edema, inhibition of cell mobility, myocardial tissue damage, and cellular aging phenomena. Malondialdehyde is generated as a result of lipid peroxidation and can be detected by complexing with thiobarbituric acid. A second procedure for detectng the products of lipid peroxides is to measure the production of hydrocarbon gases.

Dietary antioxidants can quench the radical-mediated peroxidative changes occurring in biologic systems. Their roles include modulation of the biologic aging processes, protection against ischemic heart damages, and inhibition of chemically induced carcinogenesis. Vitamin E is the most important dietary antioxidant for protection against membrane peroxidation. It acts as a free-radical scavenger after insertion into the lipid bilayer. An increase in polyunsaturated fatty acids is found in rat liver membranes with age. This increase is linked with an increased susceptibility of the membranes to lipid peroxidation. Dietary deficiency in vitamin E and selenium results in an increase in cholesterol and cholesterylester levels in the rat adrenal gland. In most instances, BHT cannot replace vitamin E in overcoming the deficiency symptoms. The same deficient group also shows a decrease in $(n-3)$ fatty acids, but the $(n-6)$ fatty acids are not altered.

Dietary supplementation of a high level of vitamin E in rats results in a decrease in the level of phospholipids in liver mitochondria, but the proportion of 18 : 2 in the phospholipids is increased. This change in membrane lipid composition may be caused by adaptation to the presence of the high level of vitamin E in the membrane. High levels of vitamin E given to rabbits fed an atherogenic diet also results in a suppression of the serum lipids, especially the cholesterol. Consequently, future studies should be directed toward examining the role of dietary antioxidants in alleviating the deleterious cellular processes occurring during aging.

References

1. Menzel DB: Nutritional needs in environmental intoxication: Vitamin E and air pollution, an example. *Environ Health Perspect* 1979; 29:105–114.
2. Britton L, Malinowski DP, Fridovich I: Superoxide dismutase and oxygen metabolism in *Streptococcus faecalis* and comparisons with other organisms. *J Bacteriol* 1978; 134:229–236.
3. Leibovitz BE, Siegel BV: Aspects of free radical reactions in biological systems: Aging. *J Gerontol* 1980; 35:45–56.
4. Fridovich I: The biology of oxygen radicals. *Science* 1978; 201:875–880.
5. Loschen G, Azzi A, Flohe L: Mitochondrial H_2O_2 formation; relationship with energy conservation. *FEBS Lett* 1973; 33:84–87.
6. Forman HJ, Boveris A: Superoxide radical and hydrogen peroxide in mitochondria, in Pryor WA (ed): *Free Radicals in Biology,* vol V. New York, Academic Press, 1982, pp 65–90.
7. Harman D: The free-radical theory of aging, in Pryor WA (ed): *Free Radicals in Biology,* vol V. New York, Academic Press, 1982; pp 255–276.
8. Sun AY, Sun GY: Dietary antioxidants and aging on membrane functions, in Moment GB (ed): *Nutritional Approaches to Aging Research.* Boca Raton, Fla, CRC Press, 1982, pp 135–156.
9. Ames BN, Cathcart R, Schwiers E, Hochstein P: Uric acid provides an antioxidant defense in humans against oxidant- and radical-caused aging and cancer: A hypothesis. *Proc Natl Acad Sci USA* 1981; 78:6858–6862.
10. McCay PB, King MM, Pitha JV: Evidence that the effectiveness of antioxidants as inhibitors of 7,12-dimethylbenz(a)anthracene-induced mammary tumors is a function of dietary fat composition. *Cancer Res* 1981; 41:3745–3748.
11. King MM, McCay P: Modulation of tumor incidence and possible mechanisms of inhibition of mammary carcinogenesis by dietary antioxidants. *Cancer Res* 1981; 43(suppl):2485–2490.
12. Logani MK, Davies RE: Lipid oxidation: Biologic effects and antioxidants—a review. *Lipids* 1980; 15:485–495.
13. Meerson FZ, Kagan VE, Kozlov YP, et al: The role of lipid peroxidation in pathogenesis of ischemic damage and the antioxidant protection of the heart. *Basic Res Cardiol* 1982; 77:465–485.
14. Vladimirov YA, Olenev VI, Suslova TB, Cheremisina ZP: Lipid peroxidation in mitochondrial membrane. *Adv Lipid Res* 1980; 17:173–249.

15. Sun AY, Sun GY: Neurochemical aspects of the membrane hypothesis of aging. *Interdiscpl Topics Gerontol* 1979; 15:34–53.
16. Lee E, Baba A, Ohta A, Iwata H: Solubilization of adenylate cyclase of brain membranes by lipid peroxidation. *Biochim Biophys Acta* 1982; 689:370–374.
17. Libe ML, Bogdanova ED, Rozenberg AE, et al: ^{3}H-Serotonin and ^{3}H-diazepam binding and lipid peroxidation in brain cell membranes. *Bull Exp Biol Med* 1981; 92:1506–1508.
18. Dudnik LB, Bilenko MV, Alesenko AV, et al: Intensification of peroxidation and changes in lipid composition in ischemic liver homogenates and subcellular fractions. *Bull Exp Biol Med* 1980; 89:556–558.
19. Chan PH, Fishman RA: Transient formation of superoxide radicals in polyunsaturated fatty acid-induced brain swelling. *J Neurochem* 1980; 35: 1004–1007.
20. Chan PH, Yurko M, Fishman RA: Phospholipid degradation and cellular edema induced by free radicals in brain cortical slices. *J Neurochem* 1982; 38:525–531.
21. Morel DW, Hessler JR, Chisolm GM: Low density lipoprotein cytotoxicity induced by free radical peroxidation of lipid. *J Lipid Res* 1983; 24:1070–1076.
22. Barber AA, Bernheim F: Lipid peroxidation: Its measurement, occurrence and significance in animal tissues. *Adv Gerontol Res* 1967; 2:355–403.
23. Downey JE, Irving DH, Tappel AL: Effects of dietary antioxidants on *in vivo* lipid peroxidation in the rat as measured by pentane production. *Lipids* 1978; 13:403–407.
24. Tappel AL: Measurement of and protection from *in vivo* lipid peroxidation, in Pryor WA (ed): *Free Radicals in Biology,* vol 4. New York, Academic Press, 1980, pp 1–25.
25. Tappel AL: Vitamin E and selenium protection from *in vivo* lipid peroxidation. *Ann N Y Acad Sci* 1980; 355:18–31.
26. Kivits GA, Ganguli-Swarttouw MA, Christ EJ: The composition of alkanes in exhaled air of rats as a result of lipid peroxidation *in vivo.* Effects of dietary fatty acids, vitamin E and selenium. *Biochim Biophys Acta* 1981; 665:557–570.
27. Tappel AL, Fletcher B, Deamer D: Effects of antioxidants and nutrients on lipid peroxidation fluorescent products and aging parameters in the mouse. *J Gerontol* 1973; 28:415–424.
28. Sun AY, Sun GY: Effects of dietary vitamin E and other antioxidants on aging process in rat brain, in Roberts J, Adelman RC, Cristofalo VJ (eds): *Pharmacological Intervention in the Aging Process.* New York, Plenum Press, 1978, pp 285–290.
29. Dillard CJ, Kunert KJ, Tappel AL: Effects of vitamin E, ascorbic acid and mannitol on alloxan-induced lipid peroxidation in rats. *Arch Biochem Biophys* 1982; 216:204–212.
30. Chan AC, Pritchard ET, Choy PC: Different effects of dietary vitamin E and antioxidants on eicosanoid synthesis in young rabbits. *J Nutr* 1983; 113:813–819.
31. Tappel AL, Dillard CJ: *In vivo* lipid peroxidation: measurement via exhaled pentane and protection by vitamin E. *Fed Proc* 1981; 40:174–178.
32. Scott ML: Advances in our understanding of vitamin E. *Fed Proc* 1980; 39:2736–2739.
33. Sevanian A, Hacker AD, Elsayed N: Influence of vitamin E and nitrogen

dioxide on lipid peroxidation in rat lung and liver microsomes. *Lipids* 1982; 17:269–277.

34. Dahlin KJ, Chan AC, Benson ES, Hegarty PVJ: Rehabilitating effect of vitamin E therapy on the ultra structural changes in skeletal muscles of vitamin-E-deficient rabbits. *Am J Clin Nutr* 1978; 31:94–99.
35. Carroll KK, Khor HT: Effects of level and type of dietary fat on the incidence of mammary tumors induced in female Sprague-Dawley rats by 7,12-DMBA. *Lipids* 1971; 6:415–420.
36. Chan PC, Head JF, Cohen LA, Wynder EL: Influence of dietary fat on the induction of mammary tumors by *N*-nitrosomethylurea: associated hormone changes and differences between Sprague-Dawley and F-344 rats. *J Natl Cancer Inst* 1977; 59:1279–1283.
37. Hopkins GJ, Kennedy TG, Carroll KK: Polyunsaturated fatty acids as promoters of mammary carcinogenesis induced in Sprague-Dawley rats by 7,12-dimethylbenz[*a*]anthracene. *J Natl Cancer Inst* 1981; 66:517–522.
38. King MM, Bailey DM, Gibson DD, et al: Incidence and growth of mammary tumors induced by 7,11-DMBA as related to the dietary content of fat and antioxidant. *J Natl Cancer Inst* 1979; 63:657–663.
39. King MM, McCay PB, Kosanke SD: Comparison of the effect of BHT on *N*-nitrosomethylurea and 7,12-DMBA in induced mammary tumors. *Cancer Lett* 1981; 14:219–226.
40. Hamelin SSt-J, Chan AC: Modulation of platelet thromboxane and malonaldehyde by dietary vitamin E and linoleate. *Lipids* 1983; 18:267–269.
41. Steiner M, Anastasi J: Vitamin E. An inhibitor of the platelet release reaction. *J Clin Invest* 1976; 57:732–737.
42. Fong JSC: Alpha-tocopherol: Its inhibition on human platelet aggregation. *Specialia* 1976; 15:639–641.
43. Steiner M: Vitamin E changes the membrane fluidity of human platelets. *Biochim Biophys Acta* 1981; 640:100–105.
44. Steiner M: Effect of alpha-tocopherol administration on platelet function in man. *Thromb Haemost* 1983; 49:73–77.
45. Hoffeld JT: Agents which block membrane lipid peroxidation enhance mouse spleen cell immune activities *in vitro*: relationship to the enhancing activity of 2-mercaptoethanol. *Eur J Immunol* 1981; 11:371–376.
46. Gavino VC, Miller JS, Ikharebha SO, et al: Effect of polyunsaturated fatty acids and antioxidants on lipid peroxidation in tissue cultures. *J Lipid Res* 1981; 22:763–769.
47. Fukuzawa K, Chida H, Tokumura A, Tsukatani H: Antioxidant effect of α-tocopherol incorporation into lecithin liposomes on ascorbic acid—Fe^{2+}-induced lipid peroxidation. *Arch Biochem Biophys* 206:173–180.
48. Lucy JA: Functional and structural aspects of biological membranes: a suggested structural role for vitamin E in the control of membrane permeability and stability. *Ann N Y Acad Sci* 1972; 203:4–11.
49. Horrocks LA, Sun GY, D'Amato RA: Changes in brain lipids in aging, in Ordy JM, Brizzee KR (eds): *Neurobiology of Aging*. New York, Plenum Press, 1975, pp 359–368.
50. Sun GY, Samorajski T: Age changes in acyl groups of phosphoglycerides from myelin isolated from the corpus callosum of the rhesus monkey. *Biochim Biophys Acta* 1973; 316:19–27.

51. Sun GY, Samorajski T: Age changes in the lipid composition of whole homogenates and isolated myelin fractions of mouse brain. *J Gerontol* 1972; 27:10–17.
52. Sun AY, Sun GY, Foudin LL: Aging in the nervous system, in Lajtha A (ed): *Handbook of Neurochemistry*, ed : 2, vol 10. New York, Plenum Press, 1984, (in press).
53. Horrocks LA, Van Rollins M, Yates AJ: Lipid changes in the aging brain, in Davison AN, Thompson RHS (eds): *The Molecular Basis of Neuropathology*. London, Edward Arnold, 1982, pp 601–630.
54. Sun GY, Foudin L: Phospholipid composition and metabolism in the developing and aging nervous system, in Eichberg J (ed): *Phospholipids in the Nervous System*. New York, Wiley, 1984, (in press).
55. Stege TE, Mischke BS, Zipperer WC: Levels of lipid peroxidation in hepatocytes isolated from aging rats fed an antioxidant-free diet. *Exp Gerontol* 1982; 17:273–279.
56. Grinna LS: Effect of dietary α-tocopherol on liver microsomes and mitochondria of aging rats. *J Nutr* 1976; 106:918–929.
57. Brenner RR: The oxidative desaturation of unsaturated fatty acids in animals. *Mol Cell Biochem* 1974; 3:41–52.
58. Sprecher H: Biochemistry of essential fatty acids. *Prog Lipid Res* 1982; 20:13–22.
59. Nervi AM, Peluffo RO, Brenner RR, Leikin AI: Effect of ethanol administration on fatty acid desaturation. *Lipids* 1980; 15:263–268.
60. Brenner RR: Nutritional and hormonal factors influencing desaturation of essential fatty acids. *Prog Lipid Res* 1982; 20:41–48.
61. Wang DL, Reitz RC: Ethanol ingestion and polyunsaturated fatty acids: Effects on the acyl-CoA desaturases. *Alcoholism: Clin Exp Res* 1983; 7:220–226.
62. Yoshida S, Inoh S, Aseno T et al: Effect of transient ischemia on free fatty acids and phospholipids in the gerbil brain: Lipid peroxidation as a possible cause of post ischemic injury. *J Neurosurg* 1980; 53:323–331.
63. Wiegand RD, Anderson RE: Determination of molecular species of rod outer segment phospholipids, in Packer L (ed): *Methods in Enzymology* vol 81. New York, Academic Press, 1983, pp 297–304.
64. Kagan VE, Shvedova AA, Novikov KN, Kozlov YP: Light-induced free radical oxidation of membrane lipids in photoreceptors of frog retina. *Biochim Biophys Acta* 1973; 330:76–80.
65. Wiegand RD, Giusto NM, Anderson RE: Lipid Changes in albino rat rod outer segments following constant illumination, in Clayton R, Heywood I, Reading H, Wright A (eds): *Biology of Normal and Genetically Abnormal Retinas*. New York, Academic Press, 1982, pp 121–128.
66. Wilson RB, Middleton CC, Sun GY: Vitamin E, antioxidants and lipid peroxidation in experimental atherosclerosis of rabbits. *J Nutr* 1978; 108:1858–1867.
67. Hermann WJ, Ward K, Faucett J: The effect of tocopherol on high density lipoprotein cholesterol. *Am J Clin Pathol* 1979; 72:848–852.
68. Stampfer MJ, Willett W, Castelli WP, et al: Effect of vitamin E on lipids. *Am J Clin Pathol* 1983; 79:714–716.

10

Membrane Changes Associated with Alcohol Use and Aging: Possibilities for Nutritional Intervention

W. Gibson Wood and R. Strong

Alcohol is consumed by a large number of adults. Although it serves as a food in some cultures (1), most individuals drink alcohol for its mood-altering effects. Unfortunately, a significant number of individuals drink large amounts of alcohol, which can result in a wide range of physical, psychologic, and social problems. In the past few years, increasing attention has been focused on alcohol consumption by elderly individuals (2–4). While the extent of alcohol problems among the elderly has not been well documented, it has been estimated that between 2% and 10% of elderly individuals have alcohol problems (5). The percentage increases significantly among the elderly in various institutional facilities (6). For some elderly individuals alcohol problems may be brought on by changes that occur with aging, eg, loss of a spouse, retirement, or isolation (7–9).

The prevalence of alcoholism and alcohol abuse declines with increasing age (10). However, aged individuals may be "at risk" for developing alcohol-related problems because of their increased susceptibility to pathologic effects stemming from chronic alcohol abuse and changes associated with aging (11). Excessive consumption of alcohol can result in pathologic changes in various organ systems of the body: liver disease, respiratory disease, gastrointestinal pathology, diseases of the nervous and cardiovascular systems (12–16). Many of those organ systems show a high morbidity with advancing age (17). Excessive drinking in an elderly individual could precipitate or exaggerate pathologic changes in these systems. The similarities between the effects of alcohol and changes that occur with aging have induced some researchers to propose that alcoholism may accelerate the aging process (18–20). Although this hypothesis is speculative, it is evident that the elderly are very vulnerable to the effects of alcohol.

Generally, aged organisms are more sensitive than younger ones to the effects of alcohol (21). This sensitivity may be expressed as greater susceptibility to alcohol-related problems such as drug–alcohol interactions, cognitive impairment, motor dysfunction, and development of dependence than is observed among younger organisms (11,22–26). The specific mechanism for the age-related sensitivity to alcohol has not been identified, but the effect of alcohol on aged brain structure and function appears to be very different from its impact on younger brains (27–29). This chapter discusses the effects of alcohol on the aged organism, with special emphasis on alcohol- and aged-induced changes in the physical and biochemical properties of brain membranes.

Human and Animal Studies

The effects of alcohol are age related. Studies on human subjects have reported that aging individuals differ in response to ethanol as measured by cognitive performance (22), blood ethanol levels (30), and (Na^+–K^+)ATPase activity (27). Older subjects (56 to 80 years of age) did not perform as well on information-processing tasks as younger subjects (20 to 55 years of age) following alcohol administration (22). Peak blood ethanol levels were higher for the older subjects; however, when young and old subjects were matched for blood ethanol levels, the performance of the older subjects was still significantly lower than that of the younger subjects. Interestingly, in the same study, the older subjects reported feeling less affected by ethanol than the younger subjects. Another study with different age groups of subjects has reported that blood ethanol levels were higher for older as compared to younger subjects. However, ethanol elimination did not differ with age (30). Age differences have been noted in the effects of alcohol on the brain. Sun and Samorajski (27) observed that brain tissue from human autopsy specimens of old individuals (67, 68, and 84 years) differed in response to ethanol from the tissue of younger individuals (19 and 34 years). This age difference was demonstrated by the greater inhibition of synaptosomal (Na^+–K^+)ATPase activity in the presence of ethanol for tissue samples from old individuals.

A general conclusion of these human studies is that aged subjects differ from younger subjects in both behavioral and biochemical responses to ethanol. This conclusion applies also to animal studies on ethanol and aging, in which there was both acute and chronic administration of ethanol (for reviews, see references 21,31,32). Age differences in animals in response to ethanol in vivo have been reported for alcohol consumption, motor function, chronic intoxication, and severity of withdrawal and ethanol-induced hypothermia. Aged animals are generally more sensitive to the intoxicating effects of ethanol (23–25), but are less responsive to its hypothermic effects (25,33).

Mechanisms of Age-Related Differences to Ethanol

The mechanism(s) for age differences in response to ethanol has not been determined. Possible mechanisms include age differences in ethanol elimination, body water levels, and brain sensitivity in response to ethanol. Both human and animal studies have shown that age differences in ethanol elimination do not play a significant role in effects of ethanol (23,30). Age differences in body water have been proposed as an explanation for the effects of ethanol on the aged organism (33–36). This explanation is based on the observation that the percentage of body water to body weight declines with increasing age (17). If ethanol dosage is based on body weight, older organisms would receive a higher dosage because they have less body water. When ethanol dose is based on estimated body water, the effect of ethanol in aged Sprague-Dawley rats is reduced (36). However, it has been reported recently that even when ethanol dose is based on estimated body water, age differences in response to ethanol are observed in Sprague-Dawley rats (33). The body water hypothesis is interesting and may account in part for the in vivo age differences in response to ethanol. This area needs much more work, which should include an appropriate animal model, more precise measures of body water, and the use of several different age groups.

Aged mice lose and regain the righting response at lower brain and blood ethanol levels than younger mice (23,24). Table 10-1 shows time at loss of the righting response, duration of loss, and blood ethanol levels at loss and regaining of the righting response of three different age groups of C57BL/6NNIA mice. Blood ethanol levels were lower at both time points and the aged mice were impaired longer. Those results support the hypothesis that ethanol may have a greater effect on brain function of aged animals.

Aged animals are more sensitive to the sedative effects of ethanol (Table 10-1) and more affected during chronic administration and withdrawal (Figs. 10-1 and 10-2), but are less sensitive to ethanol-induced hypothermia (Fig. 10-3). Those age differences were not attributable to differences in blood ethanol levels or differences in the amount consumed of an ethanol liquid diet during chronic administration. The contribution of ethanol elimination and body water do not fully explain age-

Table 10-1. Time and Blood Ethanol Levels at Loss and Regaining of the Righting Response*

Age Group (mo)	LRR† Time (min)	LRR† BEL‡ (mg/dL)	RRR† Time (min)	RRR† BEL (mg/dL)
8	1.52 ± 0.22	427 ± 33	66.37 ± 4.43	393 ± 19
18	1.43 ± 0.09	406 ± 29	72.37 ± 6.79	371 ± 11
28	1.72 ± 0.22	350 ± 22§	87.50 ± 7.53§	338 ± 20§

*Data expressed as mean ± SEM; No. = 8 for each age group.

†Loss (LRR) and regaining (RRR) of the righting response as described previously (24).

‡Blood ethanol level.

§$P < .05$ as compared with the eight-month-old group.

related differences in response to ethanol. Data from in vivo studies of humans and animals support the hypothesis that ethanol may act differently on the brain of aged organisms than on that of younger organisms (22–26). Specifically, ethanol may be acting on brain membrane structure and function differently in aged than in younger animals.

Changes in biologic membranes are associated with both ethanol administration and increasing age. The primary effects of ethanol appear to be on the cell membrane (37). Changes in cell membranes have been suggested as a basic factor in the aging process (38).

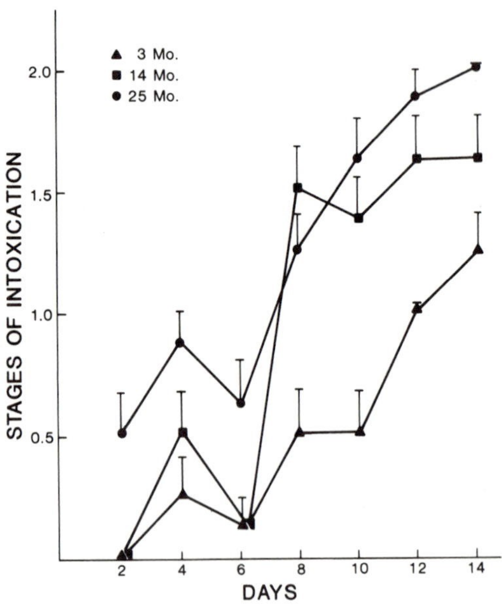

Figure 10-1. Mean ± SEM stage of intoxication for each ethanol group. Severity of intoxication is represented by an increase in the stage number. Ethanol was administered in a liquid diet for 14 days. Each point represents the mean of eight animals per age group (25).

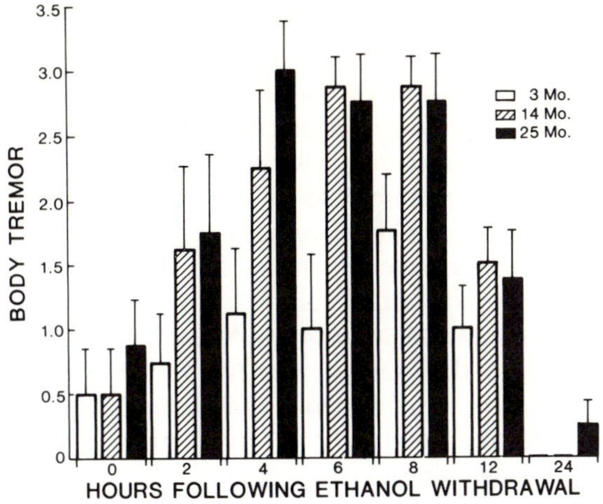

Figure 10-2. Mean ± SEM for body tremor observed during withdrawal from ethanol for each ethanol age group. Ethanol was withdrawn on Day 15 and observations for signs of withdrawal were made by two individuals who were not aware of which treatment an animal was receiving. Each point represents the mean of 8 per age group (25).

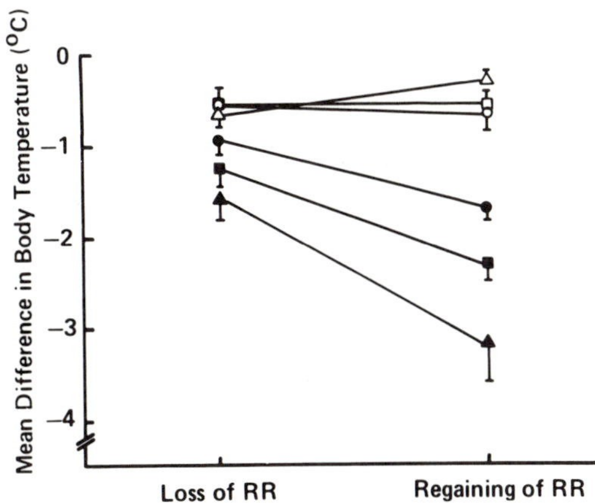

Figure 10-3. Mean ± SEM difference in body temperature at loss and regaining of the righting response for ethanol (8 month ▲——▲; 18 month ■——■; and 28 month, ●——●) and saline (8 month △——△; 18 □——□; and 28 month ○——○). Each point represents the mean of eight mice per age group (24).

Ethanol and Membranes

Ethanol fluidizes the lipid environment of membranes (37). This effect of ethanol has been observed using techniques such as electron spin resonance (39,40) and fluorescence polarization (41). A positive correlation between increased in vivo ethanol sensitivity and increased disordering of brain membranes by ethanol in vitro has been reported (42). Long-sleep lines of mice are more affected by ethanol in vivo than short-sleep lines, and there are differences when membranes from these mice are perturbed with ethanol in vitro. Membranes from long-sleep mice are more disordered by ethanol than membranes from short-sleep mice. Whereas membrane disordering is increased when ethanol is administered in vitro, membranes from animals who received ethanol in vivo chronically are resistant to this disordering effect of ethanol in vitro (39,40). Such resistance has been attributed to increased cholesterol content (43) and changes in other lipids (44,45) that may affect partitioning of ethanol into the membrane (40). Ethanol-induced disordering of the membrane may alter the mobility of membrane lipids and thus modify the function of membrane proteins and transport processes (46). Alternatively, ethanol may interact directly with membrane proteins (47–50).

One of the consequences of ethanol's disrupting the lipid environment of membranes is that it may also affect neuronal function (51). Both pre- and postsynaptic effects are described in the presence of anesthetic concentrations of ethanol, in vivo and in vitro (52,53). Ethanol causes changes in neurotransmitter uptake and release in brain tissue. These ethanol-induced effects have been observed for catecholamines, serotonin, α-aminobutyric acid, and acetylcholine (52).

Ethanol modulates the activity of certain membranebound enzymes. In particular, the activity of $(Na^+–K^+)$ATPase is affected by ethanol both in vitro and in vivo (54). The $(Na^+–K^+)$ATPase found in synaptosomal membranes may be inhibited by ethanol in vitro but the Mg-ATPase appears to be much less sensitive. While there is some question about the involvement of $(Na^+–K^+)$ATPase in ethanol intoxication and withdrawal, it has been observed that ethanol's in vitro effect is less on membranes from ethanol-tolerant versus control animals (55). Moreover, it has been proposed that ethanol may inhibit the $(Na^+–K^+)$ATPase by affecting the lipid environment of the membrane (55).

Aging and Membranes

Cell membranes are not only affected by ethanol, but also show changes with increasing age. Age-related differences in the physical properties (ie, membrane order, fluidity, phase transition) of membranes have been observed for erythrocytes, lymphocytes, and liver microsomes

(56–58). Lymphocyte membrane microviscosity has been found to increase with age in samples from human subjects ranging in age from 10 to 80 years (57). It has been reported that membrane order of rat hepatic microsomal membranes decreased with age (58). A phase transition was detected for membranes of aged rats, but not for membranes of younger rats. Age differences in erythrocyte membranes of different age groups of human subjects did not differ (56). Those results are similar to what we have found for erythrocyte membranes, synaptic plasma membranes, and microsomal membrane from different age groups of mice (28).

Age differences have been reported for the lipid composition of cell membranes. The ratio of cholesterol to phospholipid was greater for myelin from old C57BL mice (26-month-old) as compared with 3-month-old mice (59). In the same study, it was observed that there was a decrease in unsaturated acyl groups of membrane phosphoglycerides with increasing age. The cholesterol/phospholipid ratio also has been found to be higher in myelin from 19-month-old Sprague-Dawley rats than in 3-month-old rats (60).

Membrane transport processes as measured by release and reuptake of neurotransmitters are altered during aging (61). High-affinity sodium dependent uptake of glutamate, dopamine, and norepinephrine are reduced in cortex, neostriatum, and hypothalamus of aged rodents (62). However, neurotransmitter secretion from brain synaptosomes of 12-month-old mice was increased as compared with 6-month-old mice (63). Dopamine release from the neostriatum of aged rodents does not appear to be altered (64). The uptake velocity of α-aminobutyric acid (GABA) accumulation of neostriatal synaptosomes has been found to increase with age (65). Increasing age has been found to be associated with changes in cholinergic receptor binding, glutamic acid decarboxylase, and choline acetyltransferase activities (65–67).

Ethanol-Induced Changes in the Physical Properties of Membranes

In vivo ethanol sensitivity and in vitro ethanol disordering of membranes of young animals are positively correlated (42). Based on our in vivo results on aging and effects of ethanol, we predicted that there would be age differences in membrane disorder induced by ethanol. This hypothesis was examined using synaptic plasma membranes (SPM), brain microsomes, and erythrocytes from C57BL/6NNIA mice 3 to 5 months, 11 to 13 months, and 22 to 24 months. The disordering effects of ethanol (250 and 500 mmol/L) were measured using electron spin resonance (ESR) and the 5-nitroxide stearic acid spin label that reports motion near the surface of the membrane. Membranes were prepared from animals that had never been exposed to ethanol in vivo. Ethanol had a greater disordering effect on the bulk lipid environment on membranes from young animals, as compared with older animals (Figs. 10-4, 10-5, 10-6). This effect occurred at both ethanol concentrations. These age differences were not due to differences in baseline order parameters (ie, in the absence of ethanol, Table 10-2). While the ethanol concentrations were above physiologic levels, these results demonstrated that membranes from aged mice differ fundamentally in response to ethanol as compared with younger mice.

Two major questions were generated by the results on age differences in ethanol-induced membrane disorder. First, what is the mechanism (eg, lipid composition) that makes membranes from aged animals less perturbed by ethanol than younger animals? Second, it would seem that the correlation between in vivo ethanol sensitivity and in vitro ethanol membrane disordering does not apply to aged animals. In aged animals, does ethanol act differently on membrane proteins and membrane transport processes than it does in younger animals?

Changes in lipid composition have been associated with physical properties of biologic membranes. It is reasonable to hypothesize that age differences in lipid composition may affect ethanol-induced disordering of membranes. We measured the cholesterol and phospholipid content of whole brain homogenate, SPM, brain microsomes, and erythrocyte membranes. There was a significant increase in cholesterol content with increasing age (Table 10-3). The largest increase occurred in whole brain homogenate. There was a slight but significant increase observed in synaptic plasma membranes (SPM) and brain microsomes (Table 10-3). The

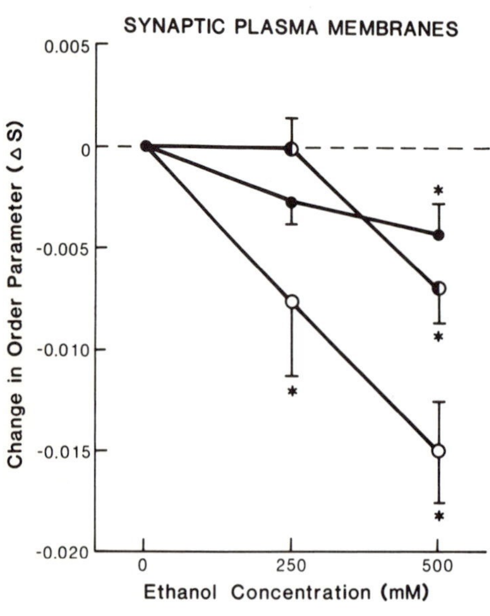

Figure 10-4. Effect of ethanol concentration on the order parameter of SPMs isolated from young (○), middle (○) and old (●) mice. The order parameter S was measured at 37.0 ± 0.2°C. ΔS = difference between the order parameter in the presence of ethanol and its baseline order parameter. An asterisk indicates a significant change ($P < .05$) in the order parameter relative to the age-related control (28).

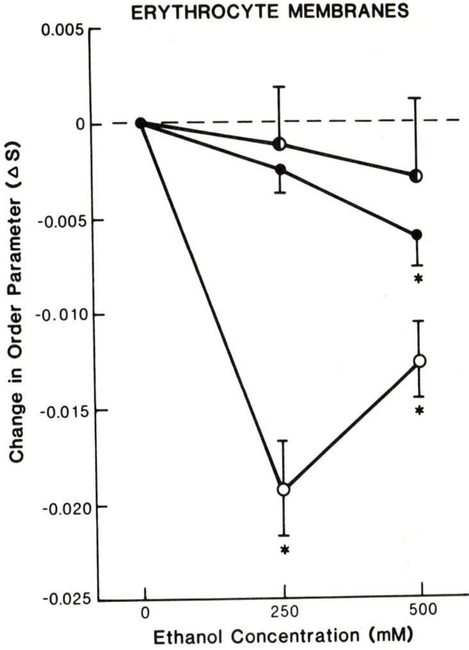

Figure 10-5. Effect of ethanol concentration on the order parameter of erythrocyte membranes isolated from young (○), middle (○), and old (●) mice. Experimental procedures were the same as in Figure 10-1 (28).

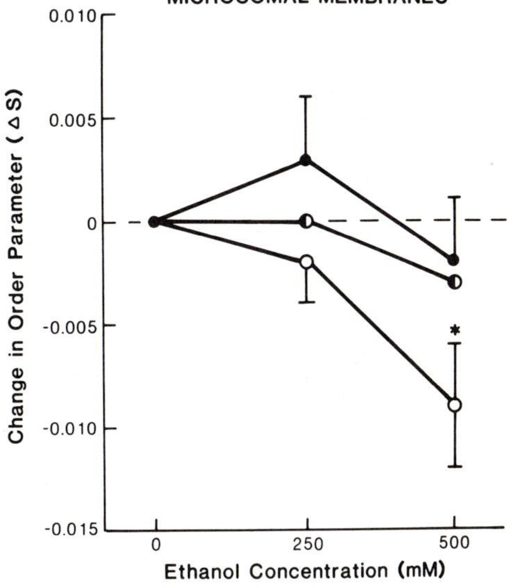

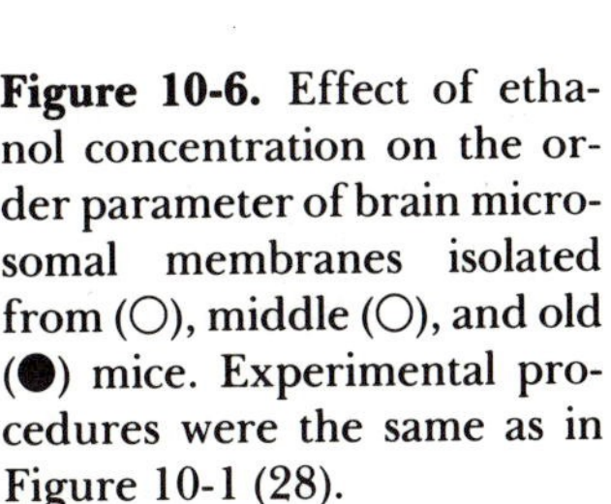

Figure 10-6. Effect of ethanol concentration on the order parameter of brain microsomal membranes isolated from (○), middle (○), and old (●) mice. Experimental procedures were the same as in Figure 10-1 (28).

Table 10-2. Baseline Membrane Order of Membranes Isolated from Three Age Groups of Mice*

Age Group (mo)	Membrane Order (S)		
	Synaptic Plasma Membranes	Brain Microsomal Membranes	Erythrocyte Membranes
Young (3–5)	0.591 ± 0.002	0.577 ± 0.001	0.607 ± 0.001
Middle (11–13)	0.594 ± 0.001	0.578 ± 0.004	0.603 ± 0.002
Old (22–24)	0.593 ± 0.001	0.573 ± 0.002	0.604 ± 0.001

*Table entries are the mean ± SEM of three preparations. Membrane order was measured at 37.0 ± 0.2°C using the 5-nitroxide spin label. Membrane order was quantitated using the order parameter *S* (28).

cholesterol to phospholipid ratio was significantly different for only whole brain homogenate. The results for cholesterol and phospholipid content, while significant, do not appear to account for our findings of age differences in ethanol-induced membrane disordering.

Another component of lipid composition associated with membranes is the distribution of saturated and unsaturated fatty acids (38). Increased saturation has been found to be associated with a "stiffening" of the membrane. We examined the fatty acid profile of total phospholipids of SPM from three age groups of mice (68). Our data indicate that, with age, there is a decrease in unsaturated fatty acids and an increase in saturated fatty acids (Table 10-4). These results are consistent with our finding that membranes from aged animals are less disordered by ethanol than the membranes of younger animals. Although these results shed some light on age differences in membrane disorder, it is clear that much more work needs to be accomplished. For example, the acyl group profile of individual phospholipids of SPM needs to be examined. In addition, studies on the turnover of phospholipids with age should be conducted.

Ethanol-Induced Changes in Membrane Function

The physical effects of ethanol on membranes from aged mice is similar to that observed in membranes from young ethanol-tolerant animals. Because ethanol effects aged organisms differently in vivo (ie, increased sedative effects) as compared with younger organisms, it may act differently on membrane proteins and membrane transport processes in the aged organism. Ethanol may be acting directly on membrane proteins and/or microdomains of lipids surrounding proteins.

An enzyme that has been studied extensively in relation to ethanol is $(Na^+–K^+)$ATPase (54). We examined the activity of $(Na^+–K^+)$ATPase in

Table 10-3. Total Cholesterol and Phospholipid Levels in Whole Brain and Membranes from Three Age Groups of Mice

Tissue*	Age† Group	Cholesterol (μmol/g brain)	Phospholipid (μmol/g brain)	Cholesterol/ Phospholipid (molar ratio)
Whole brain	Y	58.33 ± 1.10‡	77.63 ± 1.06	.751 ± .022
	M	66.70 ± 0.72§	79.43 ± 0.75	.839 ± .007‖
	O	68.63 ± 0.92§	80.56 ± 0.52	.852 ± .007§
Microsomes	Y	1.65 ± 0.12	2.60 ± 0.36	.646 ± .044
	M	1.91 ± 0.18 ‖	2.92 ± 0.29‖	.655 ± .011
	O	1.95 ± 0.17 ‖	3.00 ± 0.24§	.648 ± .010
SPM	Y	0.460 ± 0.036	0.993 ± 0.183	.480 ± .045
	M	0.580 ± 0.046‖	1.183 ± 0.206‖	.506 ± .045
	O	0.603 ± 0.081‖	1.176 ± 0.179‖	.515 ± .010
Erythrocytes	Y	0.949 ± 0.048	1.41 ± 0.102	.673 ± .017
	M	1.045 ± 0.007	1.58 ± 0.041	.661 ± .013
	O	1.006 ± 0.498	1.44 ± 0.084	.695 ± .011

*Cholesterol and phospholipid of erythrocytes expressed as μmol/mg protein.

†Y = 3–5 mo; M = 11–13 mo; O = 22–24 mo

‡Values are the mean ± SEM from three experiments in which tissue from five animals per age group was pooled (28).

§$P < .02$ as compared with youngest age group.

‖$P < .05$ as compared with youngest age group.

Table 10-4. Synaptic Plasma Membrane Phospholipid Fatty Acid Composition of Three Age Groups of Mice

Fatty Acid*	Age (mo)		
	3–5	11–13	22–24
16:0†	26.1 ± .35	28.4 ± .29	31.5 ± .81
18:0	27.2 ± .17	30.8 ± .75	33.4 ± .98
18:1	17.3 ± .12	17.1 ± .40	15.0 ± .29
20:1	1.6 ± .23	1.2 ± .23	3.1 ± .64
20:4	7.4 ± .29	6.9 ± .46	3.7 ± .12
22:4	1.7 ± .12	1.4 ± .64	—
22:6	17.2 ± .35	10.3 ± .46	13.1 ± 1.1
DBI‡	158.5	113.3	111.5
% Unsaturated	46.7	40.8	35.1

*Fatty acid composition expressed as percentage by weight of the listed fatty acids. Data expressed as mean ± SEM of three preparations for each age group (28).

†Terminology for fatty acids (number of carbon atoms' length : number of double bonds).

‡DBI = double bond index and is the sum of the products of percentage and number of double bonds of the fatty acids present.

response to identical ethanol concentrations used in our ESR studies of SPM from different age groups of mice. Age differences in (Na^+–K^+)ATPase activity in the absence of ethanol were not significant (Table 10-5). These results are in agreement with those reported by Sun and Samorajski (27). Inhibition of activity was greater at 250 mmol/L for membranes from old animals as compared with younger animals (Table 10-5). Age differences were not observed at 500 mmol/L ethanol. Similar results have been reported previously using different age groups of mice and human brain tissue (27).

Another effect of ethanol on membranes may be on membrane transport processes. Ethanol affects depolarization-dependent transport of calcium across synaptosomal membranes and the degree of membrane disorder can affect calcium transport. We have begun to examine this system, studying the effect of ethanol on calcium-dependent-depolarization induced release of GABA from synaptosomes. The GABA system was chosen because it is the most prevalent neurotransmitter in the central nervous system (69) and may play a role in the actions of ethanol (70). The use of synaptosomes to study the system were selected for several reasons. Isolated synaptosomes provide an ideal preparation to investigate drug effects because the isolation procedure eliminates direct interneuronal interactions and minimizes diffusional barriers, allowing accurate control of extracellular fluid composition (71,72). Previous studies of voltage-dependent GABA release in response to ethanol have been done on intact brain or brain tissue slices (73). In those preparations the neurotransmitter being studied in relation to ethanol is not isolated from the influence of other neuronal systems that may also be affected by ethanol.

Depolarization-induced GABA release was inhibited by ethanol and

Table 10-5. Effect of Ethanol on the (Na^+-K^+)ATPase Activity of Synaptic Plasma Membranes*

	Ethanol Concentration (%)		
Age Group (mo)	0	250 mmol/L	500 mmol/L
Young (3–5)	100	104.2 ± 0.2	63.4 ± 1.6†
Middle (11–13)	100	83.5 ± 3.4†	77.5 ± 1.3†
Old (22–24)	100	86.7 ± 0.5†	65.6 ± 1.4†

*Table entries are the mean ± SEM of (Na-$^+$-K^+)ATPase activity of three preparations per age group. (Na^+-k^+)ATPase activity was normalized by setting activity in the absence of ethanol were 434.41 ± 14.82, 482.87 ± 11.23, and 451.25 ± 39.64 nmol/L of ATP hydrolyzed/min/mg protein for young, middle, and old animals, respectively.

*Significantly less than no ethanol ($P < .05$).

Table 10-6. Inhibition of GABA Release by Ethanol: Effect of Aging on Dose–Response Characteristics*

	4 mo	14 mo	28 mo
IC_{50}† (mmol/L Ethanol)	636 ± 46	780 ± 72	1086 ± 153‡

*Each value is the mean ± SEM of four separate experiments for each age group. The IC_{50} was determined from six concentrations of ethanol (0, 125, 250, 500, 750, and 1,000 mmol/L

†IC_{50}, the concentration of ethanol required to reduce GABA release by 50% of control.

‡$P < .05$ as compared with 4-month-old group (29).

this effect was greatly attenuated in cortical synaptosomes from older mice, as compared with younger ones. Table 10-6 shows that the concentration of ethanol required to inhibit net potassium-evoked release by 50% (IC_{50}) increased with age. The IC_{50} value for the oldest age group was nearly twice that of the youngest age group. Inhibition of GABA release occurred whether depolarization was produced by potassium or veratridine (Table 10-7). The age differences in ethanol-induced inhibition of GABA release did not appear to be related to changes in the GABA neuron population with age. Accumulation of GABA or release in the absence of ethanol did not differ with age (71). Those results are consistent with earlier studies on the GABA system and age.

In addition to age differences in inhibition of GABA release by ethanol in vitro, we also found that GABA release was affected by in vivo ethanol administration and that this finding differed with age. Ethanol was administered in a liquid diet for 6 weeks to two different age groups of C57BL/6NNIA mice. GABA release of synaptosomes from young ethanol-tolerant animals was significantly greater than it was from the young pair-fed control group (Table 10-8). Interestingly, GABA release for the old ethanol and control groups did not differ, nor did the old groups differ from the young ethanol group. Chronic ethanol consump-

Table 10-7. Veratridine-Stimulated GABA Release in the Presence and Absence of Ethanol Three Age Groups of Mice*

Age Group (mo)	0	Net GABA Release 500 mmol/L Ethanol
4	213 ± 51	64 ± 11
14	262 ± 9	90 ± 22
28	228 ± 60	114 ± 20†

*Each value is the mean ± SEM of four separate experiments. Net release is depolarized CPM minus basal CPM expressed as a percentage of the basal release.

†$P < .05$ as compared with young (29).

Table 10-8. Comparison of the Effect of Chronic Ethanol Consumption on Potassium-Stimulated GABA Release in the Presence of Ethanol*

Treatment	Ethanol (mmol/L)	[^{14}C]GABA Release (% Release above Baseline) 4 mo	28 mo
Control	0	150 ± 23	144 ± 32
	500	73 ± 8	113 ± 12
Chronic ethanol	0	157 ± 13	173 ± 12
	500	128 ± 24†	144 ± 33

*Each value is the mean ± SEM of four separate experiments. The values represent the difference in [^{14}C]GABA release obtained in the presence and absence of 500 mmol/L ethanol. Animals received either an ethanol-containing liquid diet or an isocaloric liquid diet for 6 weeks (29).

†$P < .05$ as compared with young control.

tion did not affect potassium-evoked GABA release in the absence of in vitro ethanol in any age group.

The reduced effect of ethanol on synaptosomes from young ethanol-tolerant mice and aged mice would appear to be associated with an action of ethanol on the membrane. We base this conclusion on three lines of evidence. First, we found a high correlation between IC_{50}s and membrane/buffer partition coefficients of a series of *n*-alcohols, suggesting that the inhibitory effects of ethanol are mediated, in part, by the hydrophobic region of the membrane (Table 10-9). Second, several investigators have reported that membranes from ethanol-tolerant animals are perturbed less by ethanol than membranes from control groups. Finally, membranes from aged animals never exposed to ethanol are less disordered by ethanol than are membranes from young animals.

Table 10-9. Effect of in Vitro Addition of a Series of Alcohols on Potassium-Stimulated [^{14}C]GABA Release

Alcohol	P(m/b)*	IC50	r	log P(m/b) v log IC_{50}
Ethanol	0.096	636	.82	
n-Propanol	0.438	209	.94	$r = -.995$
n-Butanol	1.52	112	.94	

*Membrane/buffer partition coefficient.

†The IC_{50} was determined by linear regression of six concentrations of alcohol versus net [^{14}C]GABA release (29).

Conclusion

Membranes from aged animals respond very differently to ethanol than do membranes from younger animals. We have shown that ethanol has less of an effect on membrane disordering and inhibition of neurotransmitter release of brain tissue from aged animals, as compared with younger animals. Both of these effects have been shown in young ethanol-tolerant animals. It might be predicted from those results that aged animals never exposed to ethanol would be less affected by ethanol in vivo than younger animals. However, a general finding is that aged animals are more affected by ethanol behaviorally than younger animals. Thus, a paradox exists between the in vivo and in vitro effects of ethanol in the aged organism. One explanation is that ethanol may directly affect membrane proteins and that changes in the bulk lipid environment are ancillary to effects of proteins. Ethanol may be acting on the microdomain of lipids surrounding proteins whose physical properties are different from those of the bulk lipid. Another explanation for age differences in ethanol sensitivity may reside with the postsynaptic receptor. To date, our findings have been based on possible presynaptic mechanisms. We do not know the precise mechanism for age differences in response to ethanol in vivo. However, our studies reveal clearly that aging is associated with fundamental changes in physical and biochemical properties of membranes.

A promising area for further research on membranes and aging is to determine the extent to which alterations in membrane composition contribute to pathologic conditions associated with old age. One approach is to alter membrane composition through dietary supplementation. For example, it was recently reported that a special lipid mixture from egg yolk markedly reduced withdrawal signs of morphine-dependent mice (74). Further investigation showed that the dietary supplement was acting on the cell membrane by restoring the fluidity of the membrane to the premorphine-dependent state (ie, a less rigid membrane). Perhaps this type of intervention would be appropriate as a means of improving mental status of aged individuals, for drug-induced toxicity, or in pretreatment of elderly surgical patients.

Another area worthy of consideration is the similarity between membranes of young ethanol-tolerant animals and membranes of aged animals not exposed previously to ethanol. Courville and others have proposed that alcoholism may cause premature aging (18,75,76). This hypothesis, for the most part, has been based on autopsy data and neuropsychologic studies of young alcoholics and old nonalcoholics, in which it is difficult to control for life history variables, eg, health status, polydrug use, diet that may influence physical and behavioral status. While it is very speculative to hypothesize that alcoholism can influence the aging process, it is apparent from our results that the effects of alcohol and of aging on brain membranes are similar. Perhaps the common denominator is that changes induced by alcohol and changes that occur with aging are caused by lipid peroxidation of the cell membrane. If this should be the case, then the use of nutritional intervention (eg, the active lipid mixture mentioned previously) may be a very effective means of preventing and/or reducing the deterioration of the cell membrane.

Acknowledgments

This work was supported by the Medical Research Service of the Veterans Administration and the Geriatric Research, Education and Clinical Center of the St. Louis VA Medical Center. Appreciation is extended to Drs. James Armbrecht and Ronald Wise, who collaborated on some of the studies reported here, and to Cheryl Duff for excellent secretarial assistance.

References

1. Heath DB: In other cultures, they also drink, in Gomberg EL, White HR, Carpenter JA (eds): *Alcohol, Science and Society Revisited.* Ann Arbor, University of Michigan Press, 1982, pp 63–79.
2. Hartford JT, Samorajski T: Alcoholism in the geriatric population. *Am Geriatr Soc* 1982; 30:18–24.
3. Wood WG, Elias MF (eds): *Alcoholism and Aging: Advances in Research.* Boca Raton, FL, CRC Press, 1982.
4. Freund G, Butters N: Alcohol and aging symposium: Neurobiological interactions between aging and alcohol abuse. *Alcoholism: Clin Exp Res* 1982; 6:1–63.
5. Schuckit MA, Morrissey ER, O'Leary MR: Alcohol problems in elderly men and women. *Addict Dis* 1978; 3:405–409.
6. Barnes GM: Patterns of alcohol use and abuse among older Persons in a household population, in Wood WG, Elias MF (eds): *Alcoholism and Aging: Advances in Research.* Boca Raton, FL, CRC Press, 1982, pp 4–15.
7. Rathbone-McCuan E, Bland J: A treatment typology for the elderly alcohol abuser. *J Am Geriatr Soc* 1975; 23:553–557.
8. Rosin AJ, Glatt MM: Alcohol excess in the elderly. *Q J Stud Alcohol* 1971; 32:53–59.
9. Zimberg S: The elderly alcoholic. *Gerontologist* 1974; 14:221–224.
10. Cahalan D, Cisin IH: Drinking behavior and drinking problems in the United States, in Kissin B, Begleiter H (eds): *The Biology of Alcoholism,* vol 4. New York, Plenum Press, 1976, pp 77–115.
11. Wood WG: The elderly alcoholic: Some diagnostic problems and considerations, in Storandt M, Siegler IC, Elias MF (eds): *The Clinical Psychology of Aging.* New York, Plenum Press, 1978, pp 97–113.

12. Feinman L, Lieber CS: Liver disease in alcoholism, in Kissin B, Begleiter H (eds): *The Biology of Alcoholism,* vol 3. New York, Plenum Press, 1974, pp 303–338.
13. Lyons HA, Saltzman A: Diseases of the respiratory tract in alcoholics, in Kissin B, Begleiter H (eds): *The Biology of Alcoholism,* vol 3. New York, Plenum Press, 1974, pp 403–434.
14. Lorber SH, Dinoso VP, Chey WY: Diseases of the gastrointestinal tract, in Kissin B, Begleiter H (eds): *The Biology of Alcoholism,* vol 3. New York, Plenum Press, 1974, pp 339–357.
15. Dreyfus PM: Disease of the nervous system in chronic alcoholics, in Kissin B, Begleiter H (eds): *The Biology of Alcoholism,* vol 3. New York Plenum Press, 1974, pp 265–290.
16. Bing RJ: Cardiac metabolism: Its contributions to alcoholic heart disease and myocardinal failure. *Circulation* 1978; 58:965–971.
17. Timiras PS: *Developmental Physiology and Aging.* New York, Macmillan, 1972.
18. Courville C: *The Effects of Alcoholism on the Nervous System in Man.* Los Angeles, San Lucas Press, 1955.
19. Blusewicz MJ, Cannon WG, Dustman RE: Alcoholism and aging: Similarities and differences in neuropsychological performances, in Wood WG, Elias MF (eds): *Alcoholism and Aging:* Advances in research. Boca Rotan, FL, CRC Press, 1982, pp 48–60.
20. Parsons OA, Leber WR: Premature aging, alcoholism, and recovery, in Wood WG, Elias MF (eds): *Alcoholism and Aging: Advances in Research.* Boca Raton, FL, CRC Press, 1982, pp 80–92.
21. Wood WG, Armbrecht HJ: Behavioral effects of ethanol in animals: Age differences and age changes. *Alcoholism: Clin Exp Res* 1982; 6:3–12.
22. Robertson-Tchabo EA, Arenberg D, Vestal RE: Age differences in memory performance following ethanol infusion. Tenth International Congress of Gerontology, Jerusalem, Israel, 1975.
23. Ritzmann RF, Springer A: Age differences in brain sensitivity and tolerance to ethanol in mice. *Age* 1980; 3:15–17.
24. Wood WG, Armbrecht HJ: Age differences in ethanol-induced hypothermia and impairment in mice. *Neurobiol Aging* 1982; 3:243–246.
25. Wood WG, Armbrecht HJ, Wise RW: Ethanol intoxication and withdrawal among three age groups of C57BL/6NNIA mice. *Pharmacol Biochem Behav* 1982; 17:1037–1041.
26. Zornenster SF: Acceleration of age-related functional decline in mice following prior chronic ethanol consumption. *Soc Neuroscience* (abstract) 1983; 9:95.
27. Sun AY, Samorajski T: The effects of age and alcohol on (Na^+ + K^+)-ATPase activity of whole homogenate and synaptosomes prepared from mouse and human brain. *J Neurochem* 1975; 24:161–164.
28. Armbrecht HJ, Wood WG, Wise RW, et al: Ethanol-induced disordering of membranes from different age groups of C57BL/6NNIA mice. *J Pharmacol Exp Ther* 1983, 226:387–391.
29. Strong R, Wood WG: Membrane properties and aging: *In vivo* and *in vitro* effects of ethanol on synaptosomal GABA release. *J Pharmacol Exp Ther* 1984 (in press).
30. Vestall RE, McGuire EA, Tobin JD, et al: Aging and ethanol metabolism. *Clin Pharmacol Ther* 1977; 21:343–354.

31. Freund G: The interaction of chronic alcohol consumption and aging on brain structure and function. *Alcoholism: Clin Exp Res* 1982; 6:13–21.
32. Freund G: Interactions of aging and chronic alcohol consumption on the central nervous system, in Wood WG, Elias MF (eds): *Alcoholism and Aging: Advances in Research* Boca Raton, FL, CRC Press, 1982, pp 131–148.
33. York JL: Increased responsiveness to ethanol with advancing age in rats. *Pharmacol Biochem Behav* 1983; 19:687–691.
34. Ernst AJ, Dempster JP, Yee R, et al: Alcohol toxicity, blood alcohol concentration and body water in young and adult rats. *J Stud Alcohol* 1976; 37:347–356.
35. Wiberg GS, Trenholm HL, Coldwell BB: Increased ethanol toxicity in old rats: Changes in LD 50, *in vivo* and *in vitro* metabolism and liver alcohol dehydrogenase activity. *Toxicol Appl Pharmacol* 1970; 16:718–727.
36. York JL: Body water content, ethanol pharmacokinetics, and the responsiveness to ethanol in young and old rats. *Dev Pharmacol Ther* 1982; 4:106–116.
37. Seeman P: The membrane actions of anesthetics and tranquilizers. *Pharmacol Rev* 1972; 24:583–655.
38. Sun AY, Sun GY: Neurochemical aspects of the membrane hypothesis of aging, in von Hahn HP (ed): *Interdisciplinary Topics in Gerontology*, vol 15. Basel, S. Karger, 1979, pp 34–53.
39. Chin JH, Goldstein DB: Drug tolerance in biomembranes: A spin label study of the effects of ethanol. *Science* 1977; 196:684–685.
40. Rottenberg, H, Waring A, Rubin E: Tolerance and cross-tolerance in chronic alcoholics: Reduced membrane binding of ethanol and other drugs. *Science* 1981; 213:583–585.
41. Harris RA, Schroeder F: Ethanol and the physical properties of brain membranes: Fluorescence studies. *Mol Pharmacol* 1981; 20:128–137.
42. Goldstein DB, Chin JH, Lyon RC: Ethanol disordering of spin-labeled mouse brain membranes: Correlation with genetically determined ethanol sensitivity of mice. *Proc Natl Acad Sci USA* 1982; 79:4231–4233.
43. Chin JH, Parsons LM, Goldstein DB: Increased cholesterol content of erythrocyte and brain membranes in ethanol-tolerant mice. *Biochim Biophys Acta* 1978; 513:359–363.
44. Littleton JM, John GR, Grieve SJ: Alterations in phospholipid composition in ethanol tolerance and dependence. *Alcoholism: Clin Exp Res* 1979; 3-50–56.
45. John GR, Littleton JM, Jones PA: Membrane lipids and ethanol tolerance in the mouse. The influence of dietary fatty acid composition. *Life Sci* 1980; 27:545–555.
46. Sandermann H: Regulation of membrane enzymes by lipids. *Biochim Biophys Acta* 1978; 515:209–237.
47. Hoffman PL, Tabakoff B: Effects of ethanol on Arrhenius parameters and activity of mouse striatal adenylate cyclase. *Biochem Pharmacol* 1982; 31:3101–3106.
48. Gordon LM, Sauerheber RD, Esgate JA, et al: The increase in bilayer fluidity of rat liver plasma membranes achieved by the local anesthetic benzyl alcohol affects the activity of intrinsic membrane enzymes. *J Biol Chem* 1980; 255:4519–4527.
49. Franks NP, Lieb WR: Is membrane expansion relevant to anaesthesia? *Nature* 1981; 292:248–251.

50. Michaelis ML, Michaelis EK: Alcohol and local anesthetic effects of Na^+ dependent Ca^{2+} fluxes in brain synaptic membrane vesicles. *Biochem Pharmacol* 1983; 32:963–969.
51. Stokes JA, Harris RA: Alcohols and synaptosomal calcium transport. *Mol Pharmacol* 1982; 22:99–104.
52. Hunt WA, Majchrowicz E: Alterations in neurotransmitter function after acute and chronic treatment with ethanol, in Majchrowicz E, Noble EP (eds): *Biochemistry and Pharmacology of Ethanol,* vol 2. New York, Plenum Press, 1979, pp 167–185.
53. Tabakoff B, Hoffman PL: Alcohol and neurotransmitters, in Rigter H, Crabbe JC (eds): *Alcohol Tolerance and Dependence.* Amsterdam, Elsevier, 1980, pp 201–226.
54. Roach MK: Changes in the activity of Na^+, K^+-ATPase during acute and chronic administration of ethanol, in Majchrowicz E, Noble EP (eds): *Biochemistry and Pharmacology of Ethanol,* vol 2. New York, Plenum Press, 1979, pp 67–80.
55. Levental M, Tabakoff B: Sodium-potassium-activated adenosine triphosphatase activity as a measure of neuronal membrane characteristics in ethanol-tolerant mice. *J Pharmacol Exp Ther* 1980; 212:315–319.
56. Butterfield DA, Ordaz FE, Markesbery WR: Spin label studies of human erythrocyte membranes in aging. *J Gerontol* 1982; 37:535–539.
57. Rivnay B, Bergman S, Shinitzky M, Globerson A: Correlations between membrane viscosity, serum cholesterol, lymphocyte activation and aging in man. *Mech Ageing Dev* 1980; 12:119–126.
58. Armbrecht HJ, Birnbaum LS, Zenser TV, Davis BB: Changes in hepatic microsomal membrane fluidity with age. Exp Gerontol 1982; 17:41–48.
59. Sun GY, Samorajski T: Age changes in the lipid composition of whole homogenates and isolated myelin fractions of mouse brain. *J Gerontol* 1972; 27:10–17.
60. Malone MJ, Szoke MC: Neurochemical studies in aging brain. I. Structural changes in myelin lipids. *J Gerontol* 1982; 37:262–267.
62. Pradhan SN: Central neurotransmitters and aging. *Life Sci* 1980; 26:1643–1656.
62. Severson JA, Finch CE: Reduced dopaminergic binding during aging in the rodent striatum. *Brain Res* 1980; 192:147–162.
63. Haycock JW, White WF, McGaugh JL, Cotman CW: Enhanced stimulus-secretion coupling from brains of aged mice. *Exp Neurol* 1977; 57:873–882.
64. Thompson JM, Whittaker JR, Joseph JA: [^{3}H]Dopamine accumulation and release from striatal slices in young, mature and senescent rats. *Brain Res* 1981; 224:436–440.
65. Strong R, Gottesfeld, Z, Samorajski T: High-affinity uptake of neurotransmitters in the neostriatum: Effect of aging. *Neurobiol Aging* 1983 (in press).
66. Kubanis P, Zornetzer SF, Freund G: Memory and postsynaptic cholinergic receptors in aging mice. *Pharmacol Biochem Behav* 1982; 17:313–322.
67. Freund G: Cholinergic receptor loss in brains of aging mice. *Life Sci* 26:371–375.
68. Wood WG, Strong R, Armbrecht HJ, Wise RW: Biophysical properties of membranes from different age groups of mice. *Soc Neurosci* (abstract) 1983; 9:511.

69. Cooper JR, Bloom FE, Roth RH (eds): *The Biochemical Basis of Neuropharmacology*. New York, Oxford University Press, 1978.
70. Hunt WA: The effect of ethanol on GABAergic transmission. *Neurosci Biobehav Rev* 1983; 7:87–95.
71. Strong R, Hicks P, Hsu L, et al: Age-related alterations in the rodent brain cholinergic system and behavior. *Neurobiol Aging* 1980; 1:59–63.
72. Redburn DA, Broome D, Ferkany J, Enna SJ: Development of rat brain uptake and calcium-dependent release of GABA. *Brain Res* 157:1–9.
73. Carmichael FJ, Israel Y: Effects of ethanol on neurotransmitter release by rat brain cortical slices. *J Pharmacol Exp Ther* 1975; 193:824–834.
74. Heron DS, Shinitzky M, Samuel D: Alleviation of drug withdrawal symptoms by treatment with a potent mixture of natural lipids. *Eur J Pharmacol* 1982; 83:253–261.
75. Kleinknecht RA, Goldstein GC: Neuropsychological deficits associated with alcoholism. *Q J Stud Alcohol* 1972; 33:999–1019.
76. Ryan C, Butters N: Learning and memory impairments in young and old alcoholics: Evidence for the premature aging hypothesis. *Alcoholism: Clin Exp Res* 1980; 4:288–293.

Part III

Effect of Nutrition on Aging—Functional Ability

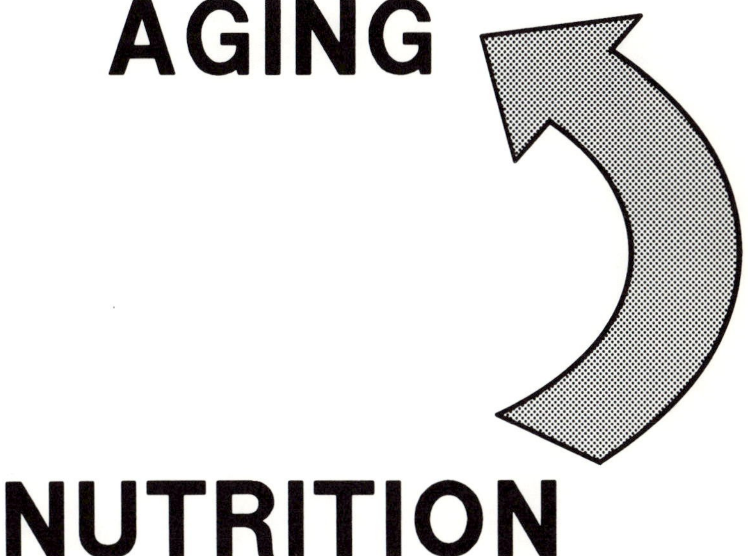

11

Calcium Supplementation and Osteoporosis

Louis V. Avioli

Osteoporosis of the senile or postmenopausal variety is defined as a skeletal disorder in which the absolute amount of bone is decreased relative to that of younger, or menstruating, individuals although the remaining bone is normal in chemical composition. Symptomatic senile or postmenopausal osteoporosis syndrome was classically considered to result from the universal loss of bone that normally attends senescence in both sexes and begins in the fourth and fifth decades of life (1,2). Recent evidence reveals that, in fact, vetebral bone loss begins in the third decade life in women (3). Although comparable decrements in the functional capacity of the heart, lungs, kidneys, and nervous tissue (ie, nerve conduction time) also attend the aging process, the decrease in bone mass may lead to significant incapacitation and result in fractures and immobilization in the aged individual, not only requiring significant hospitalization time, but also often resulting in relative inactivity and morbidity.

Incidence of Osteoporosis

The results of age-related changes in bone mass, which may actually begin in the late 20s or early 30s in women, are of considerable magnitude: approximately 6.3 million people in the United States are currently suffering from acute problems related to weakened vertebral bones. Perhaps even more significant is the fact that more than 8 million Americans today have chronic problems related to the spine, compared with 6 million reported in 1963. Moreover, past epidemiologic surveys indicate that a minimum of 10% of the female population over 50 years of age suffers from bone loss severe enough to cause hip, vertebral, or long-bone fractures (4,5); surveys performed in homes for the aged and on ambulatory individuals 50 and 75 years of age requiring medical care also disclose symptomatic (ie, back pain) osteoporosis in 15% and 50% of these populations, respectively.

Since the skeletal mass of females is normally smaller than that of males at any age, and their rate of bone loss with age is greater than that of males (1), the consequences of osteoporosis are magnified in the female, resulting in major orthopedic problems in approximately 25% to 30% of postmenopausal women. Approximately three-quarters of all deaths from falls occur in patients aged 65 and over, with a female : male fracture incidence ratio of 8 : 1. A decreased bone mass is also one of the major factors contributing to the 180,000 to 200,000 hip fractures that occur annually among women over the age of 65 (6). The rate (per 1,000 population/year) of hip fractures in white women due to minimal trauma increases from 2.0 at ages 50 to 64, to 5.0 at ages 65 to 74, to 10 at ages greater than 75. The annual incidence of femoral neck fractures in the aging female population is also high, rising rapidly from 0.13% in the seventh decade to 3.0% in the tenth. Complications of fractures of the postmenopausal female woman have produced a mortality rate of 15% to 30%, with an estimated annual cost greater than *1 billion* dollars. Currently, 32 million Americans (or 15% of the U. S. population) are 60 years of age or older. This segment of the population incerased by 8% or 9% from 1970 to 1974, although the increment of the entire U.S. population was less than half that rate. At the present rate of population growth, it is anticipated that by the year 2000, over 40 million persons will be 60 years of age or older. Obviously, at this rate of population growth, the number of individuals predisposed to either hip, femoral, forearm, or vertebrae fractures will steadily increase unless methods are developed to detect those patients at risk and appropriate preventive therapeutic measures are initiated.

Factors Contributing to Osteoporosis

Estrogen Deficiency

There is evidence that cessation of ovarian function characteristic of the menopause does result in an acceleration of age-related bone loss in some perimenopausal women that can be ameliorated by estrogen replacement (7–11). Despite these observations, there is considerable uncertainty about the role of decreasing ovarian function and estrogen deficiency in bone homeostasis and the osteoporosis–fracture syndrome in the elderly postmenopausal female. Blood estradiol, estrone, androstenedione, and follicle-stimulating and lutinizing hormones are similar in postmenopausal women with rapid bone loss when compared with women who have slow bone loss (2,26). The only consistent findings that differentiate the "rapid bone losers" from the "slow bone losers" are a decrease in serum progesterone levels and in serum testosterone and testosterone production rate (12) in the "rapid bone losers." Moreover, to date, estrogen receptors have not been demonstrated in skeletal tissue (13). The accumulated evidence suggests that the estrogenic effect on bone in perimenopausal women is most probably due (indirectly) to either an "antagonistic" effect on other bone-resorbing hormones calcitoin excess, and/or an increased efficiency in the intestinal absorption of calcium with a decrease in calcium excretion. It should be noted that obese women, who are less prone to develop symptomatic osteoporosis with vertebral and femoral fractures, have higher circulating estrogen levels and lower urinary calcium values than nonobese osteoporotic females of similar ages (14).

Calcium Deficiency

An increasing volume of data has accumulated within the last decade implicating calcium deficiency as an important factor in the development of the osteopenic postmenopausal fracture syndrome. Although dietary sources of calcium should provide sufficient calcium to maintain a positive calcium balance in the average woman, it has been well documented that the diet of the average woman is relatively deficient in calcium (15–17). In fact, the U.S. recommended daily allowance of calcium, which has been established at 800 mg/day, may prove to be inadequate to maintain the integrity of bone. Most recent dietary surveys not only reveal that at any age men ingest more calcium than women (15), but also indicate that the average woman 45 years or older ingests only 450–500 mg calcium per day. On this calcium intake, normal postmenopausal women develop a negative calcium balance greater than 40 mg/day; this degree of relative calcium loss results in a bone loss of approximately 1.5% per year (16). Elderly postmenopausal women also do not absorb oral or dietary calcium as well as younger menstruating women with higher circulating estrogens levels (16). Their intestinal adaptive efficiency to changes in calcium intake is also blunted (17) and is inadequate to maintain the homeostatic equilibrium between bone and circulating calcium that characterizes the adolescent and young-adult periods of life.

Defective renal adaptation to low calcium intakes (400–600 mg/day) with mild (but persistent) hypercalciuria most probably also contributes to the negative calcium balances (16) seen in the fracture-prone osteoporotic patients. Relative degrees of immobilization that necessarily attend senescence and peculiar dietary regimens containing excessive amounts of salt, carbohydrate, and protein are most probably contributing causes to subtle but definite increments in urinary calcium.

Age-Related Changes in Calcium-Regulating Hormones

To date, little is known about those factor(s) that modulate or condition the intestinal absorption of calcium in the senescent individual or about the relation between relative calcium deficiency and senescent bone loss (see Chapter 5). It has been established, however, that circulating levels of 1,25-dihydroxyvitamin D, the active vitamin D metabolite that stimulates calcium absorption, not only decrease with age (18,19), but are also much lower than anticipated in fracture-prone postmenopausal individuals (18,19). Moreover, serum parathyroid hormone levels also increase with age (20,21) and have been recorded as supernormal or higher in patients with advanced senile or postmenopausal osteoporosis (19,22). Increments in circulating parathyroid levels with advancing years as well as the decrease in calcitonin (a hormone that normally suppresses bone resorption) that has been reported with advancing age in some females (23–25) would obviously contribute to the age-related progressive loss of bone mass. However, these observations must be reconciled with others demonstrating low blood levels of parathyroid hormone in osteoporotic individuals (26) and similar calcitonin levels in osteoporotic patients when compared with age-matched controls (27). Because parathyroid hormone secretion is regulated primarily by the blood level of calcium, it seems reasonable to postulate that those patients with greater degrees of deficient calcium intake (and more negative calcium balance) are more prone to a senescent form of secondary hyperparathyroidism, which ultimately results in a more rapid rate of bone loss and skeletal fracture.

Calcium Supplementation

Some reports state that the administration of supplemental calcium salts to postmenopausal women in order to increase the total calcium intake to an average 1.5g/day improves calcium balance and decreases the rate of bone loss (11,16,28). Therapeutic regimens consisting of 50,000 units of vitamin D twice weekly and daily calcium supplements containing 1.5 or 2.0 g of elemental calcium have also proved effective in suppressing the accelerated bone resorption in osteoporotic patients (11,28). It seems impossible to escape conclusions that the average perimenopausal woman with a calcium intake less than 1.0–1.5 g per day is in negative calcium balance, and that this imbalance contributes to the bone loss that occurred in the previous 10 to 20 years. Moreover, recent documentation of vertebral bone loss in young ovulating women (3), who seem to be calcium deficient according to national dietary surveys (15), should lead us to reevaluate established Recommended Daily Allowance standards and begin to recommend dietary regimens with appropriate supplementation (if needed) to insure an intake of 1,200–1,400 mg of elemental calcium per day. Although we cannot replace bone tissue when it is lost, we should be able to decrease the rate of age-related bone loss with appropriate dietary surveillance and nutritional guidance.

Summary

Vertebral and femoral neck fracture syndromes and their attendant morbidity still continue to plague the lives of many postmenopausal women. The osteopenia that characterizes the "vertebral collapse" or "hip fracture" syndromes results from the gradual and progressive loss of bone mass that begins early in the fourth decade of life in all individuals and proceeds at an accelerated rate in the female population. A unified hypothesis that effectively explains the pathogenesis of the fracture-prone osteopenia state is still nonexistent, although sedentary life styles, genetic predisposition, hormonal imbalance, vitamin deficiencies, high-protein diets, caffein, and cigarette smoking have all been implicated. One of the most consistent observations, which cannot be ignored, is the inadequate calcium intake of women in the second and third decade of life and the negative calcium balance that characterizes the perimenopausal state. Nutritional adequacy with respect to this most essential skeletal ingredient is considered highly appropriate not only in any proposed therapeutic regimen for postmenopausal osteopenic females, but also in the young active, menstruating female.

References

1. Avioli LV: Osteoporosis: Pathogenesis and therapy. Avioli LV, Krane SM (eds): *Metabolic Bone Disease,* vol 1. New York, Academic Press, 1977, 307–370.
2. Avioli LV, McDonald JE, Lee SW: Influence of age in the intestinal absorption of ^{47}Ca in women and its relation to ^{47}Ca absorption in postmenopausal osteoporosis. *J Clin Invest* 1965; 44:1960–1967.
3. Riggs BL, Wahner HW, Dunn WL et al: Differential changes in bone mineral density of the appendicular and axial skeleton with aging. Relationship to spinal osteoporosis. *J Clin Invest* 1981; 67:328.
4. Lender M, Makin M, Robin G, et al: Osteoporosis and fractures of the neck of the femur. *Isr J Med Sci* 1976; 12:596–600.
5. Doyle F: Involutional osteoporosis. *Clin Endocrinol Metab* 1972; 3:143–167.

6. Stevens J, Freeman PA, Nordin BEC, Barnett E: Incidence of osteoporosis in patients with femoral neck fractures. *J Bone Joint Surg* 1962; 41B:520–527.
7. Horsman A, Gallagher JC, Simpson M, Nordin BEC: Prospective trial of oestrogen and calcium in postmenopausal women. *Br Med J* 1977; 2:789–792.
8. Hutchinson TA, Polansky JM, Feinstein AR: Postemnopausal oestrogens protect against fractures of hip and distal radius. *Lancet* 1979; 2:705–709.
9. Lindsay R, Aitken JM, Anderson JB, et al: Long-term prevention of postmenopausal osteoporosis by oestrogen. *Lancet* 1976; 1:1038–1040.
10. Riggs BL, Hodgson SF, Hoffman DL, et al: Treatment of primary osteoporosis with fluoride and calcium. Clinical tolerance and fracture occurrence. *JAMA* 1980; 243:446–449.
11. Recker RR, Saville PD, Heaney RP: Effect of estrogens and calcium carbonate on bone loss in postmenopausal women. *Ann Intern Med* 1977; 87:649–655.
12. Adlin EV, Korenman SG: Endocrine aspects of aging. *Ann Int Med* 1980; 92:429–431.
13. van Raassen HC, Poortman J, Borgard-Creutzburg IMC, et al: Oestrogen binding proteins in bone cell cytosol. *Calcif Tissue Res* 1978; 25:249–254.
14. Frumar AM, Meldrum DR, Geola F, et al: Relationship of fasting urinary calcium to circulating estrogen and body weight in postmenopausal women. *J Clin Endocrinol Metab* 1980; 50:70–75.
15. Abraham S: Dietary intake findings United States, 1971–1974. National Health Survey, Vital and Health Statistics Series 11, No. 202. US Dept of Health, Education and Welfare publication (HRA) 77-1647. Public Health Service, 1977.
16. Heaney RP, Recker RR, Saville PD: Menopausal changes in calcium balance performance. *J Lab Clin Med* 1978; 92:953–963.
17. Ireland P, Fortran JS: Effect of dietary calcium and age on jejunal calcium absorption in humans studied by intestinal perfusion. *J Clin Invest* 1973; 52:2672–2681.
18. Gallagher JC, Riggs BL, Eisman J, et al: Intestinal calcium absorption and serum vitamin D metabolites in normal subjects and osteopenic patients. *J Clin Invest* 1979; 64:729–736.
19. Okano K, Nakai R, Harasawa M: Endocrine factors in senile osteoporosis. *Endocrinol Jpn* 1979; 1:23–30.
20. Gallagher JC, Riggs BL, Jerpbak CM, et al: Effect of age on serum immunoreactive parathyroid hormone in normal and osteoporotic women. *J Lab Clin Med* 1980; 95:373–385.
21. Wiske PS, Epstein S, Bell NH, et al: Increases in immunoreactive parathyroid hormone with age. *N Engl J Med* 1979; 300:1419–1421.
22. Teitelbaum SL, Rosenberg EM, Richardson CA, et al: Histological studies of bone from normocalcemic postmenopausal osteoporotic patients with increased circulating parathyroid hormone. *J Clin Endocrinol Metab* 1976; 42: 537–543.
23. Heath H, Sizemore GW: Plasma calcitonin in normal man. Differences between men and women. *J Clin Invest* 1977; 60:1135–1140.
24. Hillgard CJ, Stevenson JC, MacIntyre I: Relative deficiency of plasma calcitonin in normal women. *Lancet* 1978; 1:961–962.

25. Shamonki IM, Fumar AM, Tataryn IV, et al: Age-related changes of calcitonin secretion in females. *J Clin Endocrinol Metab* 1980; 50:437–439.
26. Gallagher JC, Riggs BL, Eismen J, et al: Intestinal calcium absorption and serum vitamin D metabolites in normal subjects and osteoporotic patients. *J Clin Invest* 1979; 64:729–736.
27. Chestnut CH, Baylink DJ, Nelp WB, Roos BA: Basal plasma immunoreactive calcitonin in postmenopausal osteoporosis. *Metabolism* 1980; 29:559–562.
28. Nordin BEC, Horsman A, Crilly A, et al: Treatment of spinal osteoporosis in postmenopausal women. *Br Med J* 1980; (Feb 16):451–454.

12

Carbohydrate Metabolism and Diabetes in the Aged

Alan B. Silverberg

Diabetes mellitus, the most common metabolic disease, is the result of a relative or absolute lack of effective insulin action. Clinically, it is a heterogeneous disorder that involves both metabolic and vascular abnormalities (microangiopathy and macroangiopathy). The microangiopathic abnormalities are retinopathy, nephropathy, and possibly neuropathy. The macroangiopathy is identical to atherosclerosis, which affects nondiabetic individuals. The atherosclerosis occurs at a younger age and is more extensive in people with diabetes mellitus.

Diabetes is the third leading cause of death in the United States (approximately 300,000 deaths per year). There are 600,000 new cases of diabetes in the United States each year and at this rate the total number of diabetics will double in 15 years. The prevalence of diabetes mellitus Type II is 10 times the prevalence of Type I diabetes. Type II diabetes is the form of diabetes for which the geriatric population is at risk. The possibility of developing diabetes appears to double with each decade of life. Diabetes occurs more frequently in females than in males. Diabetes is also a leading cause for hospital admissions; its economic impact is estimated to be 8 billion dollars (1,2).

The vascular complications of diabetes mellitus result in significant morbidity. Blindness is 25 times more prevalent in diabetics than in the general population. Similarly, renal disease is 17 times, gangrene 20 times, myocardial infarction 2 times, and cerebral vascular accident 2 times more prevalent in individuals with diabetes mellitus. In decreasing order of incidence, the causes of death in diabetics are:

1. Myocardial infarction
2. Renal failure
3. Cerebrovascular disease
4. Ischemic heart disease, and
5. Infections (2–5)

There is increasing evidence that the hyperglycemia resulting from poorly controlled diabetes mellitus plays a pivotal role in the pathogenesis of the microvascular complications (6,7). It is hoped that with long-term glucose control the incidence, progression, and severity of retinopathy, nephropathy, and neuropathy will be reduced, thereby significantly decreasing the excess morbidity and mortality associated with diabetes.

Management strategies should be established to improve the care of patients with diabetes mellitus and reduce the morbidity of this disease and its health care costs. Some of the new technics in diabetes management (home glucose monitoring and open-loop insulin infusion devices) are expensive and, if universally used, will result in higher health care expenses for people with diabetes. Geriatric individuals often have limited incomes and thus may not be in a position to afford the latest technologic advances in diabetes care. Two aspects of diabetes care that are inexpensive and accessible to everyone are diet therapy and exercise.

The vast majority (80%–90%) of Type II diabetics are obese. Dietary therapy is the cornerstone of diabetes management in Type II diabetes and therefore in the geriatric population with diabetes. This chapter will focus on dietary therapy of diabetes mellitus.

Classification of Diabetes Mellitus

In 1979 a new classification for diabetes mellitus and glucose intolerance was published (8). The categories in this classification are as follows:

1. Diabetes mellitus (DM)
   a. Type I: Insulin-dependent diabetes mellitus (IDDM)
   b. Type II: Noninsulin-dependent diabetes mellitus (NIDDM)
2. Impaired glucose tolerance (IGT)
3. Gestational diabetes (GDM)
4. Previous abnormality of glucose tolerance
5. Potential abnormality of glucose tolerance

Patients with Type I diabetes have insulinopenia, are ketosis prone under basal conditions, and have the onset of disease usually prior to age 30. In addition, this type is associated with a nonobese body habitus, certain HLA types (eg, DR3, DR4, B8, and B15), circulating islet cell antibodies, other autoimmune endocrine diseases, and certain virus infections (eg, mumps and Coxsackie) (9,10).

Individuals with Type II diabetes usually have the onset of their disease after age 40 years, are not ketosis prone under basal conditions, and are almost always obese (80%–90%). There is no HLA type association, but there is a high concordance rate in twins. Circulating insulin levels in Type II diabetes may be normal, increased, or decreased. Since the geriatric population is primarily at risk for Type II diabetes, the dietary therapy to be discussed will primarily apply to this type of patient (9,10).

Impaired glucose tolerance (IGT) is mild glucose intolerance between normal and diabetic. Individuals with IGT are at increased risk for atherosclerosis, but are not at increased risk for the microangiopathic changes that occur with diabetes.

Pathogenesis of NIDDM

The pathogenesis of Type II diabetes mellitus may involve impaired β-cell function and/or impaired insulin action at target cells. Which factor is primary in the pathogenesis is still unclear, but in individual patients one factor may predominate. Data that support abnormal insulin secretion are

1. Absence of the first phase insulin response to glucose and, therefore, a delayed insulin secretory response to a glucose load
2. Decreased sensitivity of insulin secretory response to a glucose challenge
3. Decreased total insulin secretory capacity

Evidence for abnormal insulin action includes a decreased number of insulin receptors at target cells and postreceptor defects in insulin action in target tissues (11–14). In addition, Permutt and others (15–17) have shown that Type II diabetes is associated with DNA heterogeneity near the 5′ end of the human insulin gene. This genetic variability is manifested by deletions or insertions (the most common is a 1,600 base insertion—85% of all the insertional alleles) in a region where control for insulin gene transcription may be located. The relative risk for Type II diabetes, if a single 1,600 base insertion is present, is 1.9; the relative risk is 10-fold greater if both alleles have 1,600 base insertions. Thus far the effect of these deletions or insertions on insulin gene transcription is unknown. They do provide a valuable genetic marker for NIDDM.

Glucose Tolerance and Aging

When the new classification for diabetes mellitus was published in 1979, standardized conditions for the oral glucose tolerance test were also suggested (8). The test should be done in the morning after a 10- to 16-hour fast. After a fasting blood sugar is drawn, a 75-g glucose load is given and additional venous plasma glucose samples obtained at half-hour intervals for two hours. The test should only be done on ambulatory individuals who have had an unrestricted diet (high in carbohydrates: > 150 g) and have exercised for three days prior to the test.

Glucose tolerance changes as an individual ages. The changes are more marked in the postprandial glucoses than in the fasting blood sugar. The fasting blood sugar concentration only increases by 1mg/100 mL/decade after age 50. The one-hour postprandial glucose increases by 9.5 mg/100 mL/decade over age 50. The two-hour postprandial glucose increases by 5.3 mg/100 mL (18,19).

In addition to aging, there are other factors that may affect glucose tolerance by altering normal biochemistry and physiology. The dose and concentration of the glucose load, the time of day, the diet prior to the test, and the hours of fasting prior to the test are minimized or eliminated as significant factors by following the recommendations suggested previously. Other factors include gastrointestinal abnormalities (malabsorption and postgastrectomy syndrome), chronic disease states (eg, liver or renal insufficiency), active stress or disease (eg, fever, myocardial infarction or stroke), ingestion of certain drugs (eg, caffeine, hypnotics, salicylates, benzothiadiazene, diuretics, and alcohol) and endocrine conditions (eg, growth hormone or thyroid hormone or glucocorticoid excesses or deficiencies). The geriatric individual is more likely to be affected by factors that alter normal biochemistry and physiology (20).

The possible mechanisms for the age-related decrease in glucose tolerance are

1. Defect in insulin secretion
2. Decreased peripheral tissue responsiveness to insulin
3. Augmented basal hepatic glucose production
4. Impaired suppression of hepatic glucose production, or
5. Impaired hepatic glucose uptake

DeFronzo (18) utilized a hyperglycemic clamp technic to measure glucose metabolism by young (20–29 years) individuals (9.4 ± 0.2 mg/kg • min), middle-aged (30–49 years) individuals (7.2 ± 0.2 mg/kg • min), and geriatric (50–74 years) individuals (6.2 ± 0.3 mg/kg • min). There was a significant age-related decrease in glucose metabolism ($r = -.677$, $P < .001$). The decreases in glucose metabolism could not be explained by changes in insulin secretion with aging. A euglycemic insulin clamp study on the same individuals revealed glucose metabolism rates of 7.5 ± 0.2 mg/kg • min, 6.5 ± 0.2 mg/kg • min, and 5.4 ± 0.2 mg/kg • min for young, middle-aged, and elderly individuals, respectively. DeFronzo felt that his experimental results supported the hypothesis that the decreased glucose tolerance of aging was related to tissue unresponsiveness to insulin.

Jackson et al (21) studied forearm glucose uptake during 100-g oral glucose tolerance tests in healthy males from ages 19 to 83 years. Peripheral glucose uptake in the elderly subjects was one-third the uptake in younger individuals. There was no change in monocyte insulin receptor numbers or affinity with aging. The impaired glucose uptake was therefore felt to be due to a postreceptor defect in insulin action.

Fink et al (22) used the euglycemic glucose clamp technique to show that elderly subjects (mean age 69 ± 1) have a decrease in the maximal rate of glucose disposal and a rightward shift in the insulin action dose–response curve. Glucose disposal rate for elderly subjects was 151 ± 17 mg/m²/min and 247 ± 12 mg/m²/min for the nonelderly (mean age 37 ± 2 years) subjects. Insulin binding to isolated fat cells and monocytes was not affected by increasing age.

Rowe et al (23) did a series of euglycemic insulin clamp studies (20 mU/m²/min to 200 mU/m²/min) in two populations of healthy nonobese males: (1) young (22–37 years old) and (2) old (63–77 years old). The dose–response curves for the insulin-mediated glucose infusion rates are illustrated in Figure 12-1. The maximal glucose infusion rate was the same in both age groups. The dose–response curve was shifted to the right for the elderly subjects. They also showed no effect of age on insulin binding to receptors on circulating monocytes. Their data are consistent with previous studies in showing an age-related decline in sensitivity of peripheral tissues to insulin. However, their data differ from that of Fink et al in that the maximal tissue responsiveness is not altered by increasing age.

In summary, the pathogenesis of glucose intolerance of aging involves

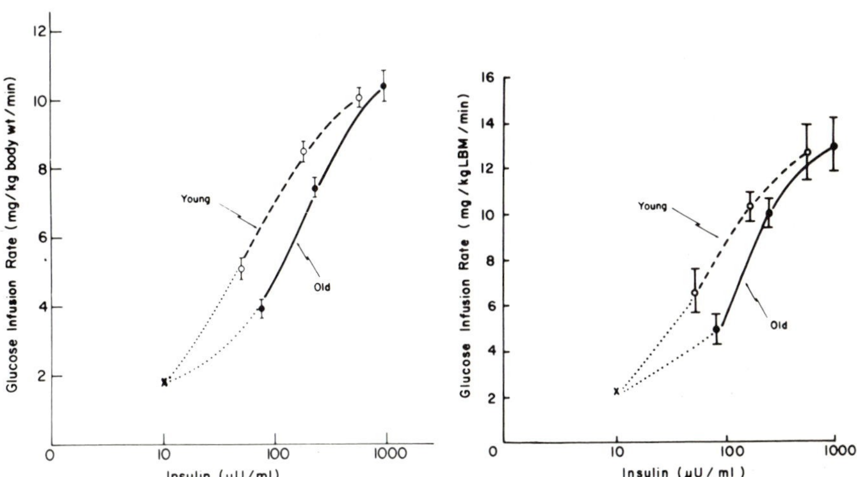

Figure 12-1. Dose–response curves for insulin-mediated whole body glucose infusion rates in young (---) and old (—) subjects. *Left panel:* glucose disposal is expressed as mg/kg body wt. *Right panel:* glucose infusion rates are normalized for lean body mass. The figure shows an age-associated decrease in sensitivity of peripheral tissues to insulin without a change in maximal tissue responsiveness. From Rowe et al (23), with permission of the publisher.

a decrease in sensitivity of peripheral tissues to insulin. This insulin resistance appears to be caused by a postreceptor defect in target tissue insulin action.

Criteria for Diabetes Mellitus in Nonpregnant Adults

The current criteria for diabetes mellitus in nonpregnant adults are as follows:

1. Fasting plasma glucose ⩾ 140 mg% on several occasions
2. Sustained elevated plasma glucose values during the oral glucose tolerance test (two-hour sample ⩾ 200 mg% and one other value ⩾ 200 mg% between the 0 time and two-hour samples), or
3. Classic symptoms of diabetes and unequivocal elevation of the plasma glucose

The criteria for impaired glucose tolerance (IGT) are

1. Fasting plasma glucose < 140 mg%
2. In an oral glucose tolerance test one value between 0 time and two hours ⩾ 200 mg%, and
3. A two-hour sample of 140–199 mg%.

Normal plasma glucose values in nonpregnant adults are

1. Fasting plasma glucose ⩽ 115 mg%
2. In an oral glucose tolerance test the two-hour value is < 140 mg% and no value between 0 time and two hours is ⩾ 200 mg% (8).

Management of Noninsulin-Dependent Diabetes Mellitus

The treatment modalities available for the management of diabetes mellitus, Type II, are

1. Diet
2. Exercise
3. Insulin, and
4. Oral hypoglycemic agents

The primary modality is dietary because the majority of people with NIDDM are overweight. Dietary therapy is noninvasive, inexpensive, and readily available to all individuals with diabetes. It may be the most successful treatment modality of the four because it attacks the basic problem, obesity, and thus decreases insulin resistance. Dietary therapy also improves insulin secretion, may reduce risk factors that are associated with macroangiopathy, and decreases the severity of hyperglycemia.

Simple diet instruction may not be successful unless it is accompanied by behavior modification (4,5,13,24).

Exercise is also inexpensive, readily available, and definitely beneficial in decreasing insulin resistance and improving glucose tolerance. There are no long-term controlled studies of the effects of exercise in diabetes. The beneficial efforts of short-term exercise or physical training include weight decrease, improved insulin sensitivity and glucose tolerance, decreased cholesterol and triglyceride levels, increased high density lipoproteins, weight loss, improved myocardial function, and decreased pulse rate and blood pressure (24). Before the geriatric individual begins any exercise program he or she should be assessed for cardiovascular status. It is probably unreasonable to expect all individuals with NIDDM or obesity to undergo strenuous physical training. But a daily exercise program consisting of walking should aid in glucose control, weight reduction, and insulin sensitivity (see also Chapter 19).

Insulin is sometimes needed to control hyperglycemia in NIDDM. There is evidence to suggest that insulin is the medication of choice in the management of NIDDM when dietary therapy has not been completely successful. Scarlett et al (25) have shown that insulin treatment decreased insulin resistance in people with NIDDM. Control of the plasma glucose in Type II diabetes has also been shown to improve endogenous insulin secretion in response to a carbohydrate challenge (26,27).

Oral hypoglycemic agents are the last treatment modality and probably the most controversial aspect of NIDDM treatment. Sulfonylureas enhance endogenous insulin secretion and in some instances improve insulin action at the target cell by modifying some postreceptor aspects of intracellular metabolism (13,28,29). The sulfonylureas available in the United States are tolbutamide, chlorpropamide, acetohexamide, and tolazamide. The second-generation sulfonylureas have been used in other countries for a number of years, but they have not received final FDA approval for release in the United States. Some of these agents are glyburide, glipizide, glybornuride, and glidazide (30). Glyburide (Diabeta® or Micronase®) and Glipizide (Glucatrol®) will be available in the United States in 1984. They are metabolized by the liver to nonactive compounds, and they have a duration of action of 24 hours. Important criteria in selecting a sulfonylurea for the treatment of the geriatric patient with diabetes are half-life and metabolism. Long-acting drugs increase the likelihood of severe sustained hypoglycemia if the individual does not or cannot eat. Renal function is decreased in elderly individuals and this may also contribute to the risk of hypoglycemia.

The basic principles for managing the geriatric patient with diabetes mellitus are identical to those for the nonelderly diabetic population. Glucose control should be as close to normal as possible throughout the day without unacceptable restrictions on life style and increased risk of severe hypoglycemia.

Dietary Management of NIDDM

The goals of diet modification in diabetes therapy are to provide good nutrition and normal growth for children, to achieve and maintain normal body weight for height and age, to correct metabolic abnormalities toward normal with or without additional treatment modalities, and to prevent or delay the onset of complications of diabetes. The current dietary recommendations by the American Diabetes Association were published in 1979 (31) and were reviewed and compared with the British and Canadian dietary recommendations in 1982 (32).

Since the approximate frequency of Type II diabetes in the United States is ten times that for Type I diabetes and obesity is present 80%–90% of the time in Type II diabetes, weight reduction is considered the primary therapy. Achievement of weight reduction is to be accomplished by a hypocaloric diet and regular exercise. The composition of the diet should be carbohydrate: 50%–60%; fat: 25%–30%; and protein: 10%–20%. Because a significant portion of individuals with diabetes mellitus also have hypertension, some restriction in salt intake is recommended for persons with diabetes and no other medical problems. Complex carbohydrates and carbohydrates that contain high concentrations of natural fiber are recommended. A ratio of 1 : 1 polyunsaturated to saturated fats and cholesterol restriction to less than 300 mg per day is also considered important to avoid an additional risk factor for coronary artery disease. Regularity of meals, day-to-day consistency of meals, and consistency in the amounts and distribution of carbohydrates are important for the individual who needs insulin therapy. The amount of protein in the diet can be estimated by multiplying 0.8 g protein times the normal weight (kg) for height and age (31–33).

The energy requirements of the individual patient play a direct role in the determination of dietary calories consumed per day. An approximate formula is as follows:

1. Weight reduction and/or sedentary life style: 20–25 kcal/kg normal weight for height and age
2. Normal weight and/or moderate activity: 30–35 kcal/kg normal weight for height and age
3. Active life style: 40–45 kcal/kg normal weight for height and age

Another formula for determining dietary calories is 6.6, 11, or 22 times normal weight (kg) for height and age for sedentary, moderate, or strenuous activity, respectively, plus 22 times normal weight for height and age (kg). In the geriatric individual caloric intake should be reduced to compensate for decreased lean body mass, resting metabolic rate, and physical activity. For moderately active elderly individuals, calories should be decreased by 5% per decade between 40 and 59 years, by 10%

between 60 and 69 years, and by an additional 10% for those older than 70 years (33).

There is no magic formula for achieving success in dietary management of the patient with Type II diabetes. It is important to have a physician knowledgeable in diabetes management, a dietician skillful enough to tailor a diet to an individual's financial, social, ethnic, and personal idiosyncrasies, and an education program flexible enough to help patients from all levels of educational background. The patient should be seen regularly by the health-care professionals involved in the diabetic management for reviews, revisions, and reeducation of the therapeutic interventions (33,34)

Carbohydrate Content of the Diabetic Diet

Does a diet in which 50%–70% of the daily calories are derived from carbohydrates aggravate postprandial hyperglycemia or complicate diabetes management if insulin or oral hypoglycemia agents are needed? What types of carbohydrates should be included in the diabetic diet?

A high-carbohydrate diet preceding an oral glucose tolerance test results in more efficient clearing of the oral glucose load than a low-carbohydrate diet preceding the test. The mechanism for this increased insulin sensitivity is not clear. There do appear to be sex differences in insulin delivery rates when a diet is changed from a low-carbohydrate diet to a high-carbohydrate one. An increase in carbohydrate content of 60% results in an increase of 8% (males) and 59% (females) in the insulin delivery rate to peripheral tissues. It is not known whether insulin requirements of diabetic males and females differ if the carbohydrate content of the diet changes (35).

An increase in the carbohydrate concentration of the diabetic diet has an advantageous effect on serum lipids. Fasting triglycerides and cholesterol decrease when an individual is changed from a low- to a high-carbohydrate diet (33).

The form and type of carbohydrate have an effect on the postprandial glucose concentration. It seems logical that if a person with diabetes ingested glucose or sucrose (a disaccharide composed of glucose and fructose), the postprandial glucose concentration would be higher than if an isocaloric portion of a complex carbohydrate (eg, starch) was eaten, but recent data have shown this to be incorrect. Bantle et al (36) administered a mixed meal of 700 calories to nondiabetics, Type I diabetics, and Type II diabetics. The mixed meal consisted of 49% carbohydrate, 18% protein, and 33% fat. Twenty-five percent of the total calories consisted of a different test carbohydrate (glucose, fructose, sucrose, potato starch, or wheat starch). Within each subject group the postpran-

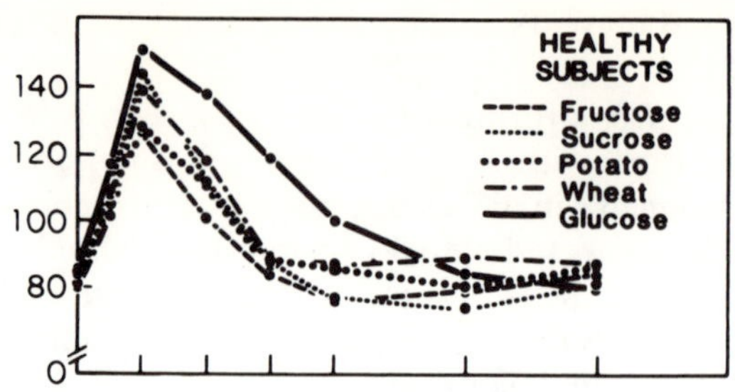
HEALTHY
SUBJECTS
Fructose
Sucrose
Potato
Wheat
Glucose
140
120
100
80
0

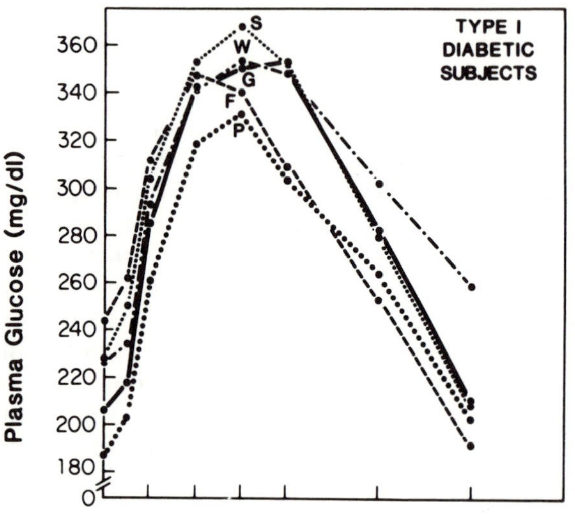
TYPE I
DIABETIC
SUBJECTS
S
W
G
F
P
Plasma Glucose (mg/dl)
360
340
320
300
280
260
240
220
200
180
0

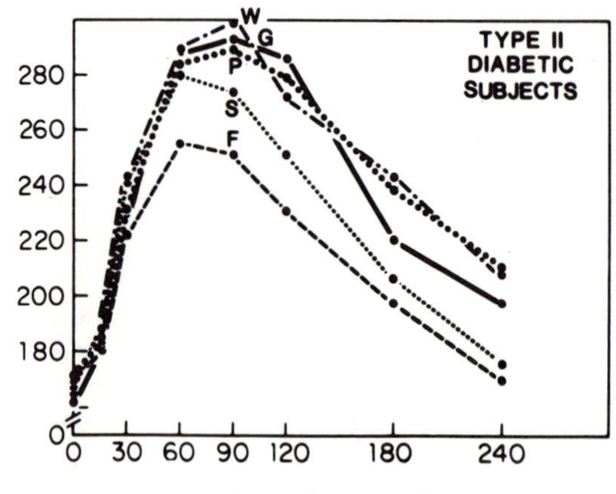
TYPE II
DIABETIC
SUBJECTS
W
G
P
S
F
280
260
240
220
200
180
0
0 30 60 90 120 180 240
Time (minutes)

A

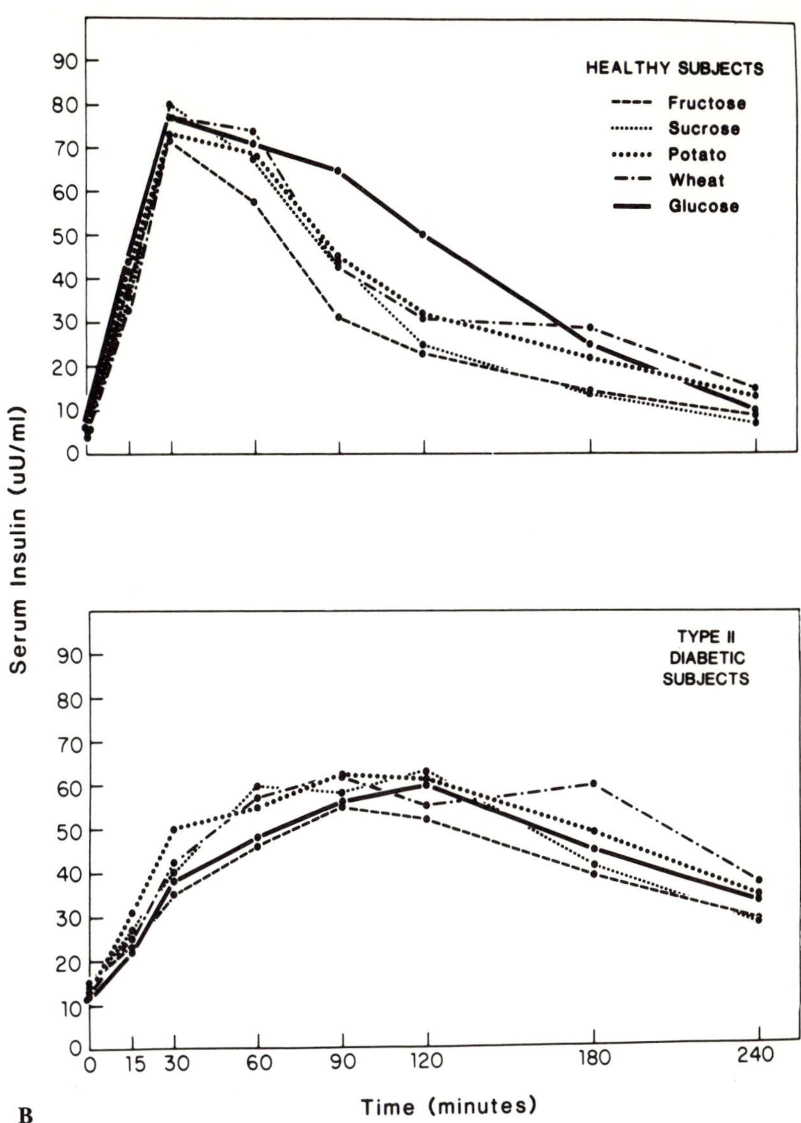

Figure 12-2. Mean plasma concentrations of glucose (**A**) before and after five test meals in individuals who are normal (*top*), who have diabetes mellitus, type I (*middle*) and who have diabetes mellitus, type II (*bottom*). Mean serum concentrations of insulin (**B**) before and after the same test meals in normal subjects (*top*) and subjects with diabetes mellitus, type II (*bottom*). From Bantle et al (36), with permission of the publisher.

Table 12-1. Glycemic Index of Foods*

100%	*40%–49%*
Glucose	Spaghetti (whole meal)
Maltose	Peas (dried)
80%–90%	Potato (sweet)
Honey	Oranges
Potatoes (instant mashed)	*30%–39%*
Carrots	Milk
Cornflakes	Yoghurt
70%–79%	Butter beans
Bread (whole meal)	Apples (Golden Delicious)
Rice (white)	Ice cream
Potato (new)	Tomato soup
60%–69%	*20%–29%*
Bread (white)	Lentils
Rice (brown)	Fructose
Bananas	Kidney beans
Raisins	*10%–19%*
50%–59%	Soya beans
Spaghetti (white)	Peanuts
Potato chips	
Peas (frozen)	
Sucrose	

*Adapted from references 38, 39, 40, 41 and 42.

$$\text{Glycemic index} = \frac{\text{Area under 2-hr blood–glucose response curve for food}}{\text{Area under 2-hr blood–glucose response curve for equivalent amount of glucose}} \times 100$$

dial glycemic response was not significantly different for each of the five test carbohydrates. The serum insulin response in nondiabetic and Type II diabetic subjects was also not significantly different for each of the test meals. Thus, simple carbohydrates, when consumed in a mixed meal, do not appear to aggravate postprandial hyperglycemia (36,37) (see Fig. 12-2).

The glycemic index is defined as the area under the two-hour blood–glucose response curve for food divided by the area under the two-hour blood–glucose response curve for an equivalent amount of glucose times 100 (38, 39). In Table 12-1 the glycemic index for a variety of foods is listed. The form and physical state of the food help determine the glycemic index. Whole meal bread has a glycemic index of 70%–79% and white bread 60%–69%. Similar differences occur with white (70%–79%) and brown (60–69%) rice, potatoes (80%–90%) and potato chips (50%–59%), and frozen (50%–59%) and dried (40%–49%) peas. Puréed foods produce higher glycemic indices than the same foods nonpuréed. Cooking a vegetable may also alter its glycemic index. Legumes, the richest source of natural fiber, produce the lowest glycemic indices. The glycemic index may have value in dietary planning (40–42).

Fiber and the Diabetic Diet

The major sources of fiber in the diet are fruits, vegetables, cereal grains, nuts, and whole-grain flours. Dietary fiber consists of various nonnutritive substances such as cellulose, hemicellulose, lignin, pectin, and gums. Plant fibers can be divided into three types:

1. Structural fibers (eg, cellulose, lignin, hemicelluloses, and pectin)
2. Gums and mucilages (eg, gum arabic, gum acacia, and guar gum), and
3. Storage polysaccharides (eg, guar gum)

Plant fibers can also be classified by their water solubility. Cellulose, lignin, and hemicelluloses are water-insoluble fibers. Pectins, hemicelluloses, gums, mucilages, algal polysaccharides, and storage polysaccharides are water soluble (43). Fibers alter gastrointestinal physiology. Table 12-2 summarizes the physiologic properties that are altered by the ingestion of nonabsorbable plant fibers (44).

Plant fibers decrease the postprandial glucose increment in normal

Table 12-2. Physiologic Actions of Fiber as it Passes Along the Gastrointestinal Tract*

Physico-chemical Properties	Type of Fiber	Modifying
Gel formation	Pectin Mucilages	Gastric emptying Mouth to cecum transit Small intestinal absorption
Water-holding capacity	Polysaccharides Lignins	Mouth to rectum transit Fecal weight Intraluminal pressure Fecal electrolytes
Matrix formation		Fecal bacterial metabolism
Bile–acid adsorption	Lignin Pectin	Fecal steroids Cholesterol turnover
Cation exchange	Acidic polysaccharides	Fecal minerals
Antioxidant	Lignin	Free radical formation and action
Digestibility	Polysaccharides	Energy availability Chemical environment of colon Other physicochemical properties

*Reprinted from Eastwood MA, Kay RM (44), with permission of the publisher.

Table 12-3. Plant Fiber and Carbohydrate Metabolism

1. Decreased postprandial glucose increment (NL and DM*).
2. Decreased postprandial insulin increment (NL and DM).
3. Decreased glycosuria (DM).
4. Decreased exogenous insulin dose or oral hypoglycemic agent.
5. Slower absorption of carbohydrate:
   a. Delayed gastric emptying.
   b. Gel-forming properties.
   c. Altered intestinal transit time.
6. Viscous fibers (guar, tragacanth, konjac mannan, pectin) are most effective in flattening the postprandial glycemia (NL and DM).
7. High-carbohydrate diets improve glucose intolerance (NL and DM).
8. A glucose load taken with guar will result in improved tolerance to a 2nd glucose load without guar 4 hr later.

*NL = normal; DM = diabetes mellitus

and diabetic individuals. Associated with this decreased glycemic response is decreased glycosuria in diabetics, decreased postprandial insulin increments in normals and diabetics, and decreased dose of exogenous insulin or oral hypoglycemic drug. The more viscous fibers (guar, tragacanth, konjac mannan, and pectin) are more effective in depressing the glucose increment after a meal. Another interesting and, as yet, unexplained feature of plant fibers is that their effect on the postprandial glucose increment is long lasting. A glucose load taken with guar will result in improved tolerance to a second glucose load given without guar four hours later (Table 12-3) (33,38,43,45).

Insoluble plant fibers are relatively ineffective in lowering serum cholesterol, but water soluble fibers have been shown to decrease serum cholesterol by 10%–15%. Fasting triglyceride values are unchanged by plant fibers, but the postprandial triglyceride values are decreased (Table 12-4) (43,45–49).

Despite the benefits of high-fiber diets, there are drawbacks. Currently there is no information on the long-term benefits or risks to a high-fiber diet. Flatulence and increased stool bulk and bowel movement frequency are readily noticeable effects of a high-fiber diet. Plant fibers may interfere with the absorption of the trace minerals and some B vitamins. Thus, long-term use of a high-fiber diet may result in deficiencies of zinc, calcium, copper, iron, magnesium, and vitamins B_6 and B_{12} (50,51). The increased bulk of the diet could cause gastric or intestinal obstruction in a susceptible host. Purified plant fibers make food unpalatable and there are no acceptable preparations available for clinical use now. A reasonable goal would be to ingest 25–40 g of natural fiber from the foods that make up the carbohydrate portion of the diabetic diet (Table 12-5) (32,33).

Table 12-4. Plant Fiber and Lipid Metabolism

1. Insoluble plant fibers are relatively ineffective in lowering serum cholesterol.
2. Water-soluble fibers have some cholesterol-lowering effect (10%–15%).
3. Wheat bran or pectin do not change fasting serum triglyceride values, but decrease postprandial values.
4. High-carbohydrate diets (with or without fiber) do not increase triglycerides or cholesterol.

Table 12-5. Adverse Effects of High-Fiber Diets

1. Severe flatulence.
2. Possible loss of trace minerals (zinc, calcium, copper, iron and magnesium).
3. Possible decrease in B_6, B_{12}, and folic acid.
4. Increase in stool bulk and bowel movement frequency.
5. Intestinal or gastric obstruction.
6. No knowledge of the long-term effects of high-fiber diets.
7. Purified fibers make food unpalatable and no acceptable preparation is available for clinical use.

Summary

The geriatric patient who develops diabetes mellitus has a number of special problems. The geriatric patient has to adjust to a new chronic disease and the medical management of the disease. Diabetes may be one of several diseases that the individual has and this results in polypharmacy and the possibility of drug–drug interactions. Compliance with the new diabetic regimen may be a problem because of lifelong habits and eating patterns, psychosocioeconomic problems, and age-related or diabetic visual impairment. Diabetes is a common disease in the elderly, but we must be careful not to overdiagnose or overtreat it. Hypoglycemia secondary to insulin or oral hypoglycemic agents may produce more morbidity for the geriatric patient. On the other hand, a complication of poor control or severe stress on good control is nonketotic hyperosmolar coma.

The management of Type II diabetes mellitus involves weight reduction to normal weight for height and age, exercise, and sometimes insulin or oral hypoglycemic drugs. The diet should consist of 50%–60% of the calories derived from carbohydrates that are complex rather than refined. Increased dietary fiber to 25 g/day may be beneficial, but the long risks or benefits need to be investigated.

References

1. What is diabetes? in Krall LP (ed): *Joslin Diabetes Manual.* Philadelphia, Lea & Febiger, 1978, pp 3–39.

2. Podolsky S: Preface, in Podolsky S (ed): *Clinical Diabetes: Modern Management.* New York, Appleton-Century-Crofts, 1980, pp xvii–xx.
3. Levin ME: Medical evaluation and treatment, in Levin ME, O'Neal LW (eds): *The Diabetic Foot,* ed 3. CV Mosby, St. Louis, 1983, pp 1–60.
4. Horwitz DJ: Diabetes and aging. *Am J Clin Nutr* 1982; 36:803–808.
5. Poplin LE: Diabetes that first occurs in older people. *Nutrition Today* 1982; 9/10:4–13.
6. Skyler JS: Complications of diabetes mellitus: Relationship to metabolic dysfunction. *Diabetes Care* 1979; 2:499–509.
7. Davidson MB: The case for control in diabetes mellitus. *West J Med* 1978; 129:193–200.
8. National Diabetes Data Group: Classification and diagnosis of diabetes mellitus and other categories of glucose intolerance. *Diabetes* 1979; 28:1039–1057.
9. Arky RA: Prevention and therapy of diabetes mellitus. *Nutr Rev* 1983; 41:165–173.
10. Skyler JS, Cahill GF: Diabetes mellitus: Progress and directions. *Am J Med* 1981; 70:101–104.
11. Skyler JS: Type II diabetes: Toward improved understanding and rational therapy. *Diabetes Care* 1982; 5:447–449.
12. Weir GC: Non-insulin dependent diabetes mellitus: Interplay between B-cell inadequacy and insulin resistance. *Am J Med* 1982; 73:461–464.
13. Reaven GM: Therapeutic approaches to reducing insulin resistance in patients with noninsulin-dependent diabetes mellitus. *Am J Med* 1983; 74 (suppl):109–112.
14. DeFronzo RA, Ferrannini E: The pathogenesis of non-insulin-dependent diabetes. *Medicine* 1982; 61:125–140.
15. Permutt MA, Rotwein P: Analysis of the insulin gene in noninsulin-dependent diabetes. *Am J Med* 1983; 75 (suppl) 1–7.
16. Owerbach D, Nerup J: Restriction fragment length polymorphism of the insulin gene in diabetes mellitus. *Diabetes* 1982; 31:275–277.
17. Bell GI, Karam JH, Ruller WJ: Polymorphic DNA region adjacent to the 5′ end of the human insulin gene. *Proc Natl Acad Sci USA* 1981; 78:5759–5763.
18. DeFronzo RA: Glucose intolerance and aging. *Diabetes Care* 1981; 4:493–501.
19. Horwitz DL: Diabetes and aging. *Am J Clin Nutr* 1982; 36:803–808.
20. Seltzer HS: Prime considerations in diagnosis and treatment, in Podolsky S (ed): *Clinical Diabetes: Modern Management.* New York, Appleton-Century-Crofts, 1980, pp 47–66.
21. Jackson RA, Blix PM, Matthews JA, et al: Influence of ageing on glucose homeostasis. *J Clin Endocrinol Metab* 1982; 55:840–848.
22. Fink RI, Kolterman OG, Griffin J, Olefsky JM: Mechanisms of insulin resistance in aging. *J Clin Invest* 1983; 71:1523–1535.
23. Rowe JW, Minaker KL, Pallotta JA, Flier JS: Characterization of the insulin resistance of aging. *J Clin Invest* 1983; 71:1581–1587.
24. DeFronzo RA, Ferrannini E, Koivisto V: New concepts in the pathogenesis and treatment of noninsulin-dependent diabetes mellitus. *Am J Med* 1983; 74 (suppl):52–81.
25. Scarlett JA, Gray RS, Griffin J, et al: Insulin treatment reverses the insulin resistance of type II diabetes mellitus. *Diabetes Care* 1982; 5:353–363.
26. Kosaka K, Kuzuya T, Akanuma Y, Hagura R: Increase in insulin response

after treatment of overt maturity-onset diabetes is independent of the mode of treatment. *Diabetologia* 1980; 18:23–28.

27. Hidaka H, Nagulesparan M, Klimes I, et al: Improvement of insulin secretion but not insulin resistance after short-term control of plasma glucose in obese type II diabetes. *J Clin Endocrinol Metab* 1981; 54:217–222.
28. Judzewitsch RG, Pfeifer MA, Best JD, et al: Chronic chlorpropamide therapy of non insulin-dependent diabetes augments basal and stimulated insulin secretion by increasing islet sensitivity to glucose. *J Clin Endocrinol Metab* 1982; 55:321–328.
29. Kolterman OG, Prince MJ, Olefsky JM: Insulin resistance in noninsulin-dependent diabetes mellitus: Impact of sulfonylurea agents in vivo and in vitro. *Am J Med* 1983; 74 (suppl):82–101.
30. Podolsky S, Krall LP, Bradley RF: Treatment of diabetes with oral hypoglycemic agents, in Podolsky S (ed): *Clinical Diabetes: Modern Management.* New York, Appleton-Century-Crofts, 1980, pp 131–172.
31. Nuttall FQ, Brunzell JD: Principles of nutrition and dietary recommendations for individuals with diabetes mellitus. *Diabetes* 1979; 28:1027–1030.
32. Arky R, Wylie-Rosett J, El-Beheri B: Examination of current dietary recommendations for individuals with diabetes mellitus. *Diabetes Care* 1982; 5:59–63.
33. Ensinck JW, Bierman EL: Dietary management of diabetes mellitus. *Ann Rev Med* 1979; 30:155–170.
34. Hadden DR: Food and diabetes: The dietary treatment of insulin-dependent and non-insulin-dependent diabetes. *Clin Endocrinol Metab* 1982; 11:503–524.
35. Nuttall FQ: Diet and the diabetic patient. *Diabetes Care* 1983; 6:197–207.
36. Bantle JB, Laine DC, Castle GW, et al: Postprandial glucose and insulin responses to meals containing different carbohydrates in normal and diabetic subjects. *N Engl J Med* 1983; 309:7–12.
37. Crapo PA, Reaven G, Olefsky J: Plasma glucose and insulin responses to orally administered simple and complex carbohydrates. *Diabetes* 1976; 25:741–747.
38. Jenkins DJA: Lente carbohydrate: A newer approach to the dietary management of diabetes. *Diabetes Care* 1982; 5:634–641.
39. Jenkins DJA, Taylor RH, Wolever TMS: The diabetic diet, dietary carbohydrate and differences in digestibility. *Diabetologia* 1982; 23:477–484.
40. Collier G, O'Dea K: Effect of physical form of carbohydrate on the postprandial glucose, insulin, and gastric inhibitory polypeptide responses in type 2 diabetes. *Am J Clin Nutr* 1982; 36:10–14.
41. Ionescu-Tirgoviste C, Popa E, Sintu E, et al: Blood glucose and plasma insulin responses to various carbohydrates in type 2 (non-insulin-dependent) diabetes. *Diabetologia* 1983; 24:80–84.
42. Jenkins DJA, Tolever TMS, Jenkins AL, et al: Glycemic response to wheat products: Reduced response to pasta but no effect of fiber. *Diabetes Care* 1983; 6:155–159.
43. Anderson JW, Chen W-JL: Plant fiber: Carbohydrate and lipid metabolism. *Am J Clin Nutr* 1979; 32:346–363.
44. Eastwood MA, Kay RM: An hypothesis for the action of dietary fiber along the gastrointestinal tract. *Am J Clin Nutr* 1979; 32:364–367.
45. Anderson JW, Ward K: Long term effects of high-carbohydrate high-fiber

diets on glucose and lipid metabolism: A preliminary report on patients with diabetes. *Diabetes Care* 1978; 1:77–82.

46. Taskinen M-R, Nikkila EA, Ollus A: Serum lipids and lipoproteins in insulin-dependent diabetic subjects during high-carbohydrate, high-fiber diet. *Diabetes Care* 1983; 6:224–230.
47. Ullrich IH, Albrink MJ: Lack of effect of dietary fiber on serum lipids, glucose and insulin in healthy young men fed high starch diets. *Am J Clin Nutr* 1982; 36:1–9.
48. Ray TK, Mansell KM, Knight KC, et al: Long-term effects of dietary fiber on glucose tolerance and gastric emptying in noninsulin-dependent diabetic patients. *Am J Clin Nutr* 1983; 37:376–381.
49. Barnard RJ, Massey MR, Cherney S, et al: Long term use of a high-complex-carbohydrate, high-fiber, low-fat diet and exercise in the treatment of NIDDM patients. *Diabetes Care* 1983; 6:268–273.
50. Anderson JW, Ferguson SK, Karounos D, et al: Mineral and vitamin status on high-fiber diets: Long term studies of diabetic patients. *Diabetes Care* 1980; 3:38–40.
51. Hollenbeck CB, Leklem JE, Riddle MC, Connor WE: The composition and nutritional adequacy of subject selected high carbohydrate low fat diets in insulin-dependent diabetes mellitus. *Am J Clin Nutr* 1983; 38:41–51.

13

Nutritional Intervention During Immunologic Aging: Past and Present

S. Jill James and Takashi Makinodan

In the last two decades, the dynamic interaction between nutritional status, resistance to disease, and immunologic vigor has been firmly established in various epidemiologic, clinical, and laboratory investigations. In the 1960s, numerous field studies of undernourished children strongly suggested that the increased morbidity and mortality associated with common infections was due to a synergistic interaction between malnutrition and infection. These clinical observations of apparent immunodeficiency secondary to undernutrition have since expanded into the interdisciplinary science of nutritional immunology, with a focus on the specific interaction of defined nutrients in the multifaceted web of immune defense.

Both clinical and experimental investigations have confirmed that thymus-dependent cell-mediated immunity is consistently more vulnerable to chronic nutritional imbalances than antibody-dependent humoral immunity. Coincidentally, those T-cell functions most sensitive to given nutritional perturbations are precisely those that have been established to decline with age in the individual. The progressive T-cell dysfunction with advanced age has been implicated in the etiology of many of the chronic degenerative diseases of the elderly, including arthritis, cancer, vascular injury, and autoimmune-immune complex diseases, as well as a pronounced increased susceptibility to infectious disease. The exacerbating role of a concomitant nutritional deficiency in the aging immune system, or the possible attentuating role of nutritional intervention during progressive immunosenescence, is a provocative, although relatively unexplored area of research.

This review of nutrition and immune function, which will be more interpretive than encylopedic, will be prefaced by a review of the simultaneous and independent changes in nutritional needs and immunologic vigor that occur over the aging spectrum from periods of growth to senescence. Recent studies documenting nutritional modulation of cell-mediated immunity will then be evaluated, including clinical and experimental protein-calorie deprivation, dietary lipid interactions, and specific micronutrient deficiencies. Finally, directions for future research will be discussed, based on recent advances in cellular immunology, in order to determine those points proximal to effector cell function that are critically affected by a given nutritional intervention.

Implications of Age-Related Changes in Immune Function and Nutritional Needs

Both immune function and nutritional requirements vary simultaneously and independently with age. At both extremes of the age spectrum and at times of physiologic stress, immunologic and nutritional vulnerability interface critically in terms of host resistance to disease.

Neonatal Changes

Immunologic

Immunologic vigor during the neonatal and early growth period is suppressed secondary to maturational changes in lymphoid tissue. The thymus gland, responsible for T-cell maturation and differentiation, has been shown to be functionally and morphologically immature at birth in humans and mice, reaching a functional peak around puberty. Thereafter, progressive involution of thymic tissue precedes a continuing decline in T-cell-dependent immune response (1). Possible mechanisms for suboptimal immune capacity in early life have been recently reviewed (2). Maturational changes may involve (a) an increase in the number of the most limiting type of immune cell involved in an antibody response (ie, either T cells, B cells, or macrophages); (b) a shift in the proportion of regulator cells with enhancing or suppressing activities; or (c) maturational changes in immune cells that alter their performance efficiency. T-helper cell activity appears to be deficient in newborn mice and to mature slowly, reaching a functional maximum around 8 to 10 weeks of age (3).

Reduced helper cell activity may be accompanied by increased suppressor cell activity in the neonate. Thus, Sato and Makinodan (4) have shown that newborn thymic adherent cell cultures release factors that inhibit the maturation of precursor cells into mitogen-responsive cells. Age-related change in mitogen responsiveness in mice has also been documented by Hori, Perkins, and Halsall (5). Maturational increases in mitogen response is dramatic from birth to 1 month of age, reaching functional maturity at 8 months, followed by a progressive decline with advancing age.

These experimental studies suggest that immune function is suboptimal after birth and during early growth, secondary to maturational changes in lymphoid cells.

Nutritional

Superimposed on the period of lymphoid maturation are increased nutritional demands (per Kg) required to support overall growth and development. Clinical consequence of the combined nutritional and immunologic vulnerability in terms of resistance to disease may depend on adequate nutritional status. In the human infant, nutritional deprivation during gestation has been associated with low birth weight, lymphocytopenia, and impaired cell-mediated immunity, which may persist for months or even years (6). Normal thymic growth and development are suspended in early childhood malnutrition, so that a derangement in thymic-dependent lymphocyte subpopulations might be anticipated. In general, the total number of circulating lymphocytes remains normal in malnutrition; however, T cells are markedly decreased with no change in B-cell numbers (7). This would imply that immature lymphocytes with neither B nor T-cell markers would be increased. Consistent with this concept, Chandra (8) has reported an increase in "null" cells in peripheral blood in undernourished children. The level of circulating thymic hormone is also reduced from normal in these children, and this may underlie the shift to more immature, undifferentiated lymphocytes.

It would appear that a critical combination of suppressed or delayed immunocompetence with nutritional vulnerability during early growth and development can act synergistically to magnify susceptibility to disease. It is also likely that the severity and duration of nutritional deficiency required to critically suppress immune reactivity, whether naturally occurring in human populations or experimentally induced, would be significantly less if imposed during immunologic immaturity. In this regard, Chandra (8) has recently reviewed the clinical evidence suggesting a synergistic relationship between undernutrition and infection during infancy and early childhood in underdeveloped countries. It is concluded that immunodeficiency secondary to malnutrition contributes significantly to the increase in morbidity and mortality due to common infection in this age group. Therefore, it would appear that the interpretation of nutritional intervention studies on immune activities must necessarily be *qualified in terms of age*.

Changes with Old Age

Immunologic

At the opposite end of the aging spectrum, immunologic vigor is again less than optimal due to senescent changes, primarily in T-cell-dependent immune function. Because thymic involution precedes the progressive decrease in T-cell-dependent immune responsiveness, morphologic and functional changes in the thymus have been implicated in the decline. Atrophic changes with advanced age have been described in thymic epithelial tissue (9), which is the site of thymic hormone synthesis required for T-lymphocyte differentiation. The percentage of immature lymphocytes within the thymus and also in the peripheral blood increases with age, suggesting that the aging thymus loses its ability to induce differentiation of prethymic lymphocytes (10).

There is substantial evidence indicating that the relative proportions of T-cell subpopulations shift with age. In humans as well as mice, an impaired capacity to produce interleukin (IL)-2, a T-cell growth factor, has been established in aged lymphocytes (11), suggesting that T-cell proliferation is reduced. In addition, IL-1, the cytokine released from activated macrophages, which is required for stimulation of IL-2 synthesis in T cells, has also been shown to be reduced with age in mice (12). Changes in suppressor-cell activity with age have been contradictory; however, the work of Webb and Nowowiejski (13) has confirmed that splenic macrophages can activate suppressor-cell populations via endogenous prostaglandin (PG) synthesis. Goodwin and Messner (14) have demonstrated a significant increase in sensitivity to PGE in elderly human T cells and has postulated that this may partially account for the depressed cellular immune responses observed in this age group.

In summary, there is abundant evidence confirming a decline in immunologic responsiveness with advanced age, but the molecular mechanisms underlying these changes remain to be elucidated.

Nutritional

The consequence of nutritional deficiencies in elderly individuals, in whom immunocompetence is already compromised, is likely to be particularly severe in terms of resistance to disease. Several recent nutritional surveys have documented an alarming prevalence of clinical malnutrition in medical and surgical wards in this country (15). Bienia and associates (16) have assessed the prevalence and consequence of malnutrition among hospitalized elderly individuals. Clinical malnutrition was diagnosed in 61% of patients over 65 years old, compared with 28% in patients under 65. A comparison between malnourished and well-nourished elderly revealed that mortality, incidence of infection, anemia, and anergy were significantly higher in the malnourished group. Of particular interest was the finding that the incidence of these abnormalities in the well-nourished elderly individuals did not differ from incidence in the younger group, suggesting that nutritional status, and not age per se, was the more significant variable.

The nutritional needs in old age have not yet been adequately defined, despite the fact that nearly 15% of our population is over the age of 60. Estimates for nutrient requirements are largely based on extrapolation of data from studies in young adults. Senescent changes in digestive and absorptive capacities, drug–nutrition interactions, and increased prevalence of infection and catabolic illness are likely to increase specific nutrient needs in the elderly. Additional studies are needed, not only to determine nutrient requirements for the healthy elderly, but also to define nutrient requirements during disease states, as nutritional status may contribute both to susceptibility and prognosis.

The negative impact of malnutrition on the response to stress, wound healing, and host defense makes effective diagnosis especially important in elderly individuals in whom immunosenescence has independently contributed to reduced resistance to disease. As reviewed elsewhere in this book (Chapter 16), many of the standard anthropometric and biochemical indices traditionally used in the diagnosis of malnutrition are inadequate for elderly individuals because many of the age-related physiologic changes tend to overlap and vary in the same direction. Thus, for example, lean body mass is known to decline with age, rendering measurements such as midarm circumference, 24-hour urinary excretion, and creatine/height index falsely low in well-nourished elderly individuals. Nutritionists are now attempting too expand traditional indices of nutritional status to include functional assessments of nutrient-dependent response to stress. However, as with traditional measurements, the validity of a functional measurement requires that it does not vary with age, or at least that it could be related to age-specific norms.

Chandra (17) has recommended the potential of various measures of immunocompetence as possible functional indicators of general malnutrition. This approach would have the advantage of predicting disease vulnerability as well as early nutritional deficiencies. However, because of the age-related decline in these indices, the sensitivity would be low in assessment of the elderly and would require age-specific norms to be established.

In conclusion, when periods of nutritional vulnerability overlap with suboptimal immune function, whether due to maturational or senescent changes, a synergistic interaction occurs. The exaggerated susceptibility to disease at both extremes of age emphasizes the pivotal role nutritional status plays in modulating susceptibility to diseases. Nutritional intervention studies that aim to define the severity and duration of deficiency required to affect immunologic activity must be qualified in terms of age since the impact of a given deficiency can be expected to vary with the

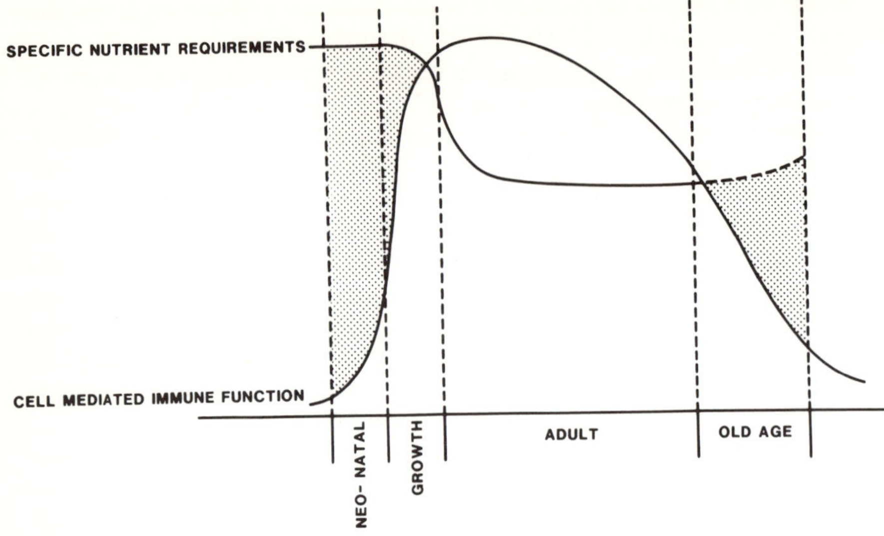

Figure 13-1. Relative changes in immune function and nutritional needs with age. At both extremes of age, when periods of nutritional vulnerability overlap with suboptimal immune function, there is an exaggerated susceptibility to disease.

age-specific changes in immune responsiveness. The simultaneous and independent changes in nutrition needs and immune function with age are schematically presented in Figure 13-1.

Nutritional Modulation of Cell-Mediated Immunity (CMI)

Acute or chronic nutritional imbalance, as an environmental variable, can critically modify cell-mediated immune response. Depending on the severity and type of nutritional deficiency, humoral immunity as well as nonspecific immune defense mechanisms, such as phagocytic cell function and complement synthesis, may also be adversely affected. However, the focus in this review will be on specific nutrient interaction with CMI.

Protein–Calorie Malnutrition (PCM)

Human Studies

Human studies of PCM, whether in children of underdeveloped countries or in hospitalized adults, have confirmed a causal association between undernutrition and secondary immunodepression leading to impaired host resistance to infection and/or physiologic stress. So consistent is this association, several studies of clinical malnutrition in medical and surgical patients have demonstrated the potential of immunologic status (eg, delayed hypersensitivity) as a predictor of clinical outcome (18,19). Response to physiologic stress (infection, trauma, surgery, catabolic disease) and nutritional status are mutually interdependent variables which can interact in two directions: (a) malnutrition can impair response to physiologic stress via secondary depression of lymphoid tissue, and (b) chronic physiologic stress can precipitate acute malnutrition via increased nutrient demands and catabolic losses. The pathophysiology of one exacerbates the other, leading to a negative synergistic and cyclic interaction which underlies increased morbidity and mortality.

The voluminous literature of human PCM and immune function has been extensively reviewed by Gross and Newberne (20). Consistent results and precise definition of immunologic derangement have proven difficult to assess in field studies for several reasons:

1. Multiple and variable nutrient deficiencies often coexist.
2. Immune responses are often evaluated after nutritional therapy has begun.
3. Assessment is often confounded by concurrent infection.
4. Degree of malnutrition (severe versus moderate, chronic versus acute) varies between studies.

Nonetheless, the general pattern indicates that cell-mediated immunity is more profoundly affected in generalized malnutrition than humoral immunity.

It must be emphasized that human PCM is a multifaceted complex syndrome involving multiple and variable nutrient deficiencies, not only in protein and energy, but in various vitamins and minerals as well. The combined deficiencies interact to consistently impair aspects of CMI at all ages with a negative impact on host resistance as previously described.

Animal Studies

Because multiple and uncontrolled variables confound immunologic evaluation in human PCM, more recent investigation has focused on the impact of single-nutrient variables on aspects of CMI in laboratory animal models, in which environmental conditions can be precisely controlled. However, extrapolation of data from animal models to human PCM should be made with caution since these univariate models are, at best, an academic approximation of a complex and multivariate condition. Nonetheless, these studies represent an important first step. Accordingly, several investigators have evaluated either protein or calorie restriction as isolated variables in an otherwise replete diet in laboratory animals (see Chapter 6). The effect of this regimen on patterns of CMI belied expectation by consistently *enhancing* T-cell-dependent responses when assessed after midlife and by significantly extending life span.

The cause for these disparate effects on CMI, depending on whether undernutrition is naturally occurring in human populations or is imposed as isolated restriction in the laboratory, is not clear. Laboratory models of PCM are restricted in protein and/or calories, but are supplemented with control levels of micronutrients. Good and associates (21) have strongly implicated the importance of micronutrient deficiencies, particularly zinc, in the etiology of depressed CMI in human malnutrition.

In attempting to dissect human PCM into its component parts, most of the controlled studies in animal models purport to investigate immunologic effects of either protein or calorie restriction independently. It should be emphasized, however, that considerable metabolic overlap exists when proteins or calories are independently restricted. For example, caloric restriction is generally imposed by feeding the restricted group one-half the quantity of diet consumed ad libitum by the control group. Since most control diets contain approximately 20% protein, the restricted animals thus receive about 10% dietary protein, which approaches the level of protein (8%) imposed in studies of chronic protein deprivation. Furthermore, metabolic alterations in response to caloric insufficiency lead to a decreased utilization of available protein. When calories are limiting, the carbon skeleton of amino acids is converted to glucose in the liver to meet priority energy requirements. It is likely, therefore, that caloric restriction is not an independent variable, but may have a component of protein deficiency as well. Conversely, dietary protein restriction, despite isocaloric adjustment of the diet, often leads to inanition, a marked reduction in food intake, as a metabolic adaptation to insufficient protein. Therefore, it is likely that a degree of caloric restriction is simultaneously imposed when protein is limiting. Such nutrition interactions are important interpretive considerations.

Caloric Restriction

The immunologic consequences of caloric restriction have been evaluated in several strains of rats and mice. Gerbase-DeLima et al (22) imposed caloric restriction on a long-lived strain of weanling mice, using a casein-based diet (14.5 calories/21% casein) by feeding the restricted group on alternate days. Various indices of T-cell function were followed throughout the life span of the animals and were observed to be uniformly *depressed* in the *early* months of restriction. However, by midlife the pattern reversed, with enhanced activity in the restricted group compared with ad libitum fed controls. The relative enhancement of T-cell function was associated with a significant increase in life span.

In 1935, McCay et al (23) observed that if the growth rate in rats was retarded in a controlled manner by withholding calories, the surviving animals lived significantly longer than ad libitum fed controls. In the early 1960s, Ross et al (24) confirmed and extended these observations. Both McCay and Ross observed significant losses to infection *early in life* in the restricted groups, which is corroborated by the early depression in CMI observed by Gerbase-DeLima et al (22). The mechanisms underlying life extension by caloric restriction have not been elucidated.

Delayed maturation and involution of thymic tissue induced by caloric deprivation has been suggested by Good et al (25) as an important determinant of life span, since rate of thymic involution has been implicated as a major factor in immunologic aging. These investigators chose to study short-lived autoimmune-prone strains of mice (NZB, NZB/NZW) as models for immunologic diseases associated with aging in humans. They found that restricted feeding of 10 calories/day (with control level of micronutrient) from weaning, regardless of variations in protein, carbohydrate, or fat in the diet, dramatically increased life span in these strains, delayed the onset of autoimmune manifestations, and enhanced indices of CMI. It is not clear, however, whether caloric restriction in autoimmune-prone strains affects life span by altering the tempo of a common aging process, or by an effect on the life-shortening disease process.

Of considerable interest, although not a focus of longevity studies, is the repeated observation of early suppression of CMI by caloric restriction during the growth period. As documented in other studies, Fernandes et al (26) similarly observed a depressed in vitro response to PHA and depressed response to sheep RBC injected in vivo during the first few months of caloric deprivation. These results suggest that the increased longevity and immunoenhancement are not univariate and appear to apply only to the surviving cohort. The vulnerability of CMI to nutritional deprivation during early growth as documented in these studies is reminiscent of our remarks earlier in the chapter. Nevertheless, after the growth period, the calorically deprived animals display increases in antigen/mitogen responsiveness, delayed deposition of lethal autoimmune complexes, increased cytotoxicity to allogeneic tumor cells, and significant extension of life span when compared with ad libitum fed animals (26).

It should be recognized that in these studies of food restriction and its effects on CMI and life span, the normal or control level of consumption is, in fact, an arbitrary definition, based on the ad libitum intake of caged animals, deprived of exercise and housed in an unvarying environment. It may be argued that under these artificial conditions, the restricted intake may be more optimal for CMI reactivity relative to the "normal" control; or alternatively that ad libitum feeding in an unnatural environment has a negative impact on life span and CMI.

The reference for caloric restriction is a diet that was designed for rapid growth, maturation, and reproductive capacity. It was never intended to promote longevity, and yet the implicit assumption in studies of caloric restriction is that life span is being extended from a normal or maximum. The high content of protein, fat, and simple sugars in the ad libitum diet undoubtedly exceeds physiologic requirements, especially as needs decline with age. Therefore, an important interpretive question is whether the reference diet is in fact *less than optimal* in terms of reflecting the genetic potential for life span in a given species. In terms of the relative immunoenhancement observed with restricted regimens, there is strong evidence that the high fat content of the control diet may be immunosuppressive, as discussed in the next section.

Lipids and Immune Function

Immunoregulatory aspects of dietary lipid composition are inherently interesting and may have particular relevance to the aging individual, in whom lipid profiles tend to increase. The immunosuppressive qualities of high dietary fat could contribute to or potentiate the natural decline in immune activity with age and conceivably exacerbate immune-related disease.

Lipids are essential for the structural and functional integrity of cell membranes. Membrane events are integrally involved in all aspects of cellular immune reactivity. Both the type and quantity of dietary lipid have been shown to modulate immune activity in several ways. First, endogenous cholesterol synthesis appears to be an essential prerequisite to DNA synthesis in lymphocyte proliferative responses in order to accommodate new membrane formation (30). Thus, if cholesterol synthesis is blocked, directly or indirectly, proliferative events are abrogated proportionately. Second, the degree of saturation of fatty acids (FA) esterified to membrane lipids can be dramatically altered by the level of FA intake. The degree of unsaturation (number of double bonds) of constituent FAs perturbs the molecular configuration and fluidity of cell membranes; increased membrane fluidity has been associated with immunosuppression (36). Third, circulating lipoproteins (LP) interact with specific membrane receptors on lymphocytes and have been shown to inhibit antigen/mitogen-induced blastogenesis (37). Although the precise biochemical interactions have yet to be elucidated, it is clear that dietary lipids have dynamic immunoregulatory effects via alterations of the cellular lipid constituents and membrane-related activity.

Cholesterol

Several studies have demonstrated that nutritionally induced hypercholesterolemia is associated with impaired host resistance to both bacterial and viral infection (27). However, the apparent immunosuppressive effects of cholesterol must be reevaluated in terms of recent evidence. Humphries (28) has recently demonstrated that the dietary cholesterol included in experimental hypercholesterolemic diets is often contaminated with auto-oxidative metabolites, which act as potent immunosuppressive agents by inhibiting sterol synthesis. In related studies, Heiniger (29) found that purified cholesterol, free of oxidized metabolites, was not immunosuppressive. Further, de novo cholesterol synthesis was shown to be an obligatory prerequisite to mitogen-stimulated DNA synthesis. Chen (30) has confirmed that endogenous cholesterol synthesis must and does precede DNA synthesis and is apparently required for new membrane synthesis. Agents that block cholesterol synthesis in vitro result in impaired mitogen responsiveness (31) and decreased cytotoxicity (32). Enhanced mitogenesis has been associated with increased levels of membrane cholesterol and relative reduction in membrane fluidity (33).

Recent studies by Broitman (34) suggest that the degree of saturation of dietary polyunsaturated fatty acids (PUFA), rather than level of serum cholesterol, correlates best with immunosuppressive activity. A 10-fold greater depression in mitogen response was observed in hypercholesterolemic rats fed PUFAs, compared with equally hypercholesterolemic rats fed saturated fats, suggesting that serum cholesterol per se was not a regulatory factor.

Polyunsaturated Fatty Acids (PUFA)

High dietary intake of PUFA can dramatically alter the composition of esterified membrane lipids. The *cis* conformation of double bonds in esterified fatty acids alters the molecular configuration of cell membrane lipid and increases membrane fluidity. A reduction in ratio of PUFA to saturated FA in the membrane or an increase in cholesterol content reduces the fluidity of the membrane. These changes have been associated with enhanced mitogen responsiveness (33) and increased cytolytic activity (32). Dynamic changes in membrane fluidity, phospholipid and cholesterol metabolism occur normally with antigen/mitogen stimulation. It has been suggested that membrane alterations induced by changes in FA composition may affect receptor aggregation, configuration, and availability for ligand binding, thereby negatively affecting immune reactivity (35).

Essential fatty acids (linoleic [18:2] and arachidonic [20:4]) are known precursors of PG; however, dietary manipulation of PG levels by increased precursor intake has been difficult to demonstrate in vivo. Nonetheless, it is tempting to postulate that dietary PUFA exert an immunosuppressive effect via increased PG synthesis, especially since availability of arachidonic acid is the rate-limiting step in PG synthesis. In support of this notion are the recent studies demonstrating that macrophage-derived PGE_2 activates suppressor cell populations (13). Increased suppressor cell activity could contribute to the immunosuppressive effects of PG precursors, particularly in older animals with increased sensitivity to PG (14).

Lipoproteins (LP)

In addition to providing a transport mechanism for hydrophobic lipids, LP have immunoregulatory properties as well. In particular, a species of low density lipoprotein (LDL), termed intermediate density lipoprotein (IDL), has been shown to have specific saturable receptors on T-cell membranes (36). The binding of IDL to these receptors has been shown to interrupt the sequence of membrane-related events initiated by PHA activation. The normal sequence of events after mitogenic stimulation includes an increase in Ca^{++} flux, arachidonic acid release, phospholipid turnover, and an elevation of cyclic GMP. Evidence presented by Harmony and Hui (36) suggests that the binding of IDL interferes with intracellular accumulation of Ca^{++}, which effectively blocks progression of events. The quantity of IDL bound to surface receptors correlated directly with a reduction in Ca^{++} accumulation intracellularly. Furthermore, internalization of IDL was not required to depress Ca^{++} flux, and the effect was independent of the cholesterol content of the bound LP.

It is apparent in reviewing these studies that abnormalities in lipid intake can reversibly affect cell-mediated immune function. The potential for therapeutic nutritional intervention, particularly for autoimmune diseases in the elderly, is an interesting consideration. It must be emphasized, however, that immunosuppressive diets high in PUFA have also been convincingly related to cancer promotion (35).

Micronutrients and Immune Function: Zinc

Inclusive review articles have recently been published which explore the experimental evidence relating each of the micronutrient to immune function (20,37). The focus here will be on the single micronutritient, zinc, since it is highly likely that zinc deficiency is a component of human malnutrition and may contribute significantly to secondary immunodeficiency. In addition to zinc, deficiencies in vitamin A and iron are most likely to contribute to secondary immunodeficiency in chronic moderate PCM.

Human Studies

According to a recent review by Sandstead (38), chronic moderate zinc deficiency in humans may be more prevalent than previously appreciated. Inadequate zinc status is most likely during early rapid growth, old age, and periods of physiologic stress, such as pregnancy, lactation, and catabolic illness. Alcoholism and malabsorptive states may also predispose to zinc deficiency.

There are no major storage sites for zinc in the body, so that when availability or intake is reduced, deficient symptoms are apparent within a few weeks. Since zinc content and availability are highest in meat protein and lowest in cereal-based diets, it is not surprising that concomitant zinc deficiency has been documented in children with PCM (39). Many of the clinical symptoms of PCM, including growth retardation, dermatitis, lymphoid hypoplasia, impaired wound healing, and immunodeficiency, mimic those observed in acrodermatitis enteropathica, a genetic disorder that impairs zinc absorption and results in severe deficiency. Golden et al (39) have demonstrated that local cutaneous application of zinc ointment to children with chronic moderate PCM resulted in significant restoration of impaired delayed hypersensitivity response.

Although isolated zinc deficiency in man is rare, severe zinc deficiency has been inadvertently produced in patients maintained on total parenteral nutrition (TPN) in which the nutrient solution was insufficient in zinc (40). Lymphocytopenia, anergy, and a profound depression of PHA response was dramatically reversed when zinc was added to the TPN solution. The importance of this study is that the single variable, zinc, was shown to reverse immunodeficiency in otherwise well-nourished humans.

Animal Studies

An adaptation to severe zinc deficiency is a pronounced reduction in food consumption (inanition). Since inanition can independently depress immune function, well-designed studies must necessarily include a pair-fed control group that is fed the same quantity of food consumed by the deficient group. However, when deficiency and inanition are severe, it is questionable whether the pair-fed animals are adequately nourished. Faraji and Swendseid (41) have circumvented problems of inanition control in rats by enteral feeding via gastric tube, so that both deficient and control animals receive an adequate quantity of diet, which varies only in zinc content.

Severe zinc deficiency imposed during rapid growth invariably results in total weight loss and lymphoid atrophy. Thymic hypoplasia is severe, with massive depletion of cortical thymocytes. Moderate zinc deficiency, on the other hand, has been shown to impair mitogen-induced blastogenesis dramatically without reducing lymphoid or body weight (42). Severity of deficiency, duration, and age appear to be interdependent variables, which must be critically considered when interpreting extent and type of immunologic impairment with nutritional intervention.

Fraker and associates (43) have shown that the spleen plaque-forming-cell response (PFC) to sheep red blood cells (a T-cell-dependent response) is markedly reduced in severe or moderate zinc deficiency in young adult mice. In these studies, the PFC response was expressed per spleen, and thus could be misleading since spleen size is invariably reduced in zinc-deficient animals. More recently, the PFC response was reevaluated in zinc-deficient rats, and when expressed per 10^6 spleen cells, differences between the groups were not significant (44). It would appear that total PFC capacity is reduced with zinc deficiency, but remaining splenocytes appear to react normally to challenge with sheep erythrocytes.

In vitro blastogenesis in response to mitogenic lectins has been shown to be significantly depressed in lymphocytes from zinc-deficient animals, despite the presence of zinc in the culture medium (45). In other studies, delayed hypersensitivity (46) and cytotoxic activity against allogenic tumor cells (45) have been shown to be impaired with zinc deficiency.

At the subcellular level, it has not been determined whether immunodeficiency with zinc deprivation is primarily due to changes in zinc-dependent enzyme activities or due to changes in cell membrane integrity or function. Enzyme and/or membrane changes may occur singly or in combination depending on the severity, duration, and age of intervention.

It is apparent that effector cell dysfunction with zinc deficiency has been well described; however, the cellular-molecular basis for dysfunction is not well understood.

Future Research: A Mechanistic Approach to Cell-Mediated Immune Dysfunction with Nutritional Intervention

For the most part, past studies have been descriptive, with emphasis on the characterization of effector response as a consequence of a given nutritional intervention. Recent advances in molecular biology and cellular immunology can now be utilized to explore the nutritional dependence of the various stages in T-cell ontogeny from bone marrow stem cell to activated peripheral cell. For example, although zinc deficiency reproducibly depresses indices of T-cell effector cell function, it is not at all clear which points along the differentiation vector are most vulnerable. The derivation and interactions of T cells and B cells are schematically presented in Figure 13-2.

The thymus is the major site in the differentiation and maturation of precursor cells into immunocompetent T lymphocytes and appears to be particularly vulnerable to nutritional imbalance. Peripheral cell dysfunction secondary to derangement in the thymic microenvironment can now be evaluated by analyzing quantitative and qualitative changes in the purified subpopulations of mature and immature thymocytes. Alterations in thymic hormone production, in terminal deoxytransferase (TdT) activ-

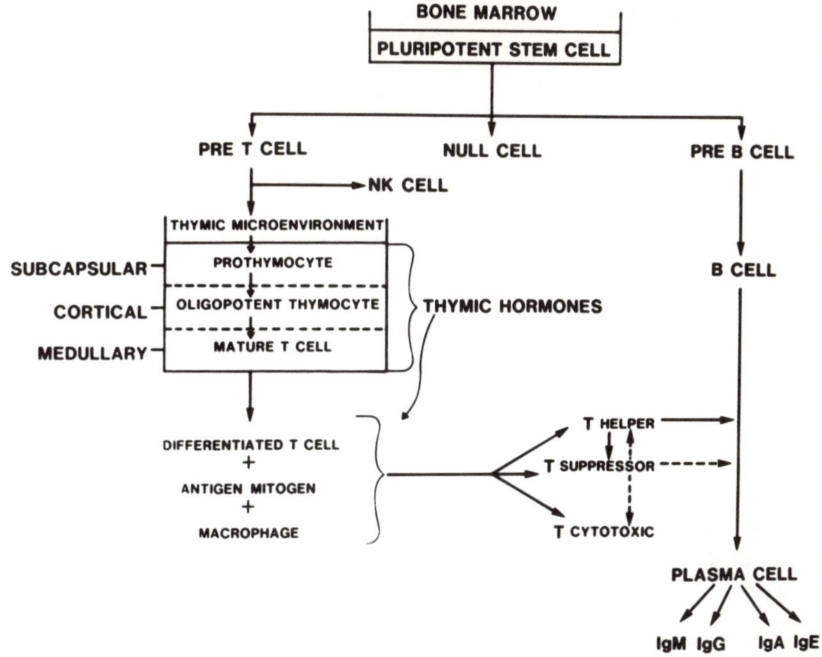

Figure 13-2. Differentiation pathways and cellular interactions between T and B lymphocytes.

ity, or in the appearance of Thy 1^{+} surface antigens by nutritional intervention would suggest a nutritional dependence in the thymic differentiation pathway.

Peripheral T cell activation is initiated by the production and release of interleukin (IL)-1 by macrophage cells. The binding of IL-1 to splenic lymphocyte receptors appears to be an absolute requirement for the differentiation of certain T lymphocytes into cells capable of producing a second mediator, IL-2. The binding of IL-2 provides a trigger for cell proliferation in subpopulations of T-helper and cytolytic cells. These rather complex interactions are diagrammed in Figure 13-3. Nutritional dependence of the proliferative response can be assessed by analyzing the release and binding of the interleukins by purified cell populations. A shift in the balance of subpopulations of T lymphocytes, specifically in T-helper and suppressor cells, may underlie nutritional modulation of CMI. In addition, technics are now available to monitor alterations in intracellular events following antigen/mitogen activation, including Ca^{++} flux, cyclic nucleotide production, and prostaglandin synthesis, which may be modified with nutritional intervention.

In summary, recent knowledge of the cellular and subcellular events

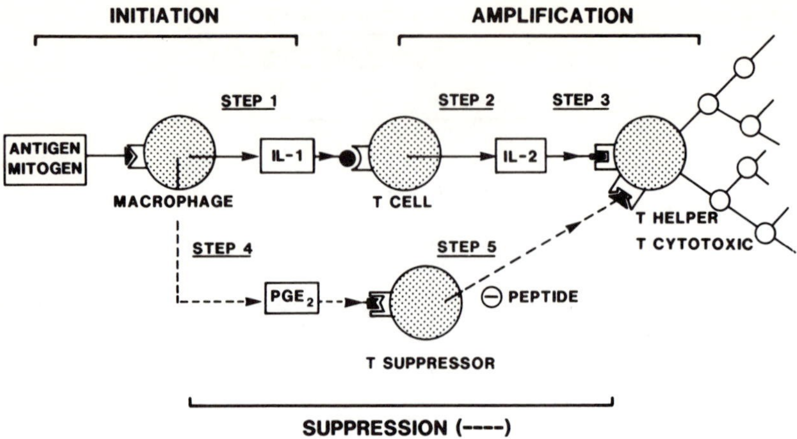

Figure 13-3. Peripheral cell interactions underlying initiation and suppression of T cell proliferative response. Note: Antigen/mitogen receptor interaction is required at each step.

which comprise intact immune response now permits a more sophisticated approach to assessing the effects of dietary manipulation at the cellular–molecular level. It is now possible to delineate which phase in the lymphocyte differentiation pathway is most susceptible to a given dietary manipulation. The potential for therapeutic intervention by dietary modulation of immune responsiveness depends on more precise elucidation at the molecular level.

Conclusion

We have reviewed the simultaneous and independent changes in immune responsiveness with age, suggesting that the sensitivity of T-cell function to a given dietary manipulation may vary with the state of immunologic maturation or senescence. The exaggerated susceptibility of humans to disease at both extremes of age, where periods of nutritional vulnerability coincide with suboptimal immune function, underscores the negative interaction between compromised nutritional status and immunocompetence. Adequate nutrition may be of pivotal importance in terms of disease prognosis, especially in the elderly, in whom immune function has already declined.

Single-nutrient modulation has been extensively documented in animal models under controlled laboratory conditions. However, these attempts to isolate the individual components of PCM are, by definition, academic approximations that cannot approach the multivariate interactions involved in the human condition. Nonetheless, an understanding of the independent contributions of individual nutrients to immune dysfunction must necessarily precede the understanding of the integrated state.

We have reviewed some of the important studies of dietary manipulation of CMI. In these studies, severity of deficiency, duration, and age of nutritional intervention appear to be interdependent variables, which must be critically considered when interpreting the extent and type of immunologic impairment.

Finally, we propose that future research effort can now extend beyond gross descriptive studies of T-cell-dependent functions by utilizing recent advances in cellular immunology and molecular biology. It is now technically possible to define nutrient interaction at the subcellular and molecular levels and in terms of T-cell ontogeny in order to delineate those points proximal to effector cell function that are most sensitive to a given nutritional deficiency.

Acknowledgments

This publication was funded in part by VA Medical Research Funds. We give special thanks to Jerry Sproul for manuscript preparation.

References

1. Makinodan T, Kay MMB: Age influence on the immune system. *Adv Immunol* 1980; 29:287–330.
2. Makinodan T, Hirokawa K, Peterson WJ, Bloom ET: Ontogeny and involution of the antibody response in mice, in Good RA (ed): *Ontogeny and Phylogeny of Immune Systems.* Japan, Iwanami Shoten, 1983.
3. Baker PJ, Morse HD, Cross SS, et al: Maturation of regulatory factors influencing magnitude of antibody response to capsular polysaccharide of type II Streptocococcus pneumoniae. *J Infect Dis* 1977; 136:820–824.
4. Sato K, Makinodan T: Age-related changes in the T cell transforming activity of factors secreted by reticulo-epithelial cells. *Proc. 5th Internat. Cong. Immunol* 1983.
5. Hori Y, Perkins EH, Halsall MK: Decline in phytohemagglutinin responsiveness of spleen cells in aged mice. *Proc Soc Exp Biol Med* 1973; 144:48–53.
6. Ferguson AC: Prolonged impairment of cellular immunity in children with intrauterine growth retardation. *J Pediatr* 1978; 33:52–56.
7. Chandra RK: Serum thymic hormone activity in protein-energy malnutrition. *Clin Exp Immunol* 1979; 38:228–230.
8. Chandra RK: Nutrition, immunity and infection: Present knowledge and future directions. *Lancet* 1983; 1:688–691.

9. Hirokawa K, Makinodan T: Thymic involution: Effect on T cell differentiation. *J Immunol* 1975; 114:1659–1664.
10. Singh J, Singh AK: Age related changes in human thymus. *Clin Exp Immunol* 1979; 37:507–511.
11. Gillis S, Kozak R, Durante M, Webster ME: Decreased production of and response to T cell growth factor by lymphocytes from aged humans. *J Clin Invest* 1981; 67:937–942.
12. Chang MP, Makinodan T, Peterson WJ, Strehler BL: Role of T cells and adherent cells in age-related decline in murine interleukin 2 production. *J Immunol* 1982; 129:2426–2430.
13. Webb DR, Nowowiejski I: Control of suppresser cell activation via endogenous prostaglandin synthesis: The role of T cells and macrophages. *Cell Immunol* 1981; 63:321–328.
14. Goodwin JS, Messner RP: Sensitivity of lymphocytes to prostaglandin E2 increases in subjects over age 70. *J Clin Invest* 1979; 64:434–439.
15. Bistrian BR, Blackburn GL, Vitale J, et al: Prevalence of malnutrition in the surgical patient. *JAMA* 1976; 235:1567–1570.
16. Bienia R, Ratcliff S, Barbour GL, Kummer M: Malnutrition in the hospitalized geriatric patient. *J Am Geriatr Soc* 1982; 30:433–436.
17. Chandra RK: Immunocompetence as a functional index of nutritional status. *Br Med Bull* 1981; 37:89–94.
18. Mullen JL, Gertper MH, Buzby GP, et al: Implications for malnutrition in the surgical patient. *Arch Surg* 1979; 114:121–125.
19. Meakins JL, Pietsch JB, Bubenick O, et al: Delayed hypersensitivity: Indicator of acquired failure of host defenses in sepsis and trauma. *Ann Surg* 1977; 186:241–249.
20. Gross RL, Newberne PM: Role of nutrition in immunologic function. *Physiol Rev* 1980; 60:188–302.
21. Schloen LH, Fernandes G, Garofalo JA, Good RA: Nutrition, immunity and cancer. Part II, Zinc, immune function and cancer. *Clin Bull* 1979; 9:63–75.
22. Gerbase-DeLima M, Liu RK, Cheney KE, et al: Immune function and survival in a long-lived mouse strain subjected to undernutrition. *Gerontologia* 1975; 21:184–202.
23. McCay CM, Crowell MF, Maynard LA: The effect of retarded growth upon the length of life span and upon the ultimate body size. *J Nutr* 1935; 10:63–79.
24. Ross MH, Lustbader E, Bras G: Dietary practices and growth responses as predictors of longevity. *Nature* 1976; 262:548–553.
25. Good RA, Fernandes G, West A: Nutrition, immunologic aging, and disease, in Singhal, Sinclair, Stiller (eds): *Aging and Immunity.* New York, Elsevier, 1979, pp 141–163.
26. Fernandes G, West A, Good RA: Nutrition, immunity and cancer. Part III: Effects of diet on the diseases of aging. *Clin Bull* 1979; 9:91–106.
27. Kos WL, Loria RM, Snodgrass MJ, et al: Inhibition of host resistance by nutritional hypercholesterolemia. *Infect Immun* 1979; 26:658–667.
28. Humphries GMK, McConnell HM: Potent immunosuppression by oxidized cholesterol. *J Immunol* 1979; 122:121–126.
29. Heiniger HJ: Cholesterol and its biosynthesis in normal and malignant lymphocytes. *Cancer Res* 1981; 41:3792–3794.

30. Chen HW: Enhanced sterol synthesis in Con A stimulated lymphocytes: Correlation with phospholipid synthesis and DNA synthesis. *J Cell Physiol* 1979; 100:147–158.
31. Meade CJ, Mertin J: Fatty acids and immunity. *Adv Lipid Res* 1978; 16:127–165.
32. Heiniger HJ, Brunner KT, Cerottini JC: Cholesterol is a critical cellular component for cytoxicity T-lymphocyte. *PNAS* 1978; 75:5683–5687.
33. Ip SHC, Abraham J, Cooper RA: Enhancement of blastogenesis in cholesterol enriched lymphocytes. *J Immunol* 1980; 124:87–93.
34. Broitman SA, Vitale JJ, Vavrousek-Jukuba E, Gottlieb LS: Polyunsaturated fat, cholesterol and large bowel tumorigenesis. *Cancer* 1977; 40:2455–2463.
35. Vitale JJ, Broitman SA: Lipids and immune function. *Cancer Res* 1981; 41:3706–3709.
36. Harmony JAK, Hui DY: Inhibition by membrane-bound low density lipoproteins of the primary inductive events of mitogen stimulated lymphocyte activation. *Cancer Res* 1981; 41:3799–3802.
37. Keusch GT, Wilson CS, Waksal SD: Nutrition, host defenses, and the immune system, in Gallin JI, Fauci AS (eds): *Advances in Host Defense Mechanisms*, vol 2. New York, Raven Press, 1982, pp 275–357.
38. Sandstead HH: Availability of zinc and its requirements in human subjects, in *Clinical, Biochemical and Nutritional Aspects of Trace Elements*. New York, Alan R Liss, 1982, pp 83–101.
39. Golden MH, Harland PS, Golden BE, Jackson AA: Zinc and immunocompetence in protein-energy malnutrition. *Lancet* 1978; 1:1226–1227.
40. Allen JI, Kay NE, McClain CJ: Severe zinc deficiency in humans: Association with a reversible T-lymphocyte dysfunction. *Ann Intern Med* 1981; 95:154–157.
41. Faraji B, Swendseid ME: Growth rate, tissue zinc levels and activity of selected enzymes in rats fed a zinc deficient diet by gastric tube. *J Nutr* 1983; 113:447–455.
42. Gross RL, Osdin N, Fong L, Newbern PM: Depressed immunological function in zinc depressed rats as measured by mitogen response of spleen, thyroid and peripheral blood. *Am J Clin Nutr* 1979; 32:1260–1265.
43. Fraker PJ, Haas SM, Leuke RW: Effect of zinc deficiency on the immune response of the young adult A/Jax mouse. *J Nutr* 1977; 107:1889–1895.
44. Carlomango MA, McMurray DN: Chronic zinc deficiency in rats: its influence in some parameters of humoral and cell-mediated immunity. *Nutr Res* 1983; 3:69–78.
45. Fernandes G, Nair M, Onoe K, et al: Impairment of cell mediated immunity functions by dietary zinc deficiency in mice. *Proc Soc Acad Sci* 1979; 76:457–461.
46. Fraker PJ, Zwickl CM, Leuke RW: Delayed type hypersensitivity in zinc deficient mice: impairment and restoration by responsivity to dinitrofluorobenzene. *J Nutr* 1982; 112:309–313.

14

Effects of Nutritional Factors on Memory Function

Arthur Cherkin

In 1982 a unique research facility opened: the U.S. Department of Agriculture's new Human Nutrition Research Center on Aging at Tufts University in Boston. A primary goal of its 50 principal investigators and 200 support personnel is to discover methods by which nutrition and other factors may delay or even prevent degenerative conditions. A degenerative condition of escalating concern is senile dementia, Alzheimer's type (SDAT), also known as primary degenerative dementia of senile onset or chronic brain syndrome. The hallmark of SDAT is memory failure because it is the earliest symptom, it occurs in all SDAT patients, and it is a major component of other serious sysmptoms, eg, confusion and disorientation. Memory failure also characterizes the so-called "reversible dementias," which can be misdiagnosed as "irreversible SDAT" (1). To what extent, if any, could memory failure be prevented, delayed, or reversed by nutritional means? Do the memory impairments observed in the young with *severe* nutritional deficiencies develop in the elderly with prolonged *subclinical* deficiencies (2,3)? Could diets be designed to improve memory, as diets are designed to control weight gain or hyptertension or diabetes?

For the purpose of this discussion, "memory" will be considered from a coarse-grained clinical point of view rather than from the fine-grained view of memory researchers. Thus, it will include the processes required to encode information into a durable memory trace and to recall information at a level that is functionally useful for carrying out independent activities of daily living. It must be kept in mind that memory processing is exceedingly complex. For example, memory can resist impairment by extremely severe insults to the brain, yet it can fail in a wide variety of ways (4), some of which are caused by apparently mild insults.

This discussion will focus upon five points. First, memory function can be impaired by specific avitaminoses, then restored by specific vitamin supplementation. Second, excessive levels of free amino acids in the brain can impair memory. Third, various dietary supplements can improve mental function in certain cases. Fourth, dietary precursors of neurotransmitters may improve memory in some demented patients. And fifth, nutrients can augment memory enhancement when combined with pharmacologic and psychologic interventions.

Vitamins

Thiamine

Deficiencies of nutrients such as niacin, cobalamin, and folate have been identified as causes of reversible dementia (1). We shall first discuss thiamine deficiency as a model of the interactions between avitaminoses and memory. When thiamine deficiency became widespread after the introduction of polished rice, severe memory failures appeared and were labeled "beriberi amnesia." One study of this condition resulted from the surrender of 32,000 British troops in Singapore in 1942. As de Wardener and Lennox (5) put it, this provided an "opportunity for placing a large number of healthy adults simultaneously on a standardized deficient diet and observing the results over a period of years." The abrupt change from normal British army rations to a diet of polished rice was followed in 6 weeks by the eruption of numerous symptoms including memory dysfunction. Of 52 patients selected for study, 61% showed memory loss for recent events. The symptomatology was complicated by dysentery in 45 cases. Keeping this in mind, the general sequence of signs and the prevalence were anorexia (88%), nausea and vomiting (57%), eye symptoms, primarily nystagmus (100%), mental changes (78%), other central nervous symptoms (11%), and signs of other forms of beriberi and vitamin deficiencies (90%). The mental changes started with anxiety (32%), followed by memory loss for recent events (61%), which progressed for 2 to 3 weeks and was followed by disorientation (46%) for time and then for place. "Memory for remote events remained excellent up to the stage of coma, except in three cases." No mention was made of aphasias; otherwise, the memory failures are grossly similar to those observed in advanced SDAT.

de Wardener and Lennox concluded that thiamine deficiency was the main etiologic factor in the symptoms they observed, as evidenced by the rapid and consistent reversal of symptoms when thiamine was administered, at an average daily dose of 2 mg by intramuscular injection. The clinical signs recovered in the same order in which they had appeared. Of 25 patients, 80% improved dramatically within two days and memory for recent events returned within two to seven days (in patients without far-advanced mental changes, where memory recovered more slowly). de Wardener and Lennox equated cerebral beriberi with Wernicke's encephalopathy on the basis of the similarity of symptoms, reversal of symptoms by thiamine, and neuropathologic evidence of hemorrhages in the mammillary bodies (6).

The limitations of controlled studies of thiamine deficiency in man are reduced by experiments on laboratory animals; these confirm the conclusions drawn from human studies. A single example is cited here (7). As seen in Figure 14-1, rats on a thiamine-deficient diet (filled circles) for 24 days began to lose their learned ability to avoid footshock in a shuttlebox; the loss progressed to more than 50% in 40 days. Oral administration of thiamine (1 mg/rat) on Day 40 and Day 41 totally reversed the loss by Day 42. Further deprivation of thiamine again caused progressive loss of the learned avoidance response; the loss was again promptly reversed within two to four days by a "normal diet." A control group of rats, pair-fed with the thiamine-deficient group to assure equal intake of all other nutrients, received also a daily oral supplement of 0.2 mg thiamine. These rats

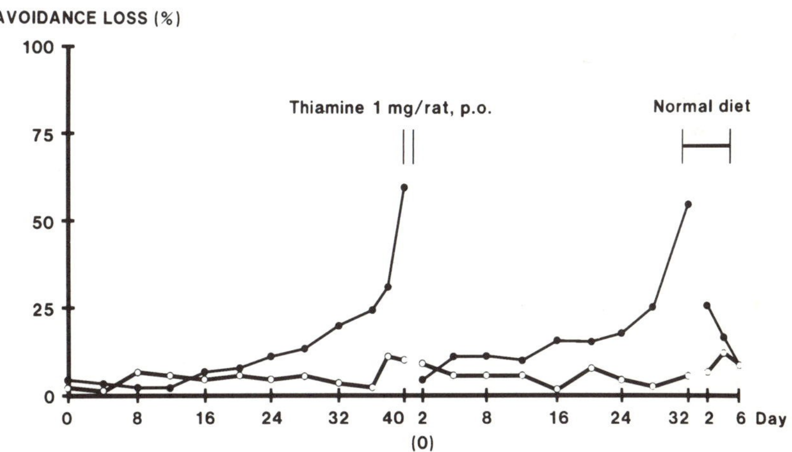

Figure 14-1. Inhibition of avoidance response in the shuttle box due to cerebral dysfunction caused by thiamine deficiency. The rats were maintained on a thiamine-deficient diet for 72 days, thiamine 1 mg/rat was administered orally on the 40th and 41st day, and from the 72nd day the animals were fed a normal diet to show recovery. See text for details of the diets. ●—●, thiamine deficient rats; ○—○, pair feeding rats. Reproduced from Yoshimura et al (7), with permission.

showed no loss of the avoidance response. The thiamine-induced reversal of avoidance loss did not occur in control groups that received supplemental riboflavin or pyridoxine, each at 1 mg/kg.

The "specificity" of thiamine in memory function may be more apparent than real. In addition to the metabolic roles of thiamine as a coenzyme throughout the body, thiamine and its phosphates have direct neurochemical activity in the central nervous system (8), interact with calcium (9) and magnesium (10), and may modulate release of acetylcholine from presynaptic nerve terminals (11). The interaction of thiamine with the brain cholinergic system suggests a possible link between beriberi amnesia (5) and senile amnesia (12).

Niacin, Pyridoxine, Cobalamin, and Folic Acid

Like thiamine, niacin is identified with a widespread deficiency disease (pellagra), which presents with a major symptom of memory failure (dementia of pellagra) that is reversible by restoring the vitamin. Serum pyridoxine in man, as measured indirectly by serum transaminase assay, declines with age but can be elevated to young adult levels within 3 weeks of pyridoxine feeding in the elderly (13). In the 3-week old rat, learning of an active avoidance task was impaired after 5 weeks of pyridoxine deficiency, then restored to normal within 1 week after a single injection of pyridoxine (50 mg/kg, i.p.) (14).

The relationship of cobalamin (vitamin B_{12}) to memory is of interest because the memory dysfunction can precede by years the hematologic or spinal cord symptoms of pernicious anemia caused by avitaminosis B_{12}. Indeed, the possibility of mental abnormality in vitamin B_{12} deficiency, in the absence of anemia, was suggested in 1905, long before the pathogenesis of pernicious anemia was understood (15). Evaluation of memory in pernicious anemia patients, using a synonym learning test, revealed abnormal short-term memory in 71%; treatment with B_{12} restored memory scores to normal within 10 to 27 days in 75% of 12 pernicious anemia patients with impaired memory (15). Strachan and Henderson (15) advised that a diagnosis of senile dementia should not be made, even in nonanemic patients, without excluding avitaminosis B_{12} by appropriate tests, among them, serum B_{12} assay.

Amino Acids

The role of amino acids as precursors of neurotransmitters (eg, of tryptophan to serotonin; tyrosine to dopamine, norepinephrine and epinephrine; and glutamic acid to γ-aminobuytyric acid) and the part these neurotransmitters play in memory function makes it inevitable that amino acids affect memory. The large distortions of plasma amino acid levels that accompany various inborn errors of metabolism (16), such as phenylketonuria, are associated with such severe mental retardation that they are unsatisfactory models of memory dysfunctions. This section will therefore limit itself to considering glutamic acid and proline. Tryptophan and tyrosine will be discussed under the topic, *precursor treatment,* below.

Glutamic Acid

During the 1950s and 1960s, a controversial literature argued the effects of glutamic acid upon human mental function, especially in mental retardation. One review concluded: "The tendency for negative findings to occur in the more adequately controlled experiments sheds doubt on the hypothesis that glutamic acid medication has a specifically beneficial effect on intellectual functioning" (17). A rebuttal review reached the opposite conclusion, as follows (18):

> A considerable amount of evidence indicates a role for glutamic acid in cognitive functioning. The sheer weight of this evidence is surprising; indeed, there is more sound experimental confirmation of the positive effects of glutamic acid than appears to exist for most of the psychotropic drugs now in common therapeutic use. The earlier judgments that glutamic acid has little behavioral effect may be considered to be based upon an incomplete or unsound analysis.

The dispute, reminiscent of today's controversies over the effectiveness of modern memory-enhancing treatments (eg, lecithin), reflects our ignorance of the mechanisms involved in normal memory processing, let alone the critical brain changes that *cause* memory failure, as opposed to merely being correlated with such failure. In any event, a preparation containing monosodium L-glutamate in combination with thiamine, riboflavin, niacin, pyridoxine, cyanocobalamin, and ferrous sulfate (Glutavite®, Crookes-Barnes Laboratories) was evaluated with generally favorable results in geriatric patients with memory dysfunction (eg, 19, 20). It may be added that the neurotoxic effects of oral glutamic acid appear to have been overemphasized, since monosodium glutamate "given with food or drinking water has never been shown to induce *any* neurotoxic effect at *any* dose, in *any* animal species, at *any* age, under *any* experimental condition tested" (21).

Other Amino Acids

Amino acids have complex effects upon learning and memory. For example, mice fasted for 24 hours declined more rapidly in avoidance performance than did fed controls (22). Feeding casein, glucose, or serine totally prevented the fast-induced impairment, whereas histidine, tyrosine, methionine, and trypotophan increased the impairment. Other amino acids had little or no effect. The positive effect of serine was attributed to its palatability and its gluconeogenic effect.

Proline

Interest in the role of proline in memory was stimulated by a new hypothesis of memory formation, which involves patterned release of intracellular glutamate during a learning experience, followed by a sequence of neuronal events leading to increased dendritic spine diameter and thus facilitation of neural transmission (23). Since L-proline (L-PRO) antagonized the glutamate effect, it was predicted that L-PRO would impair memory. This prediction has been confirmed in three animal models: chick (23, 24) goldfish (25), and mouse (26). The interesting points are as follows:

1. The amnestic effect of L-PRO is more powerful than that of electroconvulsive shock (ECS).
2. The side effects of amnestic doses of L-PRO are minimal (slight behavioral and EEG slowing for 15 minutes).
3. The amnestic effect is stereospecific, since D-PRO is not amnestic.
4. The amnestic effect is structure specific, since the lower and higher homologs of L-PRO are not amnestic.
5. L-PRO does not act either through occult brain seizures or by inhibiting brain protein synthesis.

The normal brain is protected against the amnestic effect of L-PRO by the blood–brain barrier, but if this barrier were reduced for any reason, free L-PRO in the brain could rise to an amnestic level. Recent evidence indicates that aging is accompanied by changes in the blood–brain barrier (27). A pilot study of L-PRO levels in cerebrospinal fluid, however, revealed no significant difference between 4 normal controls and 10 patients with SDAT (28).

The significance of the foregoing evidence is that a moderate increase in the brain concentration of a single nutrient can impair memory without other gross manifestations. Weakening of the blood–brain barrier for any reason places the brain at risk because nutrient molecules ordinarily excluded can penetrate into brain tissue.

Minerals

Electrolyte imbalances and acid–base disturbance are included among the causes of reversible dementia (1,29). Potassium supplementatation (48 MEQ K^+/day for 2 weeks), evaluated in a controlled double-blind, cross-over design using 46 elderly subjects, yielded negative results; memory scores on a paired-associated word learning test did not differ for subjects on potassium or placebo (29).

Current interest in dietary zinc invites mention of a suggestion that "administration of additional zinc could prevent or delay the onset of dementia in subjects genetically at risk" (30). Burnet reasons that since zinc is essential to most enzymes concerned with DNA replication, repair, and transcription, an age-associated reduced availability of zinc for enzyme synthesis could lead to a cascade of effects of impaired neuronal DNA-handling systems. The original article should be read to appreciate the rationale for this hypothesis, which offers a plausible specific unitary biochemical cause of the multiple brain changes observed in SDAT.

Dietary Supplements

Up to this point, our discussion has emphasized the relationship of severe single nutrient deficiencies to memory. In the real world, however, whenever malnutrition of the elderly occurs, mild multiple deficiencies of nutritional factors are the rule (2). To deal with these, clinical studies of complex dietary supplementation have been carried out and two examples of these will also be described. The results to date are less than encouraging.

Multiple Deficiencies

The relationship between severe nutritional deficiencies and mental impairment has been amply demonstrated by animal and clinical studies, as discussed above. Much less certain is the relationship between subclinical deficiencies and memory in the aged, especially in the understudied noninstitutionalized population. A recent study therefore correlated nutritional status with cognitive function in 260 men and women over 60 years old, living in the community (2). Significant correlations were found between memory test scores and the blood levels of riboflavin and ascorbic acid. When the bottom 5% or 10% of subjects were compared with the top 90% of subjects in terms of blood levels of specific nutrients, significant decrements in memory scores appeared for the subjects low in plasma ascorbic acid or cobalamin, but not for those low in thiamine, riboflavin, pyridoxine, or folate. When the basis of comparison was dietary intake based upon a three-day food record, significant decrements were observed for subjects low in protein, thiamine, riboflavin, niacin, pyridoxine, cobalamin, and folate.

Goodwin et al (2) properly emphasize that the correlations they observed between low blood levels of nutrients and low cognitive scores do "not mean that there is a causal relationship between nutrition and cognition." Among the sources of uncertainty is the chicken-and-egg question: Does malnutrition impair cognition or does impaired cognition induce poor dietary habits? Nevertheless, the authors suggested a controlled prospective study of the effect of vitamin supplementation on cognitive status in noninstitutionalized elderly individuals; this merits serious consideration. An editorial on the Goodwin et al study emphasizes "the critical importance of rigorous experimental design if such studies are to be meaningfully interpreted" (3). As a part of such design, careful attention should be paid to detecting subgroups of responders to vitamin supplementation, using a repeated crossover, double-blind technique (31).

Multiple Vitamin Supplementation

Suitable nutrient supplementation raises biochemical measures of nutrients in malnourished elderly to the levels found in normal young subjects, but "there is little evidence that such supplementation imparts corresponding functional benefit" (32). A longitudinal investigation of 12 hospital patients aged 71 to 84 was therefore carried out over a period of 18 weeks (32). A baseline period (Weeks 1–2) was followed by a supplementation period (Weeks 3–14), then a return to presupplement conditions (Weeks 15–18). Each subject served as his or her own control. The supplement was a malted milk drink, which provided 50% or more of the recommended daily intake of vitamins A, B_1, B_2, B_{12}, C, D, niacin, folic acid, calcium, and iron. In general, grip strength and the biochemical measures of vitamin status rose during supplementation and fell after supplementation. Mental function proved to be "extremely difficult to assess because of the many factors that affect the measurements." In any event, the scores on five mental function tests, each of which involved memory to a greater or lesser extent, did not change with supplementation.

Yeast Supplementation

The controversial literature on the effect of RNA upon memory led to an evaluation of a daily supplement of 10–15 g of dried baker's yeast in residents of homes for the aged (33). A battery of eight tests of memory function, applied at the end of the supplementation period of 4 months, revealed essentially no differences between the experimental group (N = 58) and a control group, which received a placebo bread supplement in place of the yeast. The authors suggest that the experimental period was too short for definite changes to appear, but an examination of their memory test scores indicates that six out of eight were poorer in the yeast supplement group, raising a question about prolonging such a study.

Precursor Treatment

Recent attention to dietary precursor treatment of geriatric memory dysfunction has emphasized the cholinergic system (12,34–40). Other precursors studied include the amino acids tyrosine (precursor of dopamine, norepinephrine, and epinephrine) and tryptophan or 5-hydroxytryptophan (precursors of serotonin). These will be discussed briefly, followed by a more extensive discussion of choline and lecithin.

Tyrosine and Tryptophan

A clinical trial of the combination of tyrosine with 5-hydroxytryptophan (plus carbidopa to inhibit decarboxylation of these aromatic amino acids) was attempted in 10 patients with severe dementia caused by multi-infarct dementia, Alzheimer's disease, or both (41). Neuropsychologic evaluation was completed in four patients, of whom two showed improved performance, particularly in cognition and memory, after 8 and 30 weeks of therapy. Therapy was discontinued in four patients because of side effects and in two others because of no benefit after 6–12 weeks. Overall, the results are comparable to those reported with cholinergic precursor treatment insofar as memory improvement is concerned, ie, modest improvement in a subgroup of subjects.

Choline and Lecithin

The original rationale advanced for these compounds, simply stated, is as follows (39). Acetycholine is an essential neurotransmitter for formation of the engram, the physiologic basis of long-term memory. Patients with senile dementia are deficient in brain acetylcholine. The immediate precursors of acetylcholine are choline and acetyl coenzyme A. Synthesis of acetylcholine could be increased by enlarging the concentration of brain choline, restoring acetylcholine to normal levels, and thus renewing normal memory formation. A large number of animal and clinical studies, carried out to test the prediction suggested by the rationale, have been critically reviewed (12). An example of each is described below.

Choline: Animal Study

The effect of choline on memory was evaluated in mice by comparing a choline-deficient group (<1 mg of choline per g of chow) and a choline-enriched group (12–15 mg of choline per g of chow), with a control group (1.6 mg of choline per g of chow) (42). After 4.5 months on these three choline diets, the mice (now aged 13 months) were trained on a one-trial passive avoidance task, then tested for memory retention either one day or five days after training (Fig. 14-2). The retention scores of the choline-deficient mice were significantly worse than the scores of the choline-enriched mice. Mice on the control diet had intermediate scores. Furthermore, the choline-enriched 13-month-old mice performed like normal-choline young mice (2–9 months), whereas the choline-deficient 13-month-old mice performed like normal-choline senescent mice (23–31 months).

These remarkable results support the cholinergic hypothesis of geriatric memory dysfunction (12), whether the mechanism is indeed increased formation of acetylcholine (35,39), or increased formation of dendritic spines (43), or increased fluidity of neuronal membranes, inasmuch as choline is a moiety of lecithin (phosphatidyl choline) (44), or direct action of choline (45). The latter possibility is based on the evidence that choline itself can enhance 1-week memory retention in mice when injected directly into the brain in an appropriate dose (45). A dose of 50 μg per mouse enhanced memory; lower and higher doses had less effect,

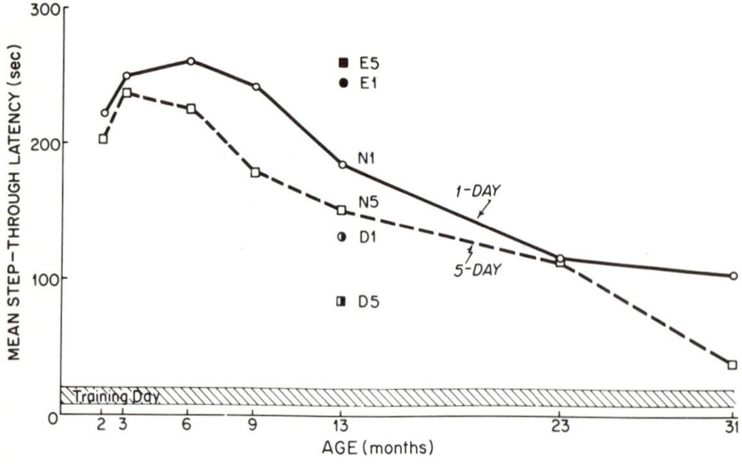

Figure 14-2. Retention of the single-trial passive avoidance task across the life spans of C57B1/6j mice. Retention is expressed as latency to reenter the rear chamber 1 day (○———○) or (5 days □– – – –□) after the training. A significant decrease in retention occurred across the life spans of mice tested either 1 day [$F(6, 108) = 6.65$, $p < .001$] or 5 days [$F(6, 113) = 7.38$, $p < .001$] after training. Because no consistent age-related differences in latency were observed on the training day (cross-hatched area), it is reasonable to assume that this behavioral deficit is not due to differences in activity or responsiveness, but probably reflects impairments in retention of the training trial. Six groups of 13-month-old mice are represented: enriched choline diet, tested for 5-day (■) or 1-day (●) retention; normal choline diet, tested for 5-day (□) or 1-day (○) retention; and deficient choline diet, tested for 5-day (◧) or 1-day (◑) retention. Data from Bartus et al (42).

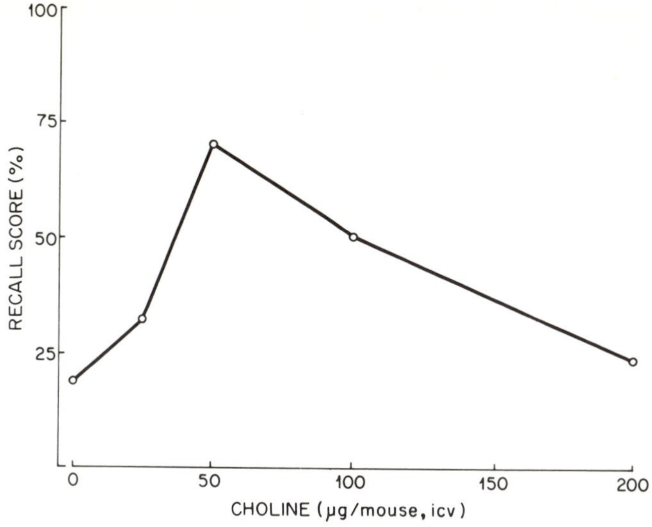

Figure 14-3. Retention of active avoidance T-maze training by 7-week old CD-1 male mice. Retention is expressed as percentage of each group ($N = 21–27$) that met the criterion for retention test performance 1 week after training. The stated doses of choline chloride were injected intracerebroventricularly, in 1.0 μL of saline, immediately after training. The recall score of the 50-μg group is significantly higher than that of the saline control group ($p < .001$, chi-square test) and of the 200-μg group ($p < .005$, chi-square test). Data from Flood et al (45).

and a dose of 200 μg per mouse actually impaired retention (Figure 14-3). It is, of course, possible that more than one of these four postulated mechanisms act upon memory formation.

Lecithin: Clinical Studies

Despite the positive results with choline or lecithin in animal studies, the results of clinical trials have been disappointing (12). Analysis of 17 clinical studies showed no improvement in 13 and only modest improvement in four. A recent report (36), however, argues that:

> published trials have been difficult to interpret because of defects in design. The numbers have been small, the cases often very severely advanced, the doses of lecithin low, or the preparations used have contained low proportions of phosphatidylcholine. Many reports have been of uncontrolled trials over a short duration and with no follow-up.

Levy et al (36) therefore launched a double-blind study of 52 early cases of Alzheimer's disease, using lecithin containing at least 90% phosphatidylcholine, at doses approaching the maximum tolerable (25 g per day), administered for 6 months, followed by lecithin-free follow-up for 6 months. Early results were analyzed for 30 subjects matched for age (74 years), age at onset of Alzheimer's disease (69 years), duration of illness (4 years), and parietal dysfunction score (22–25). The lecithin group ($N = 16$) was compared to the placebo group ($N = 14$) on eight tests, after six months of lecithin administration. The placebo group deteriorated on all eight tests; deterioration was less for the lecithin group on five tests, but the difference was significant for only the abbreviated mental test score and a paired associate learning task. Only the latter showed a significant improvement over the prelecithin score. During the follow-up period of 6 months, the group from which lecithin was withdrawn, as compared with the placebo group, deteriorated more on five tests, significantly so on three (abbreviated mental test score, paired associate learning task, and forced choice word test). Levy et al considered this "negative carry-over . . . might be due to receptor desensitisation, enzyme induction, or some other factor."

Another study of purified lecithin (95% phosphatidylcholine), conducted for 6 months in a double-blind design using 13 Alzheimer's disease patients, failed to show alleviation of the symptoms of dementia (38). Progression of the disease was slowed, however, in all but one patient. The authors suggest that "lecithin may be used more effectively in combination with other substances, such as piracetam, which may enhance or potentiate its action in the CNS."

The short-term side effects of choline, lecithin, or phosphatidylcholine and the possibility of adverse effects from long-term intakes of large amounts, have been reviewed by Wood and Allison (46). Concern with acute short-term side effects and with potential long-term effects is one motivation for our present series of experiments to develop synergistic combinations of cholinergic drug memory enhancers, which will permit reducing the effective dosage. Our studies with a mouse model to date suggest that two-drug combinations permit memory enhancement with very large dose reductions, as much as 95% (Fig. 14-4), whereas toxic effects are only additive (47). Of equal significance is the consistent finding of inverted-U dose response curves for all cholinergic drugs tested, alone or in combination (45,47), as well as for other classes of memory-enhancing compounds. This means that low doses have no effect, higher doses give increasing enhancement of memory retention, and still higher doses show decreasing enhancement. Thus, some of the negative results reported might have been brought on by excessively high doses, as well as by insufficient doses. Finally, in all cases we have tested, the high doses that do not enhance memory actually turn out to be amnestic when tested in "overtrained" mice. We have therefore suggested that a clinical trial strategy should be based on doses individualized for each patient, with double-blind crossover testing of the optimal dose and a placebo (48).

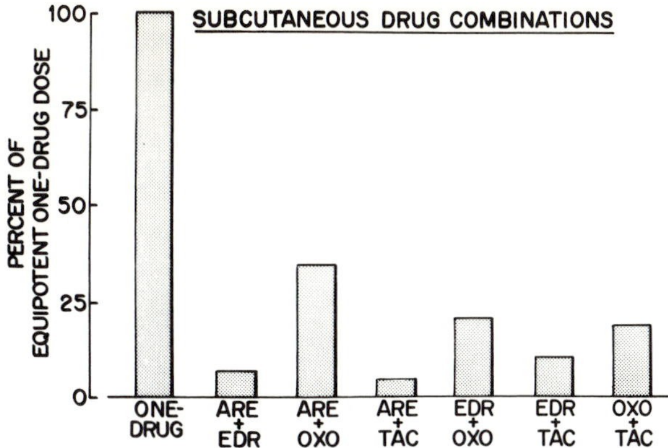

Figure 14-4. Reduced subcutaneous doses of two-drug combinations required for peak response (75% or higher recall score) in mice. The doses in each optimal combination were converted to the equipotent dose of ARE, to permit comparison. The ordinate represents the percent of the equipotent one-drug dose, normalized to 100%. The first bar refers to arecoline (ARE), or edrophonium (EDR), or oxotremorine (OXO), or tacrine (TAC), each administered by itself. Reproduced from Cherkin A, Flood JF: Remarkable synergism among memory-enhancing cholinergic drugs in mice, in: Sinex FM, and Regelson W (eds): *Intervention in the Aging Process,* Part A. New York, Alan R. Liss, 1983; pp 225–245.

Future Directions

The disappointing clinical results to date with memory enhancement by pharmacologic means have led to an appeal for more innovative drug approaches (49). The same appeal can be made in the case of nutritional approaches. We now venture upon the thin ice of advice to suggest that we need a more realistic therapeutic goal and that we should explore a multimodal approach based upon synergistic interactions.

Therapeutic Goal: Subgroups of Responders

Memory is a many-splendored thing. When we understand how a fleeting sensory input is transmuted into a durable memory trace, stored, and recalled at will, the display of that knowledge will resemble a complex metabolic map. We are only beginning to understand this phenomenon, how it becomes impaired by age-related changes in the brain, and how such impairment might be prevented, delayed, or ameliorated. With today's meager knowledge, we are unlikely to restore youthful memory function in an advanced case of senile dementia. A more realistic clinical goal would be to restore sufficient memory function to reduce the level of required care by reducing the amnesia, disorientation, confusion, wandering, and other symptoms that increase dependence upon caregivers—both in the family and in institutions. Furthermore, the improvement need not be in the majority of any group of elderly in the study population, but only in a reasonable subgroup of responders. This means abandonment of a response criterion based upon measures of central tendency in a *group*, in favor of a criterion of reproducible functional improvement in *individuals*. Because of wide individual variation, and narrow therapeutic windows in many cases, individual dose titration may be mandatory despite the difficulties and expense of such refinement.

Interactions: Multimodal Approach

The brain may be considered as a system for organizing vastly complex interactions into simple outcomes. I suggest that the research strategy of assuming a single etiology for memory failure and of manipulating a single variable has a plausible alternative, namely, that memory fails as a result of the combined effect of multiple etiologies, which call for a multiple attack. The latter includes attention to nutritional factors, where thiamine provides an instructive example. The knowledge that athiaminosis leads to amnesia and thiamine reverses the amnesia is extremely simplistic. Thiamine is involved as a coenzyme in metabolic reactions throughout the body and its monophosphate, diphosphate, and triphosphate forms are directly involved in neurochemical processes independent of its coenzyme function (8,50,51). The possibility has been suggested that athiaminosis might decrease synthesis of acetyl-CoA from pyruvate, thereby depress synthesis of brain acetylcholine, and thus explain the neurologic disturbances of athiaminosis, but experimental studies in rats have not supported this suggestion (8).

The bewildering complexity of interactions among the numerous factors that influence memory has too long delayed efforts to deal with such interactions experimentally. For example, individuals vary tremendously in their daily consumption of coffee, tea, cola beverages, tobacco, and alcoholic beverages. Although it is well established that the caffeine, nicotine, and ethanol contained in these substances can have profound effects upon memory, nutritional studies lose sight of these intakes.

The potential magnitude of such interactive factors is exemplified by our animal studies in a much less complex and more tightly controlled situation than in elderly populations living at home. For example, we find that a two-drug combination of cholinomimetics or of anticholinesterases can raise the 1-week memory retention scores of young adult mice to ceiling levels, using doses that are reduced as much as 95% from the equipotent memory-enhancing doses of each drug alone (47). We demonstrated this supra-additivity by direct injection into the brain (47), confirmed it using the subcutaneous route (52), and are now studying the oral route.

If two drugs of *similar* mechanism of action can potentiate each other's enhancement of memory so markedly, what potentiation may be expected of combinations of treatments with *different* mechanisms of action? This question calls for an answer and efforts to do so have been underway, including combinations of nutritional factors with drugs. For example, a combination of choline with piracetam (a drug considered to improve brain metabolism) was far superior to either compound alone in improving memory in aged rats (53). Curiously, the combination did not potentiate the effects of either choline or piracetam alone on brain choline or acetylcholine levels, and in some cases even reduced the single compound effects. The results were considered to "support the notion that in order to achieve substantial efficacy in aged subjects it may be necessary to reduce multiple, interactive neurochemical dysfunctions in the brain, or affect activity in more than one parameter of a deficient metabolic pathway." This sensible view has been applied in a number of clinical trials of nutrient-plus-drug combinations. For example, a small double-blind study showed that a combination of lecithin plus physostigmine (an anticholinesterase that slows the enzymatic hydrolysis of acetylcholine in the synapse) enhanced memory in patients with Alzheimer's disease under conditions where lecithin or physostigmine alone was ineffective (54). A combination of choline plus piracetam (to improve brain metabolism) improved memory storage and retrieval in a responder subgroup of elderly subjects (55).

A nutrient-plus-drug combination studied during the 1960s provided niacin plus pentylenetetrazol (PTZ). The latter is a central nervous system stimulant marketed under the trade-name Metrazol® to improve geriatric mental function. In a double-blind study of this combination, 25 geriatric outpatients received a total daily dose of 300 mg niacin plus 600 mg PTZ over a period of 4 weeks (56). A randomized control group ($N = 25$) received a placebo. The treated group improved significantly more than the placebo group on eight behavioral measures, but not on memory. However, the number of patients with a memory rating of "good" increased from one to four in the treated group but remained at zero in the placebo group. (Repeated crossovers from treatment to placebo would have revealed whether the three improved patients represented a subgroup of responders, but such a study was unfortunately not carried out.)

In another study of the niacin-PTZ combination, 29 geriatric patients with marked memory defect, and with various psychiatric diagnoses, served as their own controls; after 3 weeks of treatment, 31% of the patients had improved memory ratings (57). In addition, "48% of the patients who previously had to be assisted with their personal needs were able to take care of their personal hygiene and to attend to their personal needs alone," thus achieving the limited therapeutic goal advised above. In contradiction to the positive reports on the niacin–PTZ combination, a double-blind, placebo-controlled study of a higher daily dose (400 mg niacin plus 800 mg PTZ) had no significant effect in 40 patients with schizophrenia or dementia (58). No memory tests were carried out in this study, however, In another negative report, a single intravenous infusion of physostigmine failed to improve memory in healthy elderly subjects receiving oral lecithin (95% phosphatidyl choline, 20–26 g/day); lecithin alone or physostigmine alone had no effect in this study (59).

The multimodal approach to memory enhancement is made up of rational synergistic combinations of drugs, nutritional factors, and psychosocial interventions, including cognitive skills training, exercise, socialization, and pet animal adjuvants (48). The strategy was well-expressed as follows, for psychopharmacology in general (60):

> Now we have come to the point of asking how drugs alone compare with drugs in combination with other therapies. This necessarily brings into focus a very wide array of treatments, including family therapy, social therapy, work therapies, and many other types of rehabilitative activity. Resolving the questions raised in determining the interactions of drugs with other therapies will almost certainly become the most time-consuming, complicated, and costly of all recent ventures in psychopharmacology. There seems to be no way out but to undertake the required painstaking experimental activities for a potentially staggering number of combinations and permutations. It is a happy fact, nevertheless, that our colleagues working in this field have already made significant progress.

Devising clinically effective combinations will indeed be time consuming and complicated. For example, lecithin combined with memory training failed to show any beneficial effect upon memory in Alzheimer's disease patients treated for 2 weeks (61). Nevertheless, the positive results found with drug combinations (47) and with drug–nutrient combinations (52–54,56), described above, encourage persistence in exploring the strategy of combination therapies.

The consideration of nutrients as therapeutic agents has led to the following question, which Wurtman considers to go beyond a mere matter of terminology (39):

> When large doses of a nutrient separated from the other constituents of foods that are in its usual source, are given to people specifically to treat a disease or condition, does the nutrient thereby become a drug?

After considering the regulatory and practical consequences of such a designation, Wurtman wonders that if old people benefit from dietary enrichment in tyrosine or tryptophan or lecithin, should "their continued reliance on normal but unenriched diets be construed as constituting poor nutrition?" Since all substances included in the United States Pharmacopoeia and the National Formulary are legally defined as "drugs," and since thiamine, riboflavin, niacin, and ascorbic acid are included, the terminology question is moot. Furthermore, the borderline between a "nutritional" or "physiologic" dose and a "therapeutic" or "pharmacologic" dose might prove difficult to establish with general acceptance.

For the above reasons, a simpler and more appropriate point of view—albeit still controversial—is the orthomolecular theory advanced by Pauling (62,63) because nutritional improvement of memory in geriatric patients fits within the concept of orthomolecular psychiatry, defined as "the achievement and preservation of mental health by varying the concentration in the human body of substances that are normally present, such as the vitamins" (62,63). In view of the findings of undernutrition of many elderly, both in the community and in institutions, it would appear prudent to supplement their daily dietary intake with a multiple vitamin and mineral preparation, to reduce the risk of deficiencies of these important nutrients for normal memory function.

Summary and Conclusions

Memory failure is a major concern of the elderly and it is the hallmark of the senile dementias, which afflict 5% to 10% of those above 65 years of age. Undernutrition and malnutrition are arguably considered to be problems in 30% to 50% of the elderly, although clear nutritional standards have yet to be established for the aged population. The relationship between memory failure and undernutrition is only partly understood. The rapidly increasing elderly population calls for a better understanding of nutritional measures, which might improve memory or delay its progressive deterioration in dementias.

There is clear evidence from human and animal studies that severe deficiencies of water-soluble vitamins, eg, thiamine, niacin, pyridoxine, folic acid, or cyancobalamin, result in impaired memory, which can be restored to normal by supplying the deficient vitamin. Multiple neurobiologic changes undoubtedly accompany both the deficient and the restored vitamin status.

The possibility that excess nutrients in the brain may impair mental functions is shown by the effects of the hyperaminoacidemias. Impairment of memory by an excess of free L-proline in the brain has been demonstrated in goldfish, chick, and mouse models.

Feeding of amino acids, eg, tyrosine, tryptophan, or glutamic acid, as dietary precursors of neurotransmitters, has produced modest improvement of memory in some studies, with negative results in others. More attention has been paid to choline and lecithin, as precursors of acetylcholine. Despite promising results in some animal experiments, most clinical trials have yielded only modest improvement in memory, at best. Direct injection of choline into the brains of mice enhanced memory retention at an optimal dose, with reduced enhancement at lower or higher doses. This emphasizes the need for dose–response studies, with nutrients as well as with drugs, and may offer a partial explanation for some of the negative results reported.

In addition to dose–response studies, future investigations of the effects of nutritional factors upon memory should take into consideration: a realistic therapeutic goal, individualized optimal doses for each subject, a search for subgroups of reliable responders, and combinations of nutrients with memory-enhancing drugs and psychosocial interventions.

References

1. Task Force Sponsored by the National Institute on Aging: Treatment possibilities for mental impairment in the elderly. *JAMA* 1980; 244:259–263.
2. Goodwin JS, Goodwin JM, Garry PJ: Association between nutritional status and cognitive functioning in a healthy elderly population. *JAMA* 1983; 249:2917–2921.
3. Raskind M: Nutrition and cognitive function in the elderly. *JAMA* 1983; 249:2939–2940.
4. Weingartner H, Grafman J, Boutelle W, et al: Forms of memory failure. *Science* 1983; 221:380–382.
5. de Wardener HE, Lennox B: Cerebral beriberi (Wernicke's encephalopathy): Review of 52 cases in a Singapore prisoner-of-war hospital. *Lancet* 1947; 1:11–17.
6. Phillips GB, Victor M, Adams RD, et al: A study of the nutritional defect in Wernicke's syndrome: The effect of a purified diet, thiamine and other vitamins on the clinical manifestations. *J Clin Invest* 1952; 31:859–871.
7. Yoshimura K, Nishibe Y, Inoue Y, et al: Animal experiments on thiamine avitaminosis and cerebral function. *J Nutr Sci Vitaminol* 1976; 22:429–437.
8. Sturman JA, Rivlin RS: Pathogenesis of brain dysfunction in deficiency of thiamine, riboflavin, pantothenic acid, or vitamin B_6, in Gaull GE (ed): *Biology of Brain Dysfunction,* vol 3 New York, Plenum Press, 1975, pp 425–466.
9. Itokawa Y: Is calcium deficiency related to thiamine-dependent neuropathy in pigeon? *Brain Res* 1975; 94:475–484.
10. Traviesa DC: Magnesium deficiency: a possible cause of thiamine refractoriness in Wernicke-Korsakoff encephalopathy. *J Neurol Neurosurg Psychiatry* 1974; 37:959–962.
11. Eder L, Hirt L, Dunant Y: Possible involvement of thiamine in acetylcholine release. *Nature* 1976; 264:186–188.
12. Bartus RT, Dean III RL, Beer B, Lippa AS: The cholinergic hypothesis of geriatric memory dysfunction. *Science* 1982; 217:408–417.
13. Ranke E, Tauber SA, Horonick A, et al: Vitamin B_6 deficiency in the aged. *J Gerontol* 1960; 15:41–44.

14. Stewart CN, Coursin DB, Bhagavan HN: Avoidance behavior in vitamin B_6-deficient rats. *J Nutr* 1975; 105:1363–1370.
15. Strachan RW, Henderson JG: Psychiatric syndromes due to avitaminosis B_{12} with normal blood and marrow. *J Med* (New Series) 1965; 34:303–317.
16. Guroff G: Toxic effects of food constituents on the brain, in Wurtman RJ, Wurtman JJ (eds): *Nutrition and the Brain,* vol 4 New York, Raven Press, pp 29–77.
17. Astin AW, Ross S: Glutamic acid and human intelligence. *Psychol Bull* 1960; 57:429–434.
18. Vogel W, Broverman DM, Draguns JG: The role of glutamic acid in cognitive behaviors. *Psychol Bull* 1966; 65:367–382.
19. Gasster M: Clinical experince with L-glutavite in aged patients with behavior problems and memory deficits. *J Am Geriatr Soc* 1961; 9:370–375.
20. Whitman RM: Re-evaluation of a glutamate-vitamin-iron preparation (L-glutavite) in the treatment of geriatric chronic brain syndrome, with special reference to research design. *J Am Geriatr Soc* 1966; 14:859–870.
21. Garattini S: Evaluation of neurotoxic effects of glutamic acid, in Wurtman RJ, Wurtman JJ (eds): *Nutrition and the Brain,* vol 4. New York, Raven Press, 1979; pp 79–116.
22. Bovet D, Leathwood P, Mauron J, et al: The effects of different amino acid diets on a fast-induced performance decrement in mice. *Psychopharmacologia* 1971; 22:91–99.
23. Van Harreveld A, Fifkova E: Involvement of glutamate in memory formation. *Brain Res* 1974; 81:455–467.
24. Cherkin A, Van Harreveld A: L-proline and related compounds: Correlation of structure, amnesic potency and anti-spreading depression potency. *Brain Res* 1978; 156:265–273.
25. Riege WH, Cherkin A: Intracranial L-proline induces retrograde amnesia in goldfish. *Neurosci Abstr* 1976; 2:434.
26. Davis JL, Cherkin A: Intraventricular L-proline induces retrograde amnesia in mice. *IRCS Med Sci* 1977; 5:88.
27. Wisniewski HM, Kozlowski PB: Evidence for blood–brain barrier changes in senile dementia of the Alzheimer type (SDAT). *Ann NY Acad Sci* 1982; 396:119–129.
28. Baxter CF, Baldwin RA, Pomara N, Brinkman SD: Proline in the cerebrospinal fluid of normal subjects and Alzheimer's-disease patients, as determined with a new double-labeling assay technique. *Biochem Med* 1984; in press.
29. Burr ML, St. Leger AS, Westlake CA, Davies HEF: Dietary potassium deficiency in the elderly: A controlled trial. *Age Ageing* 1974; 4:148–149.
30. Burnet FM: A possible role of zinc in the pathology of dementia. *Lancet* 1981; 1:186–188.
31. Yesavage JA, Tinklenberg JR: Single-case study of clinical response to high-dose ergot alkaloid treatment for dementia. *Gerontology* 1981; 27:76–78.
32. Katikity M, Webb JF, Dickerson JWT: Some effects of food supplement in elderly hospital patients: A longitudinal study. *Hum Nutr: App Nutr* 1983; 37A:85–93.
33. Dalderup LM, Berend van Haard W, Keller GHM, et al: An attempt to change memory and serum composition in old people by a daily supplement of dried baker's yeast. *J Gerontol* 1979; 25:320–324.

34. Barbeau A, Growdon JH, Wurtman RJ (eds): Choline and lecithin in brain disorders. *Nutrition and the Brain,* vol 5. New York, Raven Press, 1979.
35. Blusztajn JK, Wurtman RJ: Choline and cholinergic neurons. *Science* 1983; 221:614–620.
36. Levy R, Little A, Chuaqui P, Reigh M: Early results from double blind, placebo controlled trial of high dose phosphatidylcholine in Alzheimer's disease. *Lancet* 1983; 2:987–988.
37. Mohs RC, Davis KL, Tinklenberg JR, et al: Choline chloride treatment of memory deficits in the elderly. *Am J Psychiatry* 1979; 136:1275–1277.
38. Weintraub S, Mesulam MM, Auty R, Baratz R: Lecithin in the treatment of Alzheimer's Disease. *Arch Neurol* 1983; 40:527–528.
39. Wurtman RJ: Nutrients that modify brain function. *Sci Am* 1982; 246:50–59.
40. Zeisel SH: Dietary choline biochemistry, physiology and pharmacology. *Ann Rev Nutr* 1981; 1:95–121.
41. Meyer JS, Welch KMA, Deshmukh VD, et al: Neurotransmitter precursor amino acids in the treatment of multi-infarct dementia and Alzheimer's disease. *J Am Geriatr Soc* 1977; 25:289–298.
42. Bartus RT, Dean RL, Goas JA, Lippa AS: Age-related changes in passive avoidance retention: Modulation with dietary choline. *Science* 1980; 209:301–303.
43. Mervis R, Bartus RT: Dietary choline increases dendritic spine population in aging mouse neocortex. *Soc Neurosci (Abst)* 1981; 7:370.
44. Hershkowitz M, Heron D, Samuel D, Shinitzky M: The modulation of protein phosphorylation and receptor binding in synaptic membranes by changes in lipid fluidity: Implications for ageing. *Prog Brain Res* 1982; 56:419–434.
45. Flood JF, Landry DW, Jarvik ME: Cholinergic receptor interactions and their effects on long-term memory processing. *Brain Res* 215:177–185.
46. Wood JL, Allison RG: Effects of consumption of choline and lecithin on neurological and cardiovascular systems. *Fed Proc* 1982; 41:3015–3021.
47. Flood JF, Smith GE, Cherkin A: Memory retention: Potentiation of cholinergic drug combinations in mice. *Neurobiol Aging* 1983; 4:37–43.
48. Cherkin A, Riege WH: Multimodal approach to pharmacotherapy of senile amnesias, in Cervos-Navarro J, Sarkander HI (eds): *Brain Aging: Neuropathology and Neuropharmacology Aging,* vol 21 New York, Raven Press, 1983; pp 415–435.
49. Reisberg B, London E, Ferris SH, et al: Novel pharmacologic approaches to the treatment of senile dementia of the Alzheimer's type (SDAT). *Psychopharmacol Bull* 1983; 19:220–225.
50. von Muralt A: The role of thiamine in neurophysiology. *Ann NY Acad Sci* 1962; 98:499–507.
51. Cooper J: Biochemical and physiological function of thiamine in nervous tissue. *Nature* 1963; 199:609–610.
52. Flood JF, Smith GE, Cherkin A: Memory enhancement: Supra-additive effect of subcutaneous cholinergic drug combinations in mice. *Psychopharmacology* 1984; in press.
53. Bartus RT, Dean III RL, Sherman KA, et al: Profound effects of combining choline and piracetam on memory enhancement and cholinergic function in aged rats. *Neurobiol Aging* 1981; 2:105–111.

54. Peters BH, Levin HS: Effects of physostigmine and lecithin on memory in Alzheimer's disease. *Ann Neurol* 1979; 6:219–221.
55. Reisberg B, Ferris SH, Schneck MK, et al: Piracetam in the treatment of cognitive impairment in the elderly. *Drug Dev Res* 1982; 2:475–480.
56. LaBrecque DC, Goldberg RI: A double-blind study of pentylenetetrazol combined with niacin in senile patients. *Curr Therap Res* 1967; 9:611–617.
57. Levy S: Pharmacological treatment of aged patients in a state mental hospital. *JAMA* 1953; 153:1260–1265.
58. Gabrynowicz JW, Dumbrill M: A clinical trial of leptazole with nicotinic acid and the management of psycho-geriatric patients. *Med J Australia* 1968; i: 799–802.
59. Drachman DA, Glosser G, Fleming P, Longenecker G: Memory decline in the aged: treatment with lecithin and physostigmine. *Neurology* 1982; 32: 944–950.
60. Greenblatt M (ed): *Drugs in Combination with Other Therapies.* New York, Grune & Stratton, 1975; p. viii.
61. Brinkman SD, Smith RC, Meyer JS, et al: Lecithin and memory training in suspected Alzheimer's disease. *J Gerontol* 1982; 37:4–9.
62. Pauling L: Orthomolecular psychiatry. *Science* 1968; 160:265–271.
63. Pauling L: On the orthomolecular environment of the mind: Orthomolecular theory. *Am J Psychiatry* 1974; 131:1251–1257.

15

Modifying the Effects of Environmental Chemicals by Dietary Manipulations: A Search for Hemeprotein Peroxidase Inhibitors

Bernard B. Davis and Terry V. Zenser

Exposure to chemicals appears to play a major role in the pathogenesis of a sizable portion of human diseases (1,2). For example, the chemical products of combustion in tobacco smoke may be etiologically related to one-third of all malignant disease in humans. Alcohol and tobacco combined are often factors in carcinomas of the upper respiratory tract. Exposure to chemicals may cause tissue toxicity. Both chronic and acute renal failures and a sizable portion of chronic respiratory diseases can be traced to exposure to various chemicals (1–4).

Certain aspects of chemical carcinogenesis, chemical toxicity, and the aging process may share common mechanistic pathways in that damage occurs to the structure and/or function of critical cellular molecules (2,5–7). A common pathway is also suggested by the fact that the incidence of cancer increases with age (8). In each case—aging, chemical toxicity, and chemical carcinogenesis—chemicals become activated to more reactive forms, which then inflict damage to critical cellular molecules (Fig. 15-1). Oxidant formation, lipid peroxidation, and radical generation are important contributors to these pathogenic processes (see Chapter 9). Be-

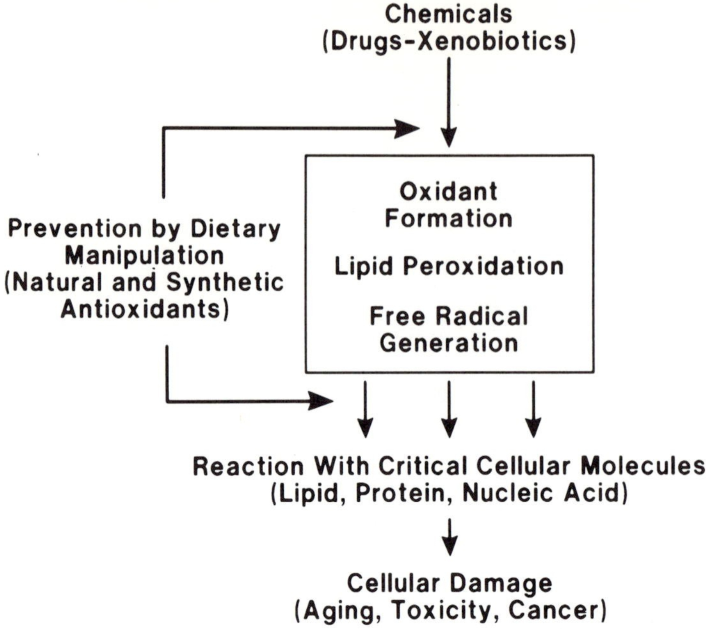

Figure 15-1. General scheme illustrating the interrelations between aging, toxicity, and cancer. The entry of chemicals can occur by mouth, skin, lung, or injection. Oxidant formation, lipid peroxidation, and free radical generation are common ingredients shared by these pathogenic processes. These ingredients react with critical cellular molecules, and initiation and/or perpetuation of cellular damage results. Production of the three common ingredients and their interactions with one another and with critical cellular molecules such as lipid, protein, and nucleic acid is complex (5–7). Specific examples of these processes are discussed relative to Figure 15-6 in the text. Dietary manipulation can prevent lipid peroxidation, oxidant formation, and free radical generation. Dietary manipulation can also prevent the latter events from altering critical cellular molecules.

cause of their common mechanistic pathways, similar prevention strategies, including dietary manipulation, are possible for certain aspects of the aging process, cancers, and toxic reactions.

Modifying Effects of Environmental Chemicals by Dietary Manipulation

Chemicals that exert pathogenic effects in areas distal from their port of entry into the body are thought to require endogenous metabolic activation. The primary activation is usually enzymatic in nature and also involves oxidative or reductive mechanisms with nonenzymatic secondary reactions (i.e., binding to macromolecules or radical generation). Understanding the entire sequence of events starting with entry and continuing through activation, initiation of adverse effects on tissues, and mechanisms of excretion permits the development of strategies for prevention. Such strategies would interfere with the metabolism of the chemical carcinogen at one or more sites in the sequence. For example, to promote detoxification over activation, endogenous compounds such as glutathione, which have the potential to promote detoxification processes, can be introduced. Inhibitors of metabolism may be either natural, as with vitamin E, or synthetic, as with ethoxyquin (Fig. 15-1). Diet supplementation with either natural or synthetic compounds provides an important means of accomplishing prevention (for review, see reference 9). Dietary factors such as lipids have been associated with an increase in certain types of cancer and other diseases of aging (5,10). Controlling intake of these factors would be a preventive measure.

Urinary Bladder Cancer

Cancer of the urinary bladder has long been associated with environmental chemicals, particularly among workers in the dye and chemical industries (11). FANFT (Fig. 15-2) is a 5-nitrofuran that causes cancer of the urinary bladder in nearly 100% of animals fed 0.2% diet of this compound for 12 weeks (12). This high incidence of tumor formation elicited by feeding FANFT makes it uniquely attractive in the design of prevention strategies by dietary manipulation. In addition, the 5-nitrofurans are a group of diverse chemical carcinogens and represent one of the largest groups of nitroaryl compounds used as human and veterinary medicines and food additives. When FANFT is fed to rats, a large proportion of the compound appears to be deformylated. ANFT is the deformylated prod-

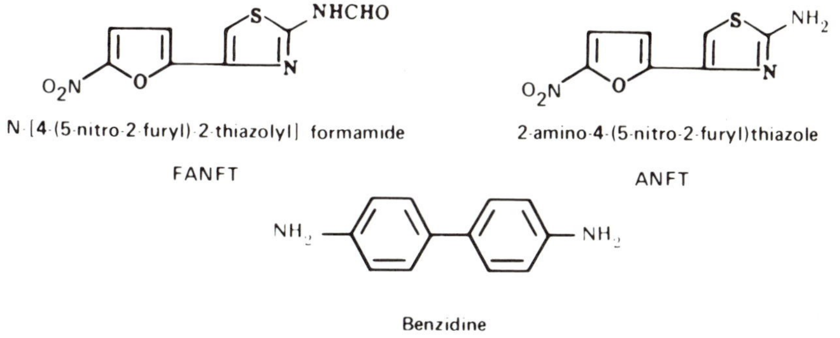

Figure 15-2. Structures of chemicals oxidized by prostaglandin hydroperoxidase.

uct of FANFT. Mutagenicity of urine from FANFT-fed rats is correlated with the urinary concentration of ANFT rather than FANFT (12). This suggests deformylation is an important step in the mechanism of FANFT-induced bladder cancer. Therefore, studies of both FANFT and ANFT metabolism are necessary.

This chapter outlines an investigation of the mechanisms involved in the initiation of FANFT-induced urinary bladder carcinoma. This investigation led to the development of a dietary prevention strategy that significantly reduced the incidence of bladder cancer. The success of these studies and the similarities of certain aspects of cancer, aging, and toxicity (Fig. 15-1) provide the molecular basis for initiating corresponding investigations in other areas.

Characteristics of Prostaglandin H Synthase

Our studies indicate that bladder prostaglandin H synthase (PHS) activates certain carcinogens and that this activation is involved in the genesis of bladder cancer by these chemical carcinogens (13,14). PHS is a hemeprotein peroxidase consisting of two separate activities: fatty acid cyclooxygenase and prostaglandin hydroperoxidase (15). Fatty acid cyclooxygenase is responsible for the initial bis-dioxygenation of the unsaturated fatty acid (Fig. 15-3). The hydroperoxidase activity is responsible for the subsequent reduction of the lipid peroxide prostaglandin G_2. This reduction results in a corresponding oxidation shown as the conversion of *A* to *B* in Figure 15-3. Prostaglandin hydroperoxidase can reduce a variety of lipid peroxides. Several procarcinogens and protoxins have been shown to be oxidized by PHS to reactive intermediates, which bind macromolecules (for review, see reference 16). Activation of procarcinogens has been attributed to the hydroperoxidase rather than the fatty acid cyclooxygenase activity of PHS (13,14,16). Subcellular localization by immunohistofluorescence has demonstrated that PHS is associated with the endoplasmic reticulum and nuclear membrane (17), making both the cytoplasm and the nucleus susceptible to damage by PHS-generated oxidants.

This review specifically addresses the action of hemeprotein peroxidase (i.e., PHS) as opposed to other peroxidases, such as the selenium-requiring glutathione peroxidase. Hemeprotein peroxidase can utilize lipid peroxides to activate certain chemicals, while glutathione peroxidase hydrolyzes and inactivates lipid peroxides, forming hydroxyacids and H_2O (5). Therefore, hemeprotein peroxidases and glutathione peroxidase could be expected to have opposing effects—the former initiating and perpetuating and the latter preventing pathogenic processes within cells.

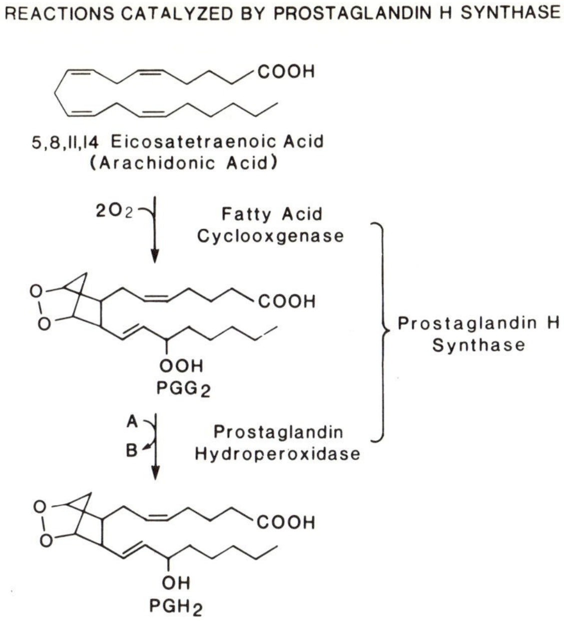

REACTIONS CATALYZED BY PROSTAGLANDIN H SYNTHASE

COOH

5,8,11,14 Eicosatetraenoic Acid
(Arachidonic Acid)

$2O_2$

Fatty Acid
Cyclooxgenase

Prostaglandin H
Synthase

O
O
COOH
OOH
PGG_2

A
B

Prostaglandin
Hydroperoxidase

O
O
COOH
OH
PGH_2

Figure 15-3. Prostaglandin H synthase (PHS) has been shown to consist of two separate activities—fatty acid cyclooxygenase and prostaglandin hydroperoxidase. Fatty acid cyclooxygenase is responsible for initial bis-dioxygenation of the unsaturated fatty acid. Arachidonic acid is the common in vivo fatty acid substrate. Arachidonic acid is metabolized to prostaglandin G_2, a 15-hydroperoxy prostaglandin cyclic endoperoxide intermediate. The hydroperoxidase activity reduces prostaglandin G_2 to the hydroxy cyclic endoperoxide prostaglandin H_2. This reduction results in a corresponding oxidation shown as the conversion of *A* to *B*. The oxidant B may then be involved in the initiation and/or perpetuation of cancer, aging, and toxicity.

Activation of Bladder Carcinogens by Prostaglandin H Synthase

Oxidative metabolism of FANFT was examined by measuring the covalent binding of [^{14}C]FANFT to microsomal protein (Table 15-1) (18). With this microsomal preparation, there was no measurable binding of FANFT to protein in the absence of added cofactors. Addition of NADPH did not cause binding. However, significant binding was detected in the presence of arachidonic acid. Both hydrogen peroxide and 15-hydroperoxy-5,8,11,13-eicosatetraenoic acid (15-HPETE), the lipid peroxide analog of arachidonic acid, supported the binding of FANFT. The nonsteroidal antiinflammatory agents aspirin and indomethacin inhibit the fatty acid cyclooxygenase, but not the hydroperoxidase compo-

Table 15-1. Effect of Different Agents on Arachidonic Acid- and Peroxide-Mediated Binding of [^{14}C]FANFT to Protein Catalyzed by Solubilized PHS*

Substrate	Addition	Concentration mmol/L	Protein Bound nmol/mg protein/min
None	—	—	nd†
NADPH	—	1.0	nd
Arachidonic acid		0.06	0.22 ± 0.01‡
	Indomethacin	0.1	nd§
	Aspirin	1.0	nd§
	Propylthioruacil	0.2	nd§
	Ethoxyquin	0.1	nd§
	Vitamin C	1.0	nd§
	Vitamin E	0.1	0.04 ± 0.01§
	Glutathione	1.0	nd§
	Allopurinol	0.25	0.19 ± 0.01
	Metyrapone	1.0	0.17 ± 0.01
	SKF-525A	0.2	0.19 ± 0.01
H_2O_2		0.2	0.09 ± 0.02
	Indomethacin	0.1	0.08 ± 0.01
	Propylthiouracil	0.2	nd§
	Ethoxyquin	0.1	nd§
	Glutathione	1.0	nd§
15-HPETE	—	0.05	0.22 ± 0.06
	Aspirin	1.0	0.20 ± 0.03

*Samples were preincubated for 2 min prior to substrate initiation of the 2-min incubation. Following ethyl acetate extraction, binding of 0.05 mmol/L FANFT to protein was assessed in 0.6 mol/L TCA precipitable material (18).

†No metabolism detected.

‡Mean ± SE with N = 3–12.

§P <.01 compared to corresponding cosubstrate value.

nent of PHS (Fig. 15-3). Thus, these drugs inhibited arachidonic acid but not peroxide-initiated binding. By contrast, propylthiouracil, a substrate for several peroxidases, including thyroid peroxidase (19), inhibited both arachidonic acid and peroxide-initiated binding. Glutathione also inhibited binding by forming a thioether conjugate of activated FANFT (data not shown). Inhibitors of xanthine oxidase (allopurinol) and mixed-function oxidases (metyrapone and SKF-525A) did not alter binding. Similar results in substrate and inhibitor specificity were noted with ANFT (20). Therefore, both ANFT and FANFT are metabolized by the hydroperoxidase component of prostaglandin H synthase.

PHS-catalyzed activation of FANFT and ANFT to bind macromolecules was compared (Table 15-2) (18). The rate of ANFT binding to protein was approximately fourfold greater than FANFT. ANFT binding to DNA was observed, but no binding of activated FANFT to DNA was detected. These results are consistent with other studies suggesting that ANFT may be a proximal carcinogen in FANFT carcinogenesis.

Table 15-2. Solubilized Ram Seminal Vesicle PHS-Catalyzed Binding of [^{14}C]FANFT and [^{14}C]ANFT to Protein and DNA*

	Protein Bound	DNA Bound
	nmol/mg protein/min	
FANFT	0.2 ± 0.01	nd†
ANFT	0.9 ± 0.03‡	0.05 ± 0.01‡§

*Binding of either 0.05 mmol/L FANFT or ANFT was initiated by addition of 0.6 mmol/L arachidonic acid (18).

†No metabolic detected, less than 0.002 nmol/mg of protein.

‡P <.01 compared with corresponding value for FANFT.

§Mean ± SE with N = 6.

The capacity of other peroxidases to metabolize ANFT was determined (Table 15-3). Of the peroxidases tested, only the hydroperoxidase component of PHS metabolized the 5-nitrofuran ANFT (21). However, all of the peroxidases tested metabolized the aromatic amine benzidine (Table 15-4). Benzidine, like FANFT, is a urinary bladder carcinogen. These results indicate that the specificity of peroxidases varies in their activation of carcinogens. They also document a possible role for peroxidases other than prostaglandin hydroperoxidase in chemical carcinogenesis.

PHS metabolism of benzidine is associated with the generation of its free radical cation (Fig. 15-4) (22). Horseradish peroxidase oxidation of benzidine results in the generation of a free radical indistinguishable from that produced by PHS oxidation. Generation of the free radical cation of benzidine by PHS is inhibited by the antithyroid (antiperoxidase) drug methimazole and ascorbic acid (vitamin C). Neither superoxide nor hydroxyl radicals appears to be involved in radical generation. The free radical cation produced by peroxidatic oxidation may be responsible for the binding of activated chemicals to macromolecules.

Peroxidases catalyze oxidation-reduction reactions. In the case of PHS, the hydroperoxidase component catalyzes the reduction of the lipid per-

Table 15-3. Peroxidase-Catalyzed Binding of [^{14}C]ANFT to Protein*

Enzyme	Substrate	Concentration mmol/L	Binding nmol/mg protein/min
Prostaglandin H synthase	15-HPETE	0.05	5.6 ± 0.6†
Horseradish peroxidase	H_2O_2	0.3	nd‡
Lactoperoxidase	H_2O_2	0.3	nd
Chloroperoxidase	H_2O_2	0.3	nd

*Experimental conditions were similar to those in Table 15-1 (21).

†Mean ± SE with N = 3.

‡No metabolism detected.

Table 15-4. Peroxidase-Catalyzed Binding of [^{14}C]Benzidine to Protein*

Enzyme	Substrate	Concentration mmol/L	Binding nmol/mg protein/ min
Prostglandin H synthase	15-HPETE	0.05	29.3 ± 3.5†
Horseradish peroxidase (10^3)‡	H_2O_2	0.3	38.5 ± 3.5
Lactoperoxidase (10^1)	H_2O_2	0.3	49.3 ± 4.4
Chloroperoxidase (10^2)	H_2O_2	0.3	12.9 ± 1.3

*Experimental conditions were similar to those in Table 15-1 (21).

†Mean ± SE with $N = 3$.

‡Activity obtained by multiplying by the factor of 10 indicated.

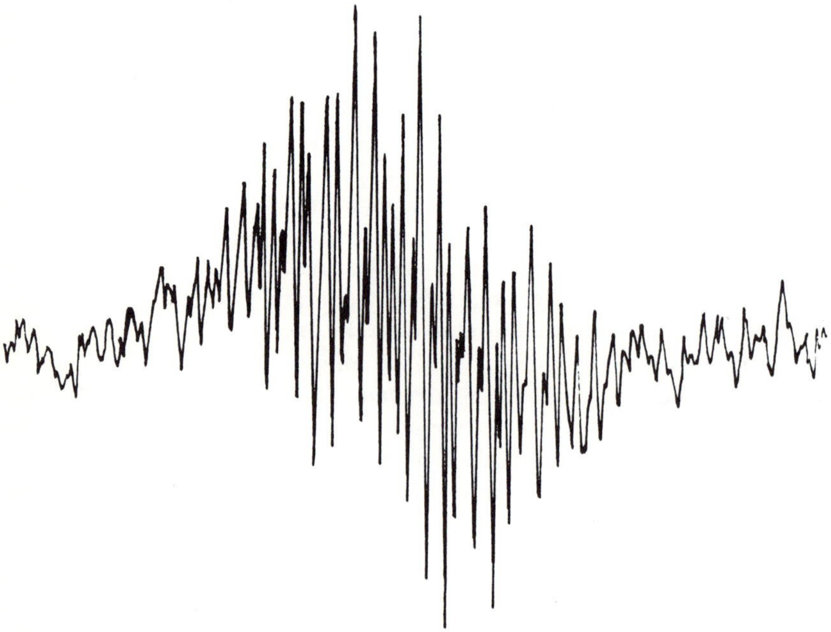

Figure 15-4. Electron spin resonance signal of a free radical species generated from the oxidation of benzidine by prostaglandin hydroperoxidase. Radical was formed at room temperature with 0.5 mmol/L benzidine, 0.5 mmol/L H_2O_2 and 0.4 mg/mL solubilized seminal vesicle microsomes in acetate buffer pH 4.2. The hyperfine structure spectra was obtained over a 100 G scan range in the region centered around g = 2. Modulation amplitude was 0.2 G, modulation frequency 100 kHz and microwave power 20 mW. Receiver gain was 3.2×10^5 with a time constant of 2 sec and scan time of 30 min. The instrument was a Varian E-109E EPR spectrometer (22).

oxide prostaglandin G_2 to prostaglandin H_2 (Fig. 15-3). This reduction must be balanced by a corresponding oxidation. The naturally occurring reducing agent is not known. Uric acid has been shown to increase prostaglandin synthesis by PHS and is a possible endogenous reducing agent. However, uric acid oxidation by PHS was not demonstrated (23). Reversible PHS oxidation of uric acid is shown in Figure 15-5. Uric acid exhibits two absorption bands with λ_{max} values at 288 nm and 230 nm. Oxidation resulted in a decrease at 288 nm and an increase at approximately 227 nm. An increased absorbance was also observed at 308–318 nm. The unstable nature of this oxidant is indicated by the disappearance of these spectral changes with time. These results are consistent with the work of Wrona and Dryhurst (24), which demonstrated reversible oxidation of uric acid by horseradish peroxidase and by electrochemical technic. These authors propose that uric acid at pH 7.0 exists as a monoanion with the primary electrochemical step being a 2e–2H$^+$ oxidation to the very unstable anionic diimine oxidant. Uric acid has been proposed by Ames et al (25) to be important as an evolutionary factor for surviving oxidant stress in mammals. In vivo uric acid content can be regulated by dietary manipulation and thus may alter the peroxidatic potential of tissues.

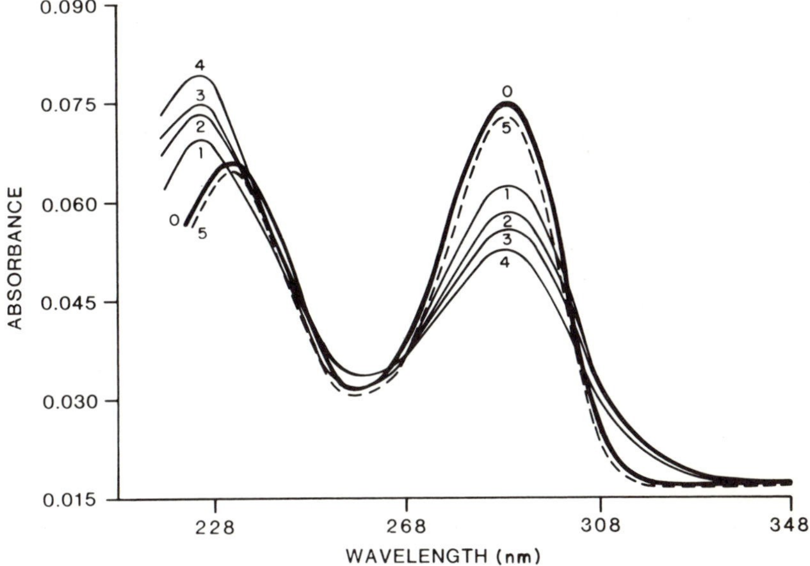

Figure 15-5. Reversible oxidation of uric acid by prostaglandin hydroperoxidase. Incubation mixtures contained 0.4 mg/mL solubilized ram seminal vesicle microsomes, 0.12 mmol/L arachidonic acid, 2.0 mmol/L uric acid, and pH 7.8 phosphate buffer. Repetitive spectral scan sweeps (numbered sequencially in the figure) were obtained with a Beckman Acta VI recording spectrophotometer.

Reduction of the Incidence of Bladder Cancer by Dietary Manipulation

The previous studies identified PHS as an enzyme with the capacity for activation of chemical carcinogens. This enzyme system (Fig. 15-3) provides a model for the development of prevention strategies.

Owing to the peroxidatic nature of PHS activation, peroxidase substrates should competitively inhibit peroxidase activation of dangerous chemicals without altering prostaglandin synthesis. Propylthiouracil, a peroxidase substrate, inhibited PHS-catalyzed activation of FANFT (Table 15-1). Propylthiouracil was also used to assess PHS activation of benzidine in renal inner medullary slices (Table 15-5). Arachidonic acid elicited a threefold increase in benzidine binding, which was inhibited by both indomethacin and propylthiouracil. However, only indomethacin inhibited prostaglandin E_2 synthesis. Effects of aspirin were similar to those of indomethacin (not shown). Propylthiouracil is thought to prevent the deleterious effects associated with carbon-tetrachloride-initiated lipid peroxidation by functioning as an antioxidant (26). Therefore, inhibition of peroxidatic activation by compounds such as propylthiouracil may have several advantages:

1. Prostaglandin synthesis is not necessarily inhibited.
2. Therefore, important prostaglandin-mediated processes are not altered.
3. Inhibition occurs with both fatty acid and lipid peroxide substrates.
4. Peroxidases, other than PHS, may also be inhibited.
5. These antiperoxidase agents can provide additional protection by functioning as antioxidants.

Our initial prevention studies used aspirin because of the extensive basic and clinical studies of its effects on PHS activity.

The capacity of kidney medullary microsomal PHS to activate benzidine was assessed following in vivo aspirin treatment (Table 15-6). Rabbits were treated with aspirin in vivo by injecting 15 mg/kg, intravenously (27). Kidneys were removed 30 minutes later from control and aspirin-treated animals. Aspirin treatment caused a significant inhibition of arachidonic-acid-dependent metabolism of benzidine. However, lipid peroxide-(15-HPETE)-dependent metabolism of benzidine was not altered. The antioxidants glutathione, propylthiouracil, and vitamin E (not shown) were effective in preventing either arachidonic-acid or lipid-peroxide-dependent metabolism. The data demonstrate that activation of procarcinogens by PHS in aspirin-treated animals can occur if lipid peroxide substrates are available. Therefore, aspirin may only partially prevent pathogenic processes involving peroxidases.

A long-term feeding study was conducted assessing the effects of coad-

Table 15-5. Effect of Propylthiouracil and Indomethacin on Archidonic-Acid-Initiated PGE_2 Synthesis and [^{14}C]Benzidine Binding by Medullary Slices*

Additions	Concentration mmol/L	PG E_2 Synthesis ng/mg wet weight	Benzidine Binding pmol/mg wet wt
None	—	3.0 ± 0.5†	4.7 ± 0.08
Arachidonic acid	0.25	22.0 ± 1.4	11.7 ± 1.0
+ Indomethacin	0.1	0.32 ± 0.02	5.4 ± 0.5
+ Propylthiouracil	0.3	22.4 ± 2.5	7.8 ± 0.8

*Slices were incubated in Krebs ringer bicarbonate buffer with 1 mg/mL each of glucose and BSA. Slices were preincubated for 30 min with a gas phase of 5% CO_2/95% N_2 with either indomethacin or propylthiouracil as indicated. Slices were then transferred to corresponding media with a gas phase of 5% CO_2/95% O_2 containing 0.25 mmol/L arachidonic acid where indicated and either 0.05 mmol/L benzidine or 0.05 mmol/L [^{14}C]benzidine. At the end of this second 30-min incubation, media were analyzed for PGE_2 content by radioimmunoassay and slices (when ^{14}C]benzidine was present) were assessed for benzidine binding.

†Mean ± SE with N = 4–6.

ministration of aspirin with FANFT on bladder tumor formation (Table 15-7) (28). Neither rats fed regular rat chow nor rats fed chow with 0.5% aspirin developed bladder carcinoma. There was an 85% incidence of bladder cancer in rats fed 0.2% FANFT for 12 weeks followed by a control diet for 57 weeks. This was significantly reduced to 37% when 0.5% aspirin was fed in combination with FANFT. These results are consistent with PHS-catalyzed initiation of FANFT-induced bladder cancer. Because previous studies have shown that FANFT is not immunosuppressive (29), it is unlikely that the effect of aspirin is mediated through the

Table 15-6. Binding of [^{14}C]Benzidine to Protein Catalyzed by Inner Medullary Microsomes Prepared from Control and Aspirin-Treated Rabbits*

	Concentration mmol/L	Control	Aspirin-Treated
		pmol/mg protein/min	
None		nd†	nd
Arachidonic Acid	0.1	338 ± 26‡	8 ± 3
+ Aspirin	2.0	10 ± 2	nd
+ Salicylate	2.0	360 ± 24	—
+ Glutathione	1.0	49 ± 5	—
15-HPETE	0.05	264 ± 18	194 ± 12
+ Aspirin	2.0	328 ± 33	198 ± 15
+ Glutathione	1.0	nd	nd

*Experimental conditions were similar to those in Table 15-1 (27).

†No metabolism detected.

‡Mean ± SE with N = 3–6.

Table 15-7. Effect of Aspirin on the Incidence of Bladder Carcinoma Induced by 12 Weeks of Feeding FANFT*

Group	No. of Rats	Carcinoma
1. 0.2% FANFT → Control diet	21	18 (86%)
2. 0.2% FANFT + 0.5% Aspirin → Control diet	27	10 (37%)†
3. 0.5% Aspirin	23	0
4. Control diet	25	0

*Rats in Groups 1 and 2 received 0.2% FANFT for 12 weeks. Rats in Group 2 received 0.5% aspirin 2 days before, during, and 1 week following FANFT diet. Rats in Group 3 received 0.5% aspirin for 13 weeks. Following the indicated treatments, rats received a control diet until the experiment was terminated at 69 weeks (23).

†Group 1 versus Group 2, $P < .001$.

immune system. The incomplete inhibition of tumor formation by aspirin may result from the presence of lipid peroxide substrates within bladder tissue. Therefore, the use of antiperoxidase drugs such as propylthiouracil instead of or in combination with aspirin may accomplish a more complete inhibition of tumor formation. These and other studies (9) demonstrate that dietary supplementation may reduce the incidence of carcinogenesis.

Conclusions

These results lead us to propose a detailed model for peroxidatic activation of environmental chemicals to oxidants that may induce cancer, cause toxic reactions in parenchymal tissues, or accelerate the aging process (Fig. 15-6). This model emphasizes only the peroxidatic pathway for eliciting these pathogenic sequela. Figure 15-1 provides a more general overview. However, the key components of Figure 15-1—lipid peroxidation, oxidant formation, and free radical generation—are also necessary factors in Figure 15-6. One consequence of lipid peroxidation is the generation of lipid peroxides. The latter are substrates for peroxidase-catalyzed activation of environmental chemicals. Oxidants (activated chemicals) produced by peroxidases may themselves be free radicals, as in the case of benzidine (Fig. 15-4). Oxidants and radicals can combine with molecules associated with membranes, cytoplasm, or nucleus, and induce and perpetuate carcinogenesis, toxicity, and aging (see Chapter 9). The model described in Figure 15-6 proposes specific sites (numbered 1 to 4) at which strategies may be developed to prevent these pathologic processes. These sites include:

1. Synthesis of peroxide substrates.
2. Activation of environmental chemicals by prostaglandin hydroperoxidase.

3. Conversion of the activated intermediate back to the parent compound.
4. Inactivation of reactive intermediate(s) by forming conjugate(s)

Specific inhibitors for each one of these sites was demonstrated for benzidine oxidation by PHS (30). Aspirin and other nonsteroidal antiinflammatory agents act at site 1a in Figure 15-6, while phenidone, a lipoxygenase inhibition, acts at site 1b. Antiperoxidase drugs, like propylthiouracil, act at site 2, regardless of the pathway (site 1a or 1b) used to generate the peroxide substrate. Ascorbic acid rapidly converts a product of benzidine oxidation—its diimine analog—back to benzidine (site 3). Glutathione forms a conjugate with an activated benzidine intermediate, preventing binding to protein and nucleic acid (site 4). Egan et al (31) have proposed that oxidation can also occur as a result of the chemical reacting with an oxidant released by PHS. In this case, the chemical is not functioning as a cofactor for PHS. This oxidation would

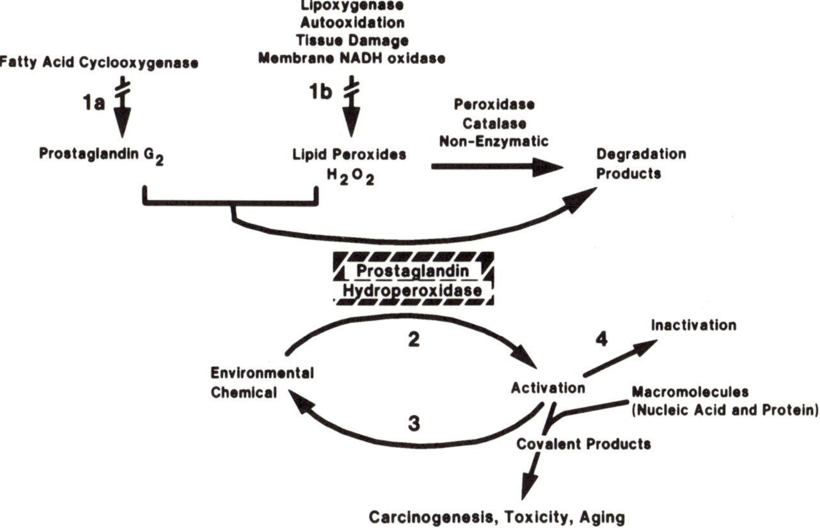

Figure 15-6. A working model based on the hypothesis that hemeprotein peroxidases such as prostaglandin hydroperoxidase are involved in the genesis of aging, carcinogenesis, and toxicity. This model proposes that environmental chemicals are metabolized within target tissues by a hydroperoxidase activity to oxidants that can covalently bind to protein and nucleic acids. This model allows one to propose specific sites (numbered 1, 2, 3, and 4) at which strategies may be developed to prevent these pathologic processes: (1) synthesis of peroxide substrates; (2) activation of environmental chemicals by prostaglandin hydroperoxidase; (3) conversion of the activated intermediate back to the parent compound; and (4) inactivation of reactive intermediate(s) by forming conjugate(s).

be inhibited by the antioxidants described above. Sites 1 to 4 are amenable to dietary manipulation.

Acknowledgments

This work was supported by the Veterans Administration, U.S. Public Health Service Grant CA-28015 from the National Cancer Institute through the National Bladder Cancer Project, and the American Cancer Society, Missouri chapter. The authors wish to thank Mrs. Cheryl Duff and Mrs. Sandy Melliere for skillful assistance in the preparation of this manuscript.

References

1. Doll R, Peto R: The causes of cancer: Quantitative estimates of avoidable risks of cancer in the United States today. *J Natl Cancer Inst* 1981; 66:1192–1308.
2. Ames BN: Dietary carcinogens and anticarcinogens: Oxygen radicals and degenerative diseases. *Science* 1983; 221:1256–1264.
3. Hook JB: Toxic responses of the kidney, in Doull J, Klaassen CD, Amdur MO (eds): *Toxicology: The Basic Science of Poisons.* New York, Macmillan, 1980, pp 232–245.
4. Ingram RH Jr: Diffuse lung disease, in Isselbaacher KJ, Adams RD, Braunwald E, et al (eds): *Principles of Internal Medicine.* New York, McGraw-Hill, 1980, pp 1235–1241.
5. Tappel AL: Protection against free radical lipid peroxidation reactions, in Roberts J, Adelman RC, Cristofalo VJ (eds): *Pharmacological Intervention in the Aging Process,* vol 97. New York, Plenum Press, 1978, pp 111–131.
6. Miller JA: Carcinogenesis by chemicals: An overview—GHA Clowes memorial lecture. *Cancer Res* 1970; 30:559–576.
7. Mason RP: Free-radical intermediates in the metabolism of toxic chemicals, in Pryor WA (ed): *Free Radicals in Biology,* vol V. New York, Academic Press, 1982, pp 161–222.
8. Pitot HC: Interactions in the natural history of aging and carcinogenesis. *Fed Proc* 1978; 37:2841–2847.
9. Slaga TJ: Cancer: Etiology, mechanisms, and prevention—A summary, in Slaga TJ (ed): *Carcinogenesis,* vol 5. New York, Raven Press, 1980, pp 243–262.
10. Hayes JR, Campbell TC: Nutrition as a modifier of chemical carcinogenesis, in Slaga TJ (ed): *Carcinogenesis,* vol 5. New York, Raven Press, 1980, pp 207–241.
11. Case RM, Hosker ME, McDonald DB, Pearson JT: Tumours of the urinary bladder in workmen engaged in the manufacture and use of certain dyestuff intermediates in the British chemical industry. *Br J Ind Med* 1954; 11:75–104.
12. Cohen SM: Toxicity and carcinogenicity of nitrofurans, in Bryan GT (ed):

Carcinogenesis, A Comprehensive Survey, vol. 4. New York, Raven Press, 1978, pp 171–231.

13. Zenser TV, Cohen SM, Mattammal MB, et al: Role of prostaglandin endoperoxide synthetase in benzidine and 5-nitrofuran-induced kidney and bladder carcinogenesis, in Powles TJ, Bockman RS, Honn KV, Ramwell P (eds): *Prostaglandins and Cancer: First International Conference,* vol. 2. New York, Alan R Liss Inc, 1982, pp 123–141.
14. Zenser TV, Cohen SM, Mattammal MB, et al: Prostaglandin hydroperoxidase-catalyzed activation of certain N-substituted aryl renal and bladder carcinogens. *Environ Health Perspect* 1983; 49:33–41.
15. Ohki S, Ogino N, Yamamoto S, Hayaishi O: Prostaglandin hydroperoxidase, an integral part of prostaglandin endoperoxide synthetase from bovine vesicular gland microsomes. *J Biol Chem* 1979; 254:829–836.
16. Marnett LJ: Polycyclic aromatic hydrocarbon oxidation during prostaglandin biosynthesis. *Life Sci* 1981; 29:531–546.
17. Rollins TE, Smith WL: Subcellular localization of prostaglandin-forming cyclooxygenase in Swiss mouse 3T3 fibroblasts by electron microscopic immunocytochemistry. *J Biol Chem* 1980; 255:4872–4875.
18. Zenser TV, Palmier MO, Mattammal MB, et al: Comparative effects of prostaglandin H synthase-catalyzed binding of two 5-nitrofuran urinary bladder carcinogens. *J Pharmacol Exp Ther* 1983; 227:139–143.
19. Taurog A: The mechanism of action of the thioureylene antithyroid drugs. *Endocrinology* 1976; 98:1031–1046.
20. Mattammal MB, Zenser TV, Davis BB: Prostaglandin hydroperoxidase-mediated 2-amino-4-(5-nitro-2-furyl)-^{14}C-thiazole metabolism and nucleic acid binding. *Cancer Res* 1981; 41:4961–4966.
21. Wise RW, Zenser TV, Davis BB: Peroxidase metabolism of the urinary bladder carcinogen 2-amino-4-(5-nitro-2-furyl)thiazole. *Cancer Res* 1983; 43: 1518–1522.
22. Wise RW, Zenser TV, Davis BB: Prostaglandin H synthase metabolism of the urinary bladder carcinogens benzidine and ANFT. *Carcinogenesis* 1983; 4:285–289.
23. Ogino N, Yamamoto S, Hayaishi O, Tokuyama T: Isolation of an activator for prostaglandin hydroperoxidase from bovine vesicular gland cytosol and its identification as uric acid. *Biochem Biophys Res Commun* 1979; 87:184–191.
24. Wrona MZ, Dryhurst G: Investigation of the enzymic and electrochemical oxidation of uric acid derivatives. *Biochim Biophys Acta* 1979; 570:371–387.
25. Ames BN, Cathcart R, Schwiers E, Hochstein P: Uric acid provides an antioxidant defense in humans against oxidant- and radical-caused aging and cancer: A hypothesis. *Proc Natl Acad Sci USA* 1981; 78:6858–6862.
26. Orrego H, Carmichael FJ, Phillips MJ, et al: Protection by propylthiouracil against carbon tetrachloride-induced liver damage. *Gastroenterology* 1976; 71:821–826.
27. Zenser TV, Mattammal MB, Rapp NS, Davis BB: Effect of aspirin on metabolism of acetaminophen and benzidine by renal inner medulla prostaglandin hydroperoxidase. *J Lab Clin Med* 1983; 101:58–65.
28. Murasaki G, Zenser TV, Davis BB, Cohen SM: Inhibition by aspirin of N-[4-(5-nitro-2-furyl)-2-thiazolyl] formamide induced bladder carcinogenesis and enhancement of forestomach carcinogenesis. *Carcinogenesis* 1984; 5:53–55.

29. Headley DB, Klopp RG, Michie PM, et al: Temporal comparisons of immune status and target organ histology in mice fed carcinogenic 5-nitrofurans and their nornitro analogs. *Cancer Res* 1981; 41:1397–1401.
30. Zenser TV, Mattammal MB, Wise RW, et al: Prostaglandin H synthase-catalyzed activation of benzidine: A model to assess pharmacologic intervention of the initiation of chemical carcinogenesis. *J Pharmacol Exp Ther* 1983; 227:545–550.
31. Egan RW, Gale PH, Baptista EM, et al: Oxidation reactions by prostaglandin cyclooxygenase-hydroperoxidase. *J Biol Chem* 1981; 256:7352–7361.

Part IV

Nutrition and Aging—Evaluation and Management

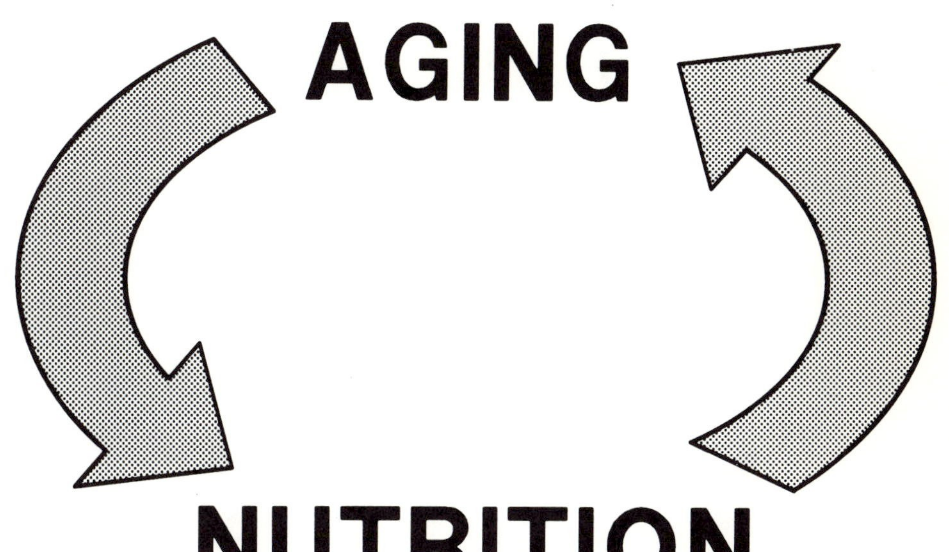

16

Nutritional Evaluation of the Institutionalized Elderly

John M. Prendergast

Longevity, Quality of Life, and the Future

The recent report of the Institute of Medicine to the National Institute of Aging (1) contained some sobering statistics concerning future demographic trends of the elderly population in the United States. We are informed that more than 50% of those who have ever been over 65 are alive today; that the age group 75 to 84 years old is growing at the fastest rate in the United States presently; and that over 23-million people, more than 11% of the population, are aged 65 and over. This figure is expected to swell to 50-million in 50 years. Over 27% of annual health care expenditures (which totaled more than 241 billion dollars in 1981) is used by the 11% of the population aged 65 and over. These statistics are in accord with a more recent report by Watkin (2), who pointed out that mortality rates for elderly Americans have been decreasing and that Gompertz's law that mortality rates for the elderly double each eight years is no longer valid (2).

The above data regulating longevity demand analysis and attention for two reasons. First, it is apparent that one or more beneficial factors are operating to extend the average length of life and a closer scrutiny of these factors and their effects on aging might help us to understand the mysteries surrounding the aging process itself. Second, and perhaps even more important to the modern-day physician and his elderly patient, a better understanding of the factors regarding longevity might significantly assist us in improving the quality of life for those who are now elderly. Such knowledge might be used to promote individual vitality and encourage independence and productivity up to the time of death. In many ways society is already experiencing the social and economic burden of an increasingly vulnerable and dependent elderly population. Failure of geriatricians and gerontologists to discover solutions that will lessen that burden may in the near future thrust upon us decisions that are more ethically distasteful than any we have ever faced.

Factors Affecting Longevity: Applicability to the Institutionalized Elderly

The more important factors among many that influence the potential for a long, productive life are contained in Table 16-1. However, in dealing with institutionalized elderly, the physician is often restricted in his choice of which factors are still manipulable. Genetic structure has already been predetermined, and it is unlikely that even future advances in genetic engineering will benefit this population. Most acquired disease states have already been established and, in some instances, they are the reason for institutionalization. While some acute problems in this population can be treated and cured, most elderly people suffer from chronic diseases, and the main treatment objective is the promotion of optimum function. Achievement of this goal requires a linkage between a holistic evaluation of individual needs and whatever resources are appropriate to optimize the patient's well-being. Intelligent environmental assessment is a critical component of this process, for successful adaptation and well-being are impossible without a congruence between the individual and his environment (3). In this regard, the value of the family (4–6) and other social support networks (7,8) cannot be underestimated either for the homebound or the institutionalized patient.

The potential benefits of exercise in correcting problems associated with the physical inactivity in old age have recently been reviewed (9,10) (see also Chapter 19). Other authors have documented the therapeutic efficacy of exercise programs in such areas as skeletal health (11), coronary disease (12), relief of tension (13), chronic bronchitis (14), and cog-

Table 16-1. Factors Affecting Longevity

1. Genetics
2. Acquired disease
3. Environmental stress
4. Exercise
5. Nutrition

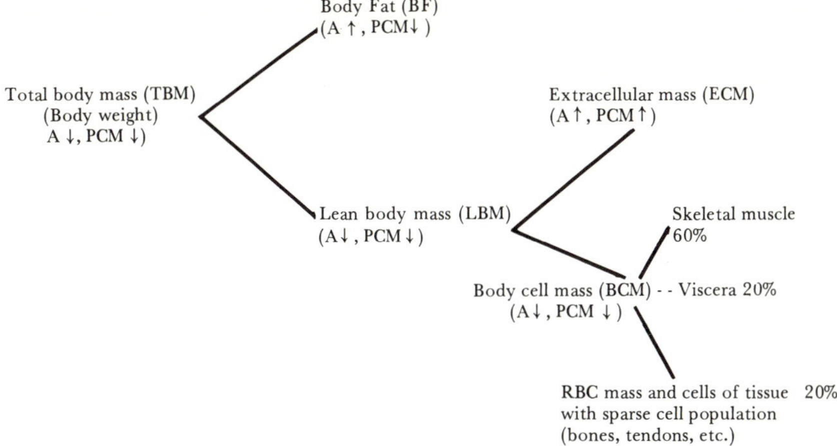

Figure 16-1. Components of body composition: Changes with Aging (A) and protein–calorie malnutrition (PCM). Adapted from Shizgal HM (24).

nitive performance (15). While many authors (16–18) contend that lifelong adherence to regular exercise programs is beneficial for health, deVries has shown that a six-week program of exercise can induce significant physiologic improvement in previously untrained elderly adults (19). However, enthusiasm for exercise as a therapeutic modality in institutionalized elderly is tempered by the work of Gutman and her associates (20), who found no distinct differences in functional parameters between test and control groups following a six-week training program in two retirement complexes. Further research aimed at determining the functional effectiveness of exercise programs for untrained, sometimes frail elderly persons is obviously needed.

The final factor affecting longevity and functional integrity is nutrition. Belloc and Breslow's classic study (21) confirmed a strong relationship between long life and healthy nutritional practices such as avoidance of overeating and excess alcohol and maintenance of consistent and regular meals. Beyond this observation one is struck by the similarities between aging itself and the results of protein–calorie malnutrition. As shown in Figure 16-1, for men, most body compartments, except body fat, respond to aging and protein–calorie malnutrition in a similar pattern. In general, this observation has now been confirmed by a number of investigators (22–24). Equally interesting is the relationship between immunity and aging and malnutrition. Both conditions are generally accepted as producing a decline in most immunologic parameters (25,26). These observations, coupled with recently published correlations between vitamin deficiency and memory dysfunction by Goodwin et al (27), makes reasonable the hypothesis that subclinical malnutrition may play a role in the aging process and in clinical deterioration. This possibility makes nutritional evaluation of the elderly, especially those in institutions, both necessary and appropriate.

Questions Regarding Nutritional Evaluation

A number of important questions have arisen in recent years concerning nutritional evaluation which have a direct bearing on any attempts at formulating a practical approach to assessment for the elderly within hospitals and nursing homes.

1. *Do the elderly differ from the rest of the population with respect to nutritional parameters?* For a number of nutritional indices, significant differences do exist between older and younger cohorts. An appreciation of this fact is critical in order to avoid serious errors in diagnosis, since standards for younger adults may not be applicable to an older population. The relationship of weight to height is an example of this problem. Data from the HANES study (28) and the Baltimore Longitudinal Study (29) have shown that weight usually peaks in the late 50s and early 60s, falling gradually thereafter. This trend is especially common in men, but seems less pronounced in women. The HANES study also showed that anthropometric values varied with age. Mid Arm Muscle Circumference (MAMC) and Arm Muscle Area (AMA) decrease with age in men but increase in women.

The aging process has a variable effect on nutritionally related biochemical and hematologic values. There is good evidence to show that a reduction in lean body mass with age causes a proportional drop in the production and excretion of creatinine (30,31). In turn the creatinine height index (32), a measure of the observed urinary excretion of a patient's creatinine during a 24-hour period as compared with a standard, will also fall. Recent studies by Mitchell and Lipschitz (33) have confirmed this decline but also have shown the limitations of this parameter in differentiating elderly controls from patients with known protein–calorie malnutrition.

Data from the HANES Preliminary Study also confirm that income and race, as well as aging, significantly affect nutritionally related values. Table 16-2 lists the percentage of persons over age 60 who had lower than normally accepted values for five commonly used nutritional parameters. From the table, it is evident that in most categories individuals with incomes below the poverty level have a higher percentage of lower than normal values than those with incomes above the poverty level. On the other hand, a higher percentage of blacks in both income brackets have low levels of hemoglobin and hematocrit. While this observation may be caused by a greater incidence of sickle cell anemia among the

Table 16-2. Percentage of Persons over Age 60 by Income and Race with Lower than Normal Values for Five Commonly Used Nutritional Parameters*

	Income Below Poverty Level		*Income Above Poverty Level*	
	White	*Black*	*White*	*Black*
Hemoglobin†	5.5	29.6	7.6	22.8
Hematocrit	13.4	47.7	16.2	27.0
Serum iron	4.0	2.2	1.3	0.8
Transferrin saturation	5.3	0.8	2.4	0.8
Serum albumin	2.2	4.8	2.5	1.9

*Data adapted from the HANES Preliminary Study.

†Lower limits of normal for males and females are as follows: Hemoglobin 14 g and 12 g; hematocrit 44 and 38 g/dL; serum iron 60 and 40 μg/100 mL; transferrin saturation <20, <15%; serum albumin <3.5 g/dL.

older black population, nutritional deficiencies in this group may also play a role in increasing the prevalence of anemia.

The levels of serum albumin in over 95% of participants was above 3.5 g/dL. This rather high percent of "normals" is interesting in that approximately 75% of subjects selected for participation in the HANES study were from "subgroups considered to have a relatively high degree of nutritional risk" (34). Either malnutrition, as defined by an albumin of less than 3.5 g/dL is relatively infrequent in this population, or the value 3.5 g/dL is a relatively low cutoff point. The latter statement may be the more appropriate, for in a recent unpublished study of 22 elderly patients either attending an ambulatory care clinic or confined to a nursing home, we found no patients who had values less than 3.5 g/dL and 19 of 22 had values over 4.0 g/dL. The three patients in the range 3.6–4.0 g/dL all suffered from significant diseases that limited nutrient intake. These observations are in agreement with other studies, which suggest that in healthy elderly people, total protein and albumin are not significantly depressed (35,36). On the other hand, Lipschitz and Mitchell have recently indicated that in the elderly, lower levels of hemoglobin, eg, 12 g/100 mL for men and 10 g/100 mL for women, were more "useful in distinguishing well from malnourished subjects" (37). Such information emphasizes the need for further investigation and verification of appropriate cutoff points for nutritional parameters in the older age group.

Further evidence that differences exist in nutritional values between young and old has resulted from the use of new, more sophisticated investigational instruments. These technics bypass indirect markers of body composition, such as albumin and skinfold measurements, and give direct measurements of individual body components. For example, in vivo neutron activation analysis allows rather precise measurements of body nitrogen, mass of muscle and nonmuscle lean tissue, lean body mass, and total protein (38). Distinct differences between younger and older cohorts have been documented, and further changes in cancer patients with presumed protein–calorie malnutrition are readily apparent (38). Other investigators have used total body conductivity to measure total body water and potassium (39); computerized axial tomography to predict more accurately the volume of liver, kidney, and spleen (40); and multiple isotope dilution technics to compute red cell mass, plasma volume, and extracellular volume (41). In the future, these rather direct means of measuring body composition may facilitate the task of determining nutritional status for both young and old.

2. *What factors increase the potential for malnutrition among elderly within institutions?* Older persons admitted to acute or chronic institutional environments are vulnerable to malnutrition because of their frail and, therefore, vulnerable conditions and the sometimes inappropriate actions and practices of providers responsible for their care.

Most elderly patients within hospitals and nursing homes have already experienced a significant depletion of physical and cognitive reserves even prior to their admission to these facilities. The aging process coupled with acute and chronic disease produces a scenario characterized by functional limitation and diminished motivation. As noted previously in Chapters 1 and 2, alteration of taste and smell depresses appetite, while a variety of psychosocial factors, such as depression, poverty, isolation, and reduced mobility, seriously impairs "coping" mechanisms. With institutionalization these deficits increase in magnitude. Also, confusion resulting from acute disease processes and/or changes in environment coupled with the depersonalization inherently associated with many institutions often change a vulnerable person into a totally dependent patient.

It is in this setting that providers sometimes fail to identify and manage the nutritional needs of the patient appropriately (41). Unconscious patients with significant metabolic demands may receive only intravenous dextrose and saline for days. Meals are missed when important radiologic or laboratory procedures require abstinence from food or attendance away from patients floors during mealtime. Food consumption is impaired by inappropriate orders, eg, nonsoft meals for patients without teeth and food trays for individuals who are restrained. Few attempts are made to understand the social and cultural background of patients, and foods are ordered without regard to ethnic tastes or appeal. Also, the valuable expertise available from dietary consultants is often not requested.

Other simple nutritional errors occur with alarming frequency in the best of hospitals and nursing homes. Charting of weight at admission and at daily intervals is often lacking. Caloric intake of frail patients is seldom monitored. Progress notes of patients on nasogastric feedings often show no evidence of an intelligent calculation of needs, of proper positioning during feedings, of regular documentation of bowel sounds, and of appropriate reaction to diarrhea. Finally, no consistent plan is made for following the efficacy of sometimes dangerous and expensive nutritional therapy.

Through these practices, caregivers often exacerbate conditions for which patients entered the health center. Lack of appropriate nutritional management becomes yet another factor fueling the downward spiral of functional deterioration. Restitution of optimum health becomes less probable, and the patient becomes either more of a burden for an already overextended nursing staff or a fatality whose death may have been premature.

3. *How valid and reliable are present techniques in diagnosing malnutrition?* The traditional approach to nutritional assessment utilizes information obtained from dietary histories and the results of anthropometric and laboratory testing to assess the nutritional status of the individual. Both of these sources of data are fraught with inaccuracies.

Beaton (42) has recently pointed out that "single, one-day observations do not characterize usual intake and cannot be used by themselves, in the probability approach to assessment of intake." His studies have shown that significant differences exist between a person's true usual intake of a nutrient source and observed intake over any single day. Repetition of measurements at different points in time improves reliability and identifies trends that direct management decisions.

The usual tests used to assess nutritional status are also imprecise. "Even the best available indicator, under the best possible conditions does not correspond exactly with malnutrition" (43). Most indicators that we use are indirect measures of more fundamental body compartments. In young, healthy adults in a steady state, a linear correlation may exist between the nutritional indicator and the compartment being evaluated eg, albumin and visceral protein or triceps skinfold and body fat (44). However, age and/or disease can seriously impair and compromise the relative precision of the indicator to compartment relationship (45). In the absence of malnutrition and without proportional change in body compartment, indicators may change in response to loss from the body eg, albumin in the nephrotic syndrome or hemoglobin in gastrointestinal bleeding; stress, eg, lymphocytes (46); or aging, eg, immune function (47,48). On the other hand, the nutritional indicators noted above are well known for the lag time between the onset of acute nutritional depletion and significant change in their values (40,50). Thus, Andres has commented that in older adults both the aging process and acute and/or chronic disease disturb the precision of "cutoff points" (51). Because aging and disease may have the same effect on a nutritional indicator as does inadequate intake of nutrients, in the elderly it is sometimes difficult to identify the precise factors responsible for indicator values outside of accepted norms. From the clinical perspective this deficit in our diagnostic acumen is important for it may cause serious overestimation of the effectiveness of nutritional supplementation in diseased patients, while at the same time it may cause delay or postponement of nutritional supplementation in those suffering from an acute or chronic deprivation of nutritional intake.

4. *Are tests more accurate than "global assessment" in predicting outcomes?* Because indicators are not consistently able to identify malnutrition (sensitivity) and at the same time to pick out the nutritionally healthy (specificity), some investigators advocate a more comprehensive approach to assessment with greater reliance on a health professional's subjective evaluation of a patient's clinical situation and environment. Using such an approach, Detsky and his colleagues (52) recently reported that the best combination of sensitivity (0.82) and specificity (0.72) was achieved with such subjective global assessment. The next best combination (0.88 and 0.45) resulted from the use of the Prognostic Nutritional Index (52,53). Both of these measures were better in identifying malnourished and healthy subjects and predicting outcome than single objective measurements, such as albumin, delayed cutaneous hypersensitivity, anthropometry, and creatinine height index.

In their concluding remarks the authors expressed doubt that it was "possible to increase the predictive properties of nutritional assessment by combining the subjective global assessment and objective tests into an index" (52). Instead, they recommended that subjective global assessment should be combined with the evaluator's expectations of the patient's hospital course based on "estimates of patient requirements for nutrition in the hospital and their expected intake" (52).

Three important points emerge from the above suggestions. First, it is encouraging that in this age of technologic advances, comprehensive assessment by a trained physician is still a valid method of evaluation. It should be noted, however, that comprehensive assessment for the purpose of "optimizing the congruence of personal characteristics and environmental resources" (3) is certainly not a new concept for students of gerontology.

A second point involves the inclusion of lab tests as part of global assessment. In this respect, various indicators and indexes might be used to initiate and/or reinforce clinical evaluations. These parameters would not act as determinants of a diagnosis, but could assist the physician in confirming his or her broader clinical impression.

Finally, it should be pointed out that although the patient population studied here was confined to the hospital, the principles outlined could be equally applied to other institutionalized populations. In nursing homes and congregate residences, nurses, dieticians, and/or nurse practitioners could assist physicians in performing comprehensive assessments and estimating the nutritional needs.

5. *Does appropriate nutritional evaluation and management affect outcomes of concurrent disease?* The goal of appropriate nutritional evaluation and management is to maintain health and improve the quality of life for those who suffer from disease. One expects that morbidity and mortality statistics would improve in those individuals whose nutritional support is adequately maintained during illness and stress. Is this assumption correct?

Through retrospective analysis of presurgical laboratory data and postsurgical outcomes, Mullen and his colleagues (53) developed the Prognostic Nutritional Index (PNI) which is a computer-generated combination of four important predictive variables used in presurgical assessment:

Prognostic Nutritional Index (%) =

$$150 - 16.6\,(\text{alb}) - 0.78\,(\text{TSF}) - 0.20\,(\text{TFN}) - 5.8\,(\text{DH})$$

In the above formula, the PNI is the risk of operative complications in an individual patient; alb equals albumin in g/100 mL; TSF equals the triceps skinfold in millimeters; TFN equals the transferrin in mg/100; and DH equals delayed hypersensitivity, graded 0 = nonreactive, 1 = <5 mm reactivity, 2 = >5 mm reactivity. The degree of risk can then be calculated as low (< 30), intermediate (30–59), and high (>60). Analysis of surgical outcomes showed a statistically significant correlation between increasing risk scores and the incidence of complications, such as major sepsis and death.

In a subsequent study of patients undergoing gastrointestinal surgery (54), these same investigators showed a statistically significant improvement in outcome when "high risk" patients underwent five to seven days of nutritional supplementation prior to surgery. No statistical difference was apparent in the "low" or "intermediate" groups (55).

While the above results could be read to imply that a subset of sick patients benefit from appropriate nutritional supplementation when another therapeutic measure (surgery) is available, the work of other investigators indicates that in some situations adequate nutritional supplementation alone is often not enough. Blackburn and his colleagues (56) recently reported on the outcomes of 229 patients who underwent complete nutritional assessment and appropriate nutritional support by the Nutritional Support Team at New England Deaconess Hospital during 1976 and 1977. The character of the population studied is significant in that most suffered from serious disease, with 49.3% of the population having cancer and the noncancer group suffering from such illness as pancreatitis (9.6%), vascular disease (9.2%), inflammatory bowel disease (7%), renal failure (2.2), and fistula (1.7%). The authors noted that patients entering the study with low nutritional indicators, eg, serum albumin values less than 3 and serum transferrin less than 170, or in an anergic state, had significantly worse outcomes (despite appropriate nutritional therapy) than those whose nutritional parameters were higher at the onset. This finding has been well corroborated by others (56–58).

While valuable in exposing the limitations of nutritional intervention in certain situations, this study raises major questions pertinent to the frail, institutionalized, elderly population. Since all 229 patients received nutritional intervention, no control groups are available to assist in determining if intervention had a significant impact on outcomes for either subset (patients with low indicators versus "normal" indicators at outset). Similarly, this study fails to identify which disease states, demographic factors, and interventions were predictive of a positive response to therapy. Finally, guidelines are needed to assist caregivers in identifying which subgroups of the elderly institutionalized population are most likely to experience complications during nutritional intervention and what steps can be taken to minimize this possibility. Because of the potential impact of the above points in terms of quality of life and fiscal effectiveness, research in those areas is necessary.

Summary of Principles for Nutritional Evaluation of Institutionalized Elderly Persons

A number of principles flow from the preceding discussion and provide the basis for a successful approach to nutritional care. It is obvious that only those evaluations that use appropriate standards for age and sex are likely to be meaningful. At the same time, the caregiver must be aware of the intrinsic limitations of most tests. While repetition of tests may improve reliability, sensitivity and specificity are best enhanced by a more holistic approach to evaluation and an awareness that factors other than malnutrition may affect nutritional indicators.

The general condition of the patient and the practices of the care team also can have a critical effect on nutritional status. Every effort must be made to identify potentially detrimental practices that might compromise the achievement of successful outcomes. In this respect, a global or comprehensive approach to both assessment and management has obvious benefits. It not only considers traditional nutritional parameters, but also takes into account the history and severity of disease processes; demographic and motivational factors; and administrative features of the present illness, eg, the effect of drugs on appetite and the timing of tests so as not to interfere with meals. Such an approach also considers the risks and complications of intervention and the likelihood that nutritional needs will be satisfied in the present institutional setting. Finally, in a truly "global" assessment of an elderly person the physician/geriatrician should be aware of the past and present functional state of the patient, physiologic reserves now available, and the impact of the present illness on both of these parameters. Although such an evaluation requires skill and intimate knowledge of the patient, it is essential in order to understand the limitations and potential of nutritional intervention.

A Practical Approach to Nutritional Evaluation of Institutionalized Elderly Persons

Table 16-3 contains the basic elements of what might be considered a practical approach to nutritional evaluation in any institutional environment.

Historical Data

Because the incidence of intellectual impairment among the elderly in some settings may reach 50% to 70% (60), it is very important to establish the reliability of historical data early in the patient encounter. When its purpose is appropriately explained to the patient, we have found the *Short Portable Mental Status Questionnaire* by Pfeiffer (61) inoffensive yet effective in identifying gross intellectual impairment.

If the patient appears to be a reliable witness and if his or her physical condition is stable, a review of *demographic and functional data* with the patient tends to establish rapport and a representative profile for deciding future management decisions. Factors assessed at this time include age, marital status, living arrangements, financial resources, social network

Table 16-3. Elements of Nutritional Evaluation

I. *Historical Data*
   - a. Cognitive evaluation
   - b. Demographic/functional data
   - c. Analysis of symptoms
   - d. Dietary history/nutritional risk measure/high risk assessment
   - e. Past medical/surgical history
   - f. Drug history
   - g. Social history
   - h. Home evaluation*
   - i. Interview family and friends

II. *Physical Evaluation*
   - a. Physical exam
   - b. Physical therapy evaluation*
   - c. Occupational therapy evaluation*
   - d. Dietary evaluation

III. *Nutritional Indicators*
   - a. Anthropometric data
   - b. Laboratory tests
   - c. Follow-up

IV. *Needs/Resources Matching*

*When available or appropriate.

relationships (62), health perception, mental health status, activities of daily living, and instrumental activities of daily living. The manner in which this information is obtained (formal versus informal) and the amount of details collected will vary with the individual physician. In general, one should attempt to establish whether the patient's social, emotional, functional, and financial resources permit access to appropriate nutritional support and will continue to do so in the future.

The next step in the historical evaluation entails an analysis of *symptoms* with which the patient now presents. Here one is particularly concerned with both symptoms related to malnutrition in general and others known to be associated with specific nutritional deficits. In an exploratory study conducted on hospitalized patients, we have found that certain symptoms on admission, eg, vomiting, diarrhea, needing help in eating, difficulty chewing, significant weight loss, food allergies, and a present history of decubitii, correlate with a poor outcome defined as a length of stay of greater than 10 days and/or death within 6 months of admission (63). Table 16-4 shows the cross-correlation of the level of nutritional risk with health outcomes. Although our initial measures were crude and the sample was small ($N = 48$), a statistically significant relationship ($X^2 = 5.6$, $P < .02$) was found between nutritional risk and health outcomes. For this reason alone, a search for and into these symptoms on admission is critical in elderly patients.

Symptoms may also provide clues to specific nutritional deficits. For example, instability and depression are associated with vitamin B_6 deficiency; joint pain and swollen gums with vitamin C deficiency; and malaise, headache, and vomiting with vitamin B_3 (pantothenic acid) deficiency (64). A number of common conditions can cause an acute disruption of zinc metabolism, precipitating a syndrome manifested by anorexia, diminished taste and smell, and reduced mentation with signs of cerebellar dysfunction (65). Muscle aches and mental dysfunction are commonly associated with potassium abnormalities (66); tetany and convulsions with hypocalcemia (67); and angina, ischemic necrosis, and ventricular instability with magnesium deficiency (68).

The *dietary history* can be helpful, although diminished recall in some

Table 16-4. Results from the Hospitalized Patients ($N = 48$) Trials Relating Nutritional Risk to Health Outcomes

	Nutritional Risk	
Health Outcomes	No Risk*	At Risk†
Good	11	12
Poor	4	21

*No evidence of any of the seven risk factors on admission.

†Evidence of one or more of the seven risk factors: $X^2 = 5.60$, $df = 1$, $P < .02$.

elderly patients may make this element less important than in the young. Asking a patient to describe a "typical meal" sometimes circumvents the problems posed by declining memory. Wolinsky et al (63) have recently described a 16-item Nutritional Risk Index, which has an impressive capacity for predicting physician, emergency room, and hospital utilization in an ambulatory population. Whether such an index will be of assistance in institutional evaluation remains to be seen.

The importance of identifying *patients at high risk* for malnutrition can not be overestimated (69). Gross overweight (weight for height above 120% of standard) or underweight (weight-for-height below 80% of standard), recent weight loss of 10% or more of body weight, having been on no oral intake for prolonged periods, protracted nutrient losses, increased metabolic needs, and certain drugs with antinutrient or anticatabolic properties can all render a patient susceptible to malnutrition. Speedy identification and treatment of these situations may reduce clinical complications and shorten length of stay.

The *past history* is important in identifying disease states and previous surgery, which have a significant impact on digestion and/or absorption and utilization of nutrients. Examples of conditions that can affect nutrient absorption and are common to an elderly population are cirrhosis, pancreatic insufficiency, malabsorption, intestinal bypass surgery, gastrectomy, and ileal resection. For a more expanded list of such conditions the reader should consult recent reviews by Butterworth (41) and Grant (64).

A detailed *drug history* is a critical element in any nutritional evaluation because of the many interactions between drugs and nutrients (41). The aging process and the older person's propensity for multiple illnesses usually exacerbate this interaction, making reduced nutritional intake and malnutrition more likely (70). Several sources provide lists of some of the more common drugs used by elderly patients, along with the nutrients affected and their mechanism of interaction and consequences (41,71).

Special attention is directed to the multiple interactions between ethanol and various nutrients. While most elderly patients readily admit to use of prescribed medications, the use and abuse of ethanol is often underestimated or denied by this age group because of the social stigma attached to alcoholism by this generation. Bloom (72) estimates that as many as three-million people over the age of 60 are alcoholics. To identify this cohort, she suggests that physicians be alert to such potential telltale clues as unexplained bruises on extremities or broken bones and sprains; prolonged seclusion or refusal to answer the door; and/or frequent use of the emergency room. Other characteristic presentations include sensory symptoms of alcoholic peripheral neuropathy, such as prickliness, burning, or numbness (73); an abnormal depressed mental state, decreased intellectual performance, and altered personality secondary to hepatic encephalopathy (74); weakness and lethargy secondary to folate-deficient anemia (75,76); and the previously mentioned symptoms associated with zinc deficiency (77). Because of the potential reversibility of most of these problems with abstinence and appropriate nutritional supplementation, it is important that health professionals make every effort to diagnose alcoholism in the elderly and arrange for rehabilitative counseling and support.

The "sociological factors which influence nutrition" and the "implications for the practitioner" have been well covered elsewhere in this text (see Chapter 1). The importance of these factors and the necessity for their investigation by the practitioner can not be overestimated. However, it should be stressed that while evaluation of the patient in an institutional setting is important, home assessment of the elderly person before and/or after institutionalization has obvious benefits (78–80). With regard to nutrition, a home visit can provide a wealth of information. One can evaluate the proximity to shops and stores and the barriers, eg, stairs and roadways, separating these from the patient's dwelling. A home visit also makes it easier to identify relationships with relatives, neighbors, and friends; investigate the presence, capacity, and content of supplies of food in cupboards and refrigerators; assess the ability of the patient to function in the familiar environment of his or her own kitchen; and judiciously note telltale clues of alcohol or drug abuse from observation of empty bottles around the dwelling or in nearby wastecans. When the information from such a visit is combined with that gained from and through *interviews with family and friends,* a much more valid data base is obtained and more appropriate and effective management decisions result.

Physical Evaluation

The physical evaluation of the elderly person is another opportunity to identify clues of adequate nutrient intake (81). Initial general inspection can often identify recent weight loss (or gain) via the fit of clothes; dehydration via reduced skin turgor; and nutritional anemia by note of excessive pallor of both skin and conjunctiva. The presence or absence of teeth, loose-fitting or painful dentures, and dysfunctional swallowing reflexes are easily observable and often reliable indicators of nutritional deficit.

As noted in Chapter 2, taste and smell are important adjuncts to appetite, and deficits in either of these sensory parameters can adversely affect nutritional status. Loss of taste and smell has been associated with a number of pathologic conditions including acute viral hepatitis (82), chronic alcoholic cirrhosis (83), and regional enteritis (84). Since all of these conditions have also been associated with zinc deficiency (65,85), it is possible that deficits in olfaction and gustation can be both a cause of malnutrition and a marker of a nutritional deficit. For this reason assessment of taste and smell should be a mandatory part of any nutritional exam.

A number of other clinical findings have been associated with nutritional deficiencies in the elderly. Easily pluckable hair is a sign of protein deficiency. Spoon-shaped nails may indicate a deficiency in dietary iron. Petechiae and purpura correlate with low intake of vitamin C and vitamin K. Glossitis may be due to deficiency of niacin, pyridoxine, or riboflavin; while bone pain and tenderness may identify low serum levels of vitamin D metabolites, calcium, or phosphorus. For a more complete listing of clinical signs and corresponding nutritional deficiencies, recent reviews by Weinsier and Butterworth are recommended (41,69).

When available and appropriate, the evaluations performed by a trained *physical therapist* and an *occupational therapist* can provide the health care team with valuable information about the functional ability of the patient to complete tasks associated with the acquisition, preparation, and consumption of proper nutrients. These assessments have particular relevance in the days preceding discharge from an acute hospital or nursing facility, especially for those patients who will live alone following deinstitutionalization. Such assessments and subsequent training sessions assist caregivers in determining the appropriate timing of discharge and identifying needs, eg, prosthetic devices, which permit successful adaptation to an independent home environment. Moreover, like predischarge cardiac rehabilitation programs, these training sessions instill confidence in elderly individuals, who are usually frightened and concerned over functional loss caused by illness. Time spent in mock kitchens, in physical therapy areas, and even on passes home with a friend or caregiver, often allays fears and enhances confidence in their own ability.

No nutritional evaluation of an elderly person within an institution would be complete without examination by a trained *dietician.* The dietician, or nutrition technician, is an indispensable participant in any multidisciplinary nutritional assessment program (86). While all patients should receive simple dietary evaluations on admission, patients at nutritional risk need more comprehensive nutritional evaluation and data collection, with recommendations for management and follow-up. Through frequent conferences and communication, physician an dietician complement each other's expertise and improve the potential for a better patient outcome.

Nutritional Indicators

As noted previously, the reliability and validity of most indicators used to assess the nutritional status of the elderly have been seriously questioned. In many instances, cutoff points that would permit differentiation between normal and malnourished elderly have not been

Table 16-5. Basic Indicators Useful in Nutritional Assessment of Institutional Elderly

Height and weight
Triceps skin fold
Mid-arm muscle circumference and area
Complete blood count*
Albumin†
Delayed hypersensitivity testing

*Should include WBC count, lymphocyte count, hemoglobin, hematocrit, and indices.
†Transferrin may also be ordered if the prognostic nutritional index is utilized.

determined. Additional problems affecting choice of indicators involve the vast size of the institutionalized population over age 65, the time constraints of staff, and the enormous costs in both acute and chronic facilities generated by intermittent lab tests. These latter three factors require that tests ordered by simple, nontime-consuming, and relatively inexpensive.

Table 16-5 contains a list of indicators which meets the above criteria. The components of this list have been tested individually and in grouped indexes in multiple clinical trials (37,47,48,52,54–58). While the ability of these indicators to predict clinical outcomes in individual situations is controversial (51), many group studies have noted a significant linear correlation between the decrement in an indicator and eventual negative outcomes (56–58). For this reason, some or all of the components of this list should be included in the total nutritional assessment of the elderly patient after appropriate standardization for age and sex.

Of the *anthropometric values,* height and weight have proven to be most valuable in our experience. The frequency with which this information is gathered will vary with the clinical situation. Stable ambulatory patients in a nursing home need weights only once per month, while sick, hospitalized elderly may require their weights taken one or more times daily. Consistent trends in weight change over time are ususally more clinically useful as a predictive factor than exaggerated daily fluctuations, which can usually be attributed to the effect of diuretics or poor weighing techniques, such as using different scales and failure to subtract the weight of wheelchairs or to recognize the effect of manual support of the patient by nursing staff. These fluctuations should require immediate reweighing, correction of errors, and education of staff.

Mitchell and Lipschitz have recently reviewed problems associated with height measurements in the elderly (33). Their work with total arm length (TAL) measurements may eventually provide clinicians with an easier, more valid tool for assessing linear growth. For the time being, necessity dictates that conventional height measurements be used, and such measurements are acceptable only when detrimental effects like kyphosis, osteoporosis, and the bedfast state are integrated into the final analysis.

Laboratory tests can be extremely helpful in evaluating the nutritional needs of institutionalized elderly. A wealth of clinical information can be gained from the complete blood count (CBC), and for this reason it has been a standard element of most clinical evaluations. From the nutritional perspective, this indicator provides potential information about metabolic stress, specific nutrient deficits, and the presence of protein–calorie malnutrition. More specifically stated, a rise in white blood count (WBC) may indicate a systemic infection, and anemia with high or low indices may be associated with B_{12} or folate deficiency when high, or Fe deficiency when low. A lymphocyte count less than 1,500 may be a clue to protein–calorie malnutrition and poor outcomes if other indicators are also low (57). While many other interpretations of the fluctuations in the CBC are possible, the value of this indicator as a warning signal can not be overestimated. Abnormalities in the CBC require the clinicians to stop, evaluate the entire clinical situation, and proceed with a management plan based on incoming data.

Certain rapid turnover transport proteins, such as prealbumin and retinol-binding protein, are "very sensitive to changes in both dietary protein and energy and respond(ed) rapidly to refeeding" (49). For this reason, they may become excellent indicators for the elderly detection of subclinical malnutrition and the long-term management and monitoring of high-risk, elderly patients receiving dietary treatment. However, at the present time, their excess cost (greater than three times that of albumin) and commercial unavailability mediate against their general usage.

Despite its deficits (50), *albumin* remains the least expensive laboratory indicator of visceral protein status presently available. An understanding of the intimate relationship between its synthesis, redistribution, and degradation clarifies the apparent discrepancy between the absence of speedy, significant decrements in serum levels following the onset of serious protein–calorie malnutrition (50). When coupled with an awareness of pathologic factors, loss of albumin in the urine or its diminished production in cirrhosis, knowledge of the physiology of albumin promotes appropriate utilization of this parameter as one of many sources of data whose correlation with other nutritional indicators are necessary before treatment plans can be formulated.

Delayed Hypersensitivity (DH) testing represents the final indicator in what might be described as a practical approach to nutritional evaluation in the elderly. An awareness of the limitations of this indicator among an older age group is critical for its successful utilization. Among factors that may influence the interpretation are the presence of other diseases that may affect cell-mediated immunity, eg, sarcoidosis, inexperience in technics of application, choice of recall antigens (87), variations regarding the definition of anergy; lack of acceptable skin turgor in some patients, and the logistical considerations associated with timely reading of results in 48 to 72 hours. If these restraints can be overcome, delayed hypersensitivity testing has obvious advantages in predicting outcomes, whether used alone in nursing homes (57) or as a part of a more extensive evaluation in an acute care setting (53–56).

After initial collection of the above anthropometric and laboratory data *follow-up evaluation* will depend on the clinical condition of the patient, the type of facility to which he or she has been admitted, and the known turnover time of various indicators. In most instances it can be assumed that the more unstable and sick the patient, the more frequently data should be collected. Thus, an elderly patient in an intensive care unit would have weight evaluated at least daily, while weights monthly or weekly might suffice for a stable elderly resident of a nursing home.

Albumin synthesis is under the control of a number of regulatory influences, including the availability of substrates, such as transfer RNA and amino acid precursors, especially tryptophan (88). Normal half life of this protein is 17 to 20 days (88). Because of large extravascular stores and diminished degradation in deficiency states, significant changes in serum levels may not occur for days following reduced nutrient intake. For this reason it is practically and financially wise to follow this indicator no more closely than at 5- to 7-day intervals. In the absence of significant infection or blood loss, the same advice applies to the frequency with which one orders the CBC.

On the other hand, an acutely ill patient needs daily calorie counts, symptom assessment, and physical examination. Close daily coordination between dietician and physician is usually in order for acute ill patients, while weekly or monthly team conferences usually suffice in more stable situations.

Needs/Resources Matching

For a variety of social and economic reasons, the focus of conventional health care is shifting from reactions to disease to maintenance and promotion of health. In no area is this mind set more important than in dealing with institutionalized elderly people. Because this portion of the population consumes an enormous percentage of health care resources, every effort must be made to prevent their deterioration and maintain their functional integrity.

The objective of the nutritional evaluation of the elderly is to identify deficits in nutritional intake which might compromise outcomes. These deficits may occur as a result of failure of individuals to receive recommended daily allowances of adequate nutrients or because recommended allowances are not sufficient. Recent investigations involving calcium metabolism, as outlined in Chapter 11, emphasize the very real possibility that the latter statement is true. Further research regarding allowances guided by more sophisticated technology is obviously needed. On the other hand, our prime present consideration is to ensure that this population is receiving recommended allowances of nutrients. To accomplish this objective, simple, valid techniques of assessment are needed.

Conclusion

In this chapter we have attempted to point out that a holistic assessment by a trained clinician (not necessarily a physician) may be the best present method for assessing nutritional need. Although we did not discuss it here, we also would suggest that the multiplicity of factors affecting needs evaluation and resource response requires cooperation and communication between various health providers working in tandom as a team. Whether in an acute care facility or in the nursing home, our experience suggests that efficiently conducted team conferences involving nurses, dieticians, physicians, social workers, physical therapists, occupational therapists, and students are a critical component of needs/resources matching, and provide the best forum for prediction of outcome. Further studies involving the influences of health care teams of actual providers on nutritional evaluation and supplementation are recommended.

References

1. Dans PE, Kerr MR: Education in gerontology and geriatrics in medical education. *N Engl J Med* 1979; 300:228–232.
2. Watkin DM: The physiology of aging. *Am J Clin Nutr* 1982; 36:750–758.
3. Lawton MP: Assessment, integration, and environments for older people. *Gerontologist* 1980; 1:38–45.
4. Sanford RA: Tolerance of debility in elderly dependents by supporters at home: Its significance for hospital practice. *Br Med J* 1975; 3:471–473.
5. Blazer D: Working with the elderly patient's family. *Geriatrics* 1978; 33:117–123.
6. Shanas E: The family as a social support system in old age. *Gerontologist* 1979; 19:173.
7. Cantor MH: Neighbors and friends. *Res Aging* 1979; 1:434–463.
8. Chappell NL: Informal support networks among the elderly. *Res Aging* 1983; 5:77–79.
9. Bortz WM: Disuse and aging. *JAMA* 1982; 248:1203–1208.
10. Kent S: Exercise and aging. *Geriatrics* 1982; 37:132–135.

11. Aloia JF: Exercise and skeletal health. *J Am Geriatr Soc* 1981; 29:104–107.
12. Morris JN, Everitt MG, Pollard R, Chaves W: Vigorous exercise in leisure time: Protection against coronary heart disease. *Lancet* 1980; 2:1207–1210.
13. deVries HA, Wiswell RA, Bulbulian R, Moritani T: Tranquilizers effect of exercise: Acute effects of moderate aerobic exercise on spinal reflex activation level. *Am J Phys Med* 1981; 60:57–66.
14. Sinclair DJM, Ingram CG: Controlled trial of supervised exercise training in chronic bronchitis. *Br Med J* 1980; 23:519–521.
15. Diesfedt HFA, Diesfedt-Grdenendijk H: Improving cognitive performance in psychogeriatric patients: The influence of physical exercise. *Age Ageing* 1977; 6:58–64.
16. Paffenbarger RS, Wing AL, Hyde RT: Physical activity as an index of heart attack risk in college alumni. *J Epidemiol Community Health* 1978; 108:161–175.
17. Magnus K, Matroos A, Strackee J: Walking, cycling or gardening with or without seasonal interruption, in relation to acute coronary events. *Am J Epidemiol* 1979; 110:724–733.
18. Clarkson PM: The effect of age and activity level on simple and choice fractionated response time. *Eur J Appl Physiol* 1978; 40:17–25.
19. deVries HA: Physiological effects of an exercise training regimen upon men aged 52–88. *J Gerontol* 1970; 25:325–336.
20. Gutmann GM, Herbert CP, Brown SR: Feldenkrais versus conventional exercises for the elderly. *J Gerontol* 1977; 32:562–572.
21. Belloc WB, Breslow L: Relationship of physical health status and health practices. *Prev Med* 1972; 1:409–421.
22. Steen B, Bruce A, Isaksson B, et al: Body composition in 70-year-old males and females in Gothenburg, Sweden. A population study. *Acta Med Scand (Suppl)* 1977; 611:87–112.
23. Borkan GA, Hults DE, Gerzof SG, et al: *J Gerontol* 1983; 38:673–677.
24. Shizgal HM: Body composition by multiple isotope dilution, in Levenson SM (ed): *Nutritional Assessment—Present Status, Future Directions and Prospects. Report of the Second Ross Conference on Medical Research.* Columbus, Ohio, Ross Laboratories, 1981, pp 94–99.
25. Toh BH, Roberts-Thomason IC, Matthews JD, et al: Depression of cell mediated immunity in old age and the immunopathic diseases, lupus erythematosus, chronic hepatitis, and rheumatoid arthritis. *Clin Exp Immunol* 1973; 14:193–202.
26. Chandra RK: Rossette-forming T lymphocytes and cell-mediated immunity in malnutrition. *Br Med J* 1974; 3:608–609.
27. Goodwin JS, Goodwin JM, Garry PJ: Association between nutritional status and cognitive function in a healthy elderly population. *JAMA* 1983; 249:2917–2920.
28. Abraham S, Lowenstein FW, Johnson CL: Preliminary findings of the first health and nutrition examination survey, United States, 1971–72: Dietary intake and biochemical findings. National Center for Health Statistics DHEW Publ. No. (HRA) 74-1219-1. Government Printing Office, 1974.
29. Elahi VK, Elahi P, Andres R, et al: A longitudinal study of nutritional intake in men. *J Gerontol* 1983; 38:162–180.

30. Forbes GB, Bruining GJ: Urinary excretion and lean body mass. *Am J Clin Nutr* 1976; 29:1359–1366.
31. Cockcroft DW, Gault MH: Prediction of creatinine clearance from serum creatinine. *Nephron* 1976; 16:31–41.
32. Viteri FE, Alvarado J: The Creatinine Height Index: Its use in the estimation of the degree of protein depletion and repletion in protein calorie malnourished children. *Pediatrics* 1970; 46:696–706.
33. Mitchell CO, Lipschitz DA: Creatinine Height Index, in Redfern DE (ed): *Assessing the Nutritional Status of the Elderly—State of the Art. Report of the Third Ross Roundtable on Medical Issues.* (Document No. 0556p.) Columbus, Ohio, Ross Laboratories, 1982, pp 28–31.
34. Nesheim RO: Public health data: Sources and limitations, in Redfern DE (ed): *Assessing the Nutritional Status of the Elderly—State of the Art. Report of the Third Ross Roundtable on Medical Issues.* (Document No. 0556p.) Columbus, Ohio, Ross Laboratories, 1982, pp 7–9.
35. Mitchell CO, Lipschitz DA: Arm length measure as an alternative to height in nutritional assessment of the elderly. Abstracted, *J Parenter Ent Nutr* 1980; 4:603.
36. Goldman R: Decline in organ function, in Rossman I (ed): *Clinical Geriatrics.* Philadelphia, J.B. Lippincott, 1979, pp 23–59.
37. Lipschitz DA, Mitchell CO: Hematological measurements in nutritional assessment of the elderly, in Redfern DE (ed): *Addressing the Nutritional Status of the Elderly—State of the Art. Report of the Third Ross Roundtable on Medical Issues.* (Document No. 0556p.) Columbus, Ohio, Ross Laboratories, 1982, pp 105–113.
38. Cohn SH, Sawitsky A, Vartsky D, et al: Body composition as measured by in vivo neutron activation analysis, in Levenson SM (ed): *Nutritional Assessment—Present Status, Future Directions and Prospects. Report of the Second Ross Roundtable on Medical Research.* Columbus, Ohio, Ross Laboratories, 1981, pp 99–102.
39. Presta E, Wang J, Harrison GC, et al: Measurement of total body electrical conductivity: A new method for estimation of body composition: *Am J Clin Nutr* 1983; 37:735–739.
40. Heymsfield SB, Fulenwider T, Nordlinger B, et al: Accurate measurement of liver, kidney, and spleen volume and mass by computerized axial tomography. *Ann Intern Med* 1979; 90:185–187.
41. Butterworth CE, Weinsier RL: Malnutrition in hospital patients: Assessment and treatment, in Goodhart RS, Shils ME (eds): *Modern Nutrition in Health and Disease.* Philadelphia, Lea & Febiger, 1980, pp 667–684.
42. Beaton GH: Evaluation of dietary intake of the elderly, in Redfern DE (ed): *Addressing the Nutritional Status of the Elderly—State of the Art. Report of the Third Ross Roundtable on Medical Issues.* (Document No. 0556p.) Columbus, Ohio, Ross Laboratories, 1982, pp 18–21.
43. Kinsell K, Harrison GG: Concepts of sensitivity and specificity: Their relevance to nutritional assessment of the elderly, in Redfern DE (ed): *Addressing the Nutritional Status of the Elderly—State of the Art. Report of the Third Ross Roundtable on Medical Issues.* (Document No. 0556p.) Columbus, Ohio, Ross Laboratories, 1982, pp 2–5.

44. Frisancho AR: Triceps skinfold and upper arm muscle size norms for assessment of nutritional status. *Am J Clin Nutr* 1974; 27:1052–1058.
45. Mitchell CO, Lipschitz DA: Detection of protein–calorie malnutrition in the elderly. *Am J Clin Nutr* 1982; 35:398–406.
46. Dale DC: Abnormalities of leucocytes, in Petersdorf RG, et al (ed): *Principles of Internal Medicine, ed.10.* New York, McGraw-Hill, 1983, p 309.
47. William H, Adler MD: Immune status and aging, in Redfern DE (ed): *Addressing the Nutritional State of the Elderly—State of the Art. Report of the Third Ross Roundtable on Medical Issues.* (Document No. 0556p.) Columbus, Ohio, Ross Laboratories, 1982, pp 42–44.
48. Roberts-Thomason TC, Whittinham S, Youngchaiyud U, MacKay IR: Aging, immune response, and mortality. *Lancet* 1974; 2:368–370.
49. Shetty PS, Jung RT, Watrasiewicz KE, James WPT: Rapid-turnover transport proteins: An index of subclinical protein-energy malnutrition. *Lancet* 1979; 1:230–232.
50. Rothschild MA, Oratz M, Schreider SS: Albumin synthesis. *N Engl J Med* 1972; 286:748–757.
51. Audres, R: Discussion: in Redfern DE (ed): *Addressing the Nutritional Status of the Elderly—State of the Art. Report of the Third Ross Roundtable on Medical Issues.* (Document No. 0556p.) Columbus, Ohio, Ross Laboratories, 1982, p 6.
52. Detsky AS, Mendelson RA, Jeejeeboy KA: A decision analysis approach to malnutrition in surgical patients, Abstracted in *Fourth Annual Meeting of Society for Medical Decision Making* et al: 1982, p 368.
53. Mullen JL, Buzby GP, Waldman MT, et al: Prediction of operative morbidity and mortality by preoperative nutritional assessment. *Surg Forum* 1979; 30:80–82.
54. Busby GP, Mullen JL, Matthews DC, et al: Prognostic Nutritional Index in gastrointestinal surgery. *Am J Surg* 1980; 139:160–167.
55. Mullen JL: Prognostic nutritional assessment, in Levenson SM (ed): *Nutritional Assessment—Present Status, Future Directions and Prospects, Report of the Second Ross Conference on Medical Research.* Columbus, Ohio, Ross Laboratories, 1981, pp 127–131.
56. Blackburn GL, Bistrian BR, Harvey K: Indices of protein-calorie malnutrition as predictors of survival, in Levenson SM (ed): *Nutritional Assessment—Present Status, Future Directions and Prospects. Report of the Second Ross Conference on Medical Research.* Columbus, Ohio, Ross Laboratories, 1981, pp 131–137.
57. Shaver HJ, Loper JA, Lutes RA: Nutritional status of nursing home patients. *J Parenter Ent Nutr* 1980; 4:367–370.
58. Seltzer MH, Bastidas JA, Cooper DM, et al: Instant nutritional assessment. *J Parenter Ent Nutr* 1979; 3:157–159.
59. Reinhardt GF, Myscofski JW, Wilkens DB, et al: Incidence and mortality of hypoalbuminemic patients in hospitalized veterans. *J Parenter Ent Nutr* 1980; 4:357–359.
60. Beck JC, Benson DF, Scheibel AB, et al: Dementia in the elderly: The silent epidemic. *Ann Intern Med* 1982; 97:231–241.
61. Pfeiffer E: A short portable mental status questionnaire for the assessment of organic brain deficit in elderly patients. *J Am Geriatr Soc* 1975; 23:433–441.
62. Coe RM, Wolinsky FD, Miller DK, Prendergast JM: Complementary and

compensatory functions in social network relationships among the elderly. *Res Aging* 1984 (in press).
63. Wolinsky FD, Coe RM, Miller DK, et al: Health services utilization among the noninstitutionalized elderly. *J Health Soc Behav* 1983; 24:325–337.
64. Grant JP, Custer PB, Thurlow J: Current techniques of nutritional assessment, in Mullen JL, Crosby LO, Rombeau JL (eds): *The Surgical Clinics of North America. Surgical Nutrition.* Philadelphia, W.B. Saunders, 1981, pp 437–463.
65. Henkin RI, Patten BM, Re PK, Bronzert DA: A syndrome of acute zinc loss. *Arch Neurol* 1975; 32:745–751.
66. Judge TG: Hypokalaemia in the elderly. *Geront Clin* 1968; 10:102–107.
67. Potts JT: Disorders of parathyroid glands, in Petersdorf RG, Adams RD, Braunwald E, et al: (eds): *Principles of Internal Medicine,* ed 10 New York, McGraw-Hill, 1983, p 1942.
68. Gubner RS: Magnesium as a physiologic calcium antagonist: A unifying view of calcium blockers. *Medical Tribune* 1983; (Oct. 12):33.
69. Weinsier RL, Butterworth CE: *Handbook of Clinical Nutrition.* St. Louis, C.V. Mosby, 1981, p 7.
70. Roe DA: Drug-induced malnutrition in geriatric patients. *Compr Ther* 1977; 3:24–28.
71. Lamy PP: Effects of diet and nutrition on drug therapy. *J Am Geriatr Soc* 1982; 30:99–112.
72. Bloom PJ: Alcoholism after sixty. *Am Fam Physician* 1983; 28:111–113.
73. Dart R, Howard L: Alcoholic peripheral neuropathy. *Nutr Rev* 1981; 39:237–238.
74. Schenker S, Henderson GI, Hoyompa AM, McCandless DW: Hepatic and Wernicke's encephalopathies: Current concepts of pathogenesis. *Am J Clin Nutr* 1980; 33:2719–2726.
75. Halstead CH: Folate deficiency in alcoholism. *Am J Clin Nutr* 1980; 33:2736–2740.
76. Lindenbaum J, Roman MJ: Nutritional anemia in alcoholism. *Am J Clin Nutr* 1980; 33:2725–2735.
77. Ressel RM: Vitamin A and zinc metabolism in alcoholism. *Am J Clin Nutr* 1980; 33:2741–2749.
78. Arcand M, Williamson J: An evaluation of home visiting of patients by physicians in geriatric medicine. *Br Med J* 1981; 283:718–720.
79. Currie CT, Moore JT, Friedman SW, Warshaw GS: Assessment of elderly patients at home: A report on fifty cases. *J Am Geriatr Soc* 1981; 29:398–401.
80. Nielsen M, Blenkner M, Bloom M, et al: Older persons after hospitalization. A controlled study of home aide service. *Am J Public Health* 1972; 62:1194–1101.
81. Skaien P: Inadequate nutrition in the elderly: A stumbling block to good health, in Wells T (ed): *Aging and Health Promotion.* Rockville, MD, Aspen Systems Corp., 1981, pp 161–166.
82. Henrin RI, Smith FR: Hyposmia in acute viral hepatitis. *Am J Med Sci* 1972; 264:401–409.
83. Burch RE, Sackin DA, Jetton MM, Sullivan JF: Decreased acuity of taste and smell in cirrhosis. *Gastroenterology* 1974; 67:781.

84. Solomons NW, Khacto KV, Sandstead HH, Rosenberg IH: Zinc nutrition in regional enteritis (RE). Abstracted, *Clin Res* 1974; 22:582a.
85. Solomons NW: Biological availability of zinc in humans. *Am J Clin Nutr* 1982; 35:1048–1075.
86. Jensen TG, Dudrick SJ: Implementation of a multidisciplinary nutritional assessment program. *J Am Diet Assoc* 1981; 79:258–266.
87. Chandra RK: Immunocompetence in nutritional assessment, in Levenson SM (ed): *Nutritional Assessment Present Status, Future Directions and Prospects. Report of the Second Ross Conference on Medical Research.* Columbus, Ohio, Ross Laboratories, 1981, pp 111–113.
88. Podolsky DK, Isselbacher KJ: Derangements of hepatic metabolism, in Petersdorf RG, Adams RD, Braunwald E, et al (eds): *Principles of Internal Medicine,* ed 10. New York, McGraw-Hill, 1983, pp 1773–1779.

17

Nutritional Management of the Elderly

Virginia M. Herrmann

Knowledge about metabolic alterations in the elderly allows health-care personnel to provide appropriate nutritional management. Age-related changes in carbohydrate (Chapter 12), protein (Chapter 3), and fat (Chapter 4) metabolism have been reviewed in this volume.

The diseases that accompany aging often have profound effects complicating the care of the elderly. Senility, organic brain syndrome, and Alzheimer's disease are frequently accompanied by lack of self-care and poor eating habits, resulting in cachexia. The elderly patient who has suffered a cerebrovascular accident may experience dysphagia and suppressed cough reflex, making eating a difficult and potentially dangerous task. Patients with severe coronary altherosclerosis may experience low cardiac output and subsequent dyspnea, which may lead to poor nutrient intake. Declining renal function in the elderly patient necessarily limits the amount of protein and possibly the amount of dietary water, sodium, and potassium that can be ingested. In these situations, nutrition unfortunately may receive low priority in the overall care being administered. With these as starting points, implementation of nutritional therapy in the elderly will be the topic of this chapter.

The Effect of Socioeconomic Factors on Nutritional Management

Eating has become a very social experience in that it predictably divides the day and provides opportunity for conversation and sharing experiences with family and friends. Eating may not be such a pleasant social experience for the elderly. For the elderly who live alone, mealtime may be a reminder of their loneliness and lack of social contacts. The elderly person who has to prepare meals for only one person may not be motivated to prepare elaborate or even adequate meals. Even mild organic brain syndrome and senility may cause some disorientation in the aged, and mealtime may simply be overlooked. More commonly, depression that is so often seen in this group of patients is frequently accompanied by anorexia and lack of interest in food or mealtime. For the elderly with arthritis, osteoporosis, or similar disabling illness, a task as apparently simple as grocery shopping or meal preparation may be extremely difficult or impossible (see also Chapter 1).

The financial income of the elderly population may vary considerably from individual to individual, but most elderly persons experience considerable cutbacks in their income. Individuals relying on Social Security or pension and retirement funds may find their incomes limited, and medication and other medical costs may absorb even more of their income than in previous years, allowing less expenditure on food. When income availability for food is limited, diets are selected that are high in carbohydrate and refined sugars. Foods that are high in protein, such as fresh fish, meat, and eggs, are often not selected because of their price. Other foods that are relatively inexpensive and may provide quantity rather than quality, such as carbohydrates, sweets, and desserts, may be selectively chosen over fresh fruits and vegetables. All of these factors tend to dilute the diet of the elderly.

Enteral Feeding—Delivery Techniques and Available Diets

Assessing the nutritional needs and establishing caloric requirements for elderly individuals has been discussed in Chapter 16. Elderly individuals who are not hospitalized and who will be eating in the home environment may need extensive counseling to ensure that their dietary intake meets their energy and protein requirements. The more difficult situation arises with the patient who is institutionalized and yet still is able to tolerate an enteral diet. Most patients in this situation receive meals on a regular schedule, ie, three times daily. Thorough dietary studies have demonstrated that hospitalized or institutionalized patients, particularly those with severe illness, will consume inadequate essential nutrients when allowed an ad libitum diet from food trays. If the elderly patient has superimposed illness or disease, this inadequate intake becomes even more significant because his or her energy and protein requirements may be greater than normal. Hypercatabolism coupled with inadequate intake makes intensive nutritional management of these patients mandatory. General guidelines for nutritional assessment and supplementation in this group of individuals are as follows (1):

1. All patients who are in a nursing home or other institutionalized form of care or a hospital require complete nutritional assessment. This should include a detailed history as well as physical examination, a history of weight loss, and calculation of the percentage of weight loss over a period of time.
2. Elderly individuals should be weighed daily or at least every other day, and an accurate record of fluid intake and output should be maintained. Patients who are on an ad libitum diet should be followed with accurate daily calorie counts initially to ensure that their intake is adequate.
3. Patients who are eating three meals a day and still taking inadequate amounts of food should be candidates for nutritional supplements or given consideration for concurrent tube feedings.
4. Patients who have suffered a weight loss of 10% or more of their total body weight should be considered for some sort of nutritional support. Maintenance of body weight is a minimal objective, and restoring weight to their previous or ideal body weight should be the goal of nutritional therapy.

After an accurate estimate of caloric and protein needs has been determined, and a decision has been made that the patient be fed an oral diet, whether by food tray or by tube feeding, it is important to decide whether the goal of nutritional therapy is weight maintenance or weight gain. Weight maintenance is achieved by meeting the metabolic requirements, that is, the energy expenditure of the patient. Weight gain, however, requires positive energy balance. An additional 1,000 Cal per day above maintenance requirements will result in a weight gain of approximately 1 kg or 2 lb per week.

Attention must also be directed to the proportion of carbohydrate and fat that the nonprotein calories will comprise. The current diet consumed in the United States consists of approximately 42 percent fat, 46 percent carbohydrates, and 12 percent protein. Our current diet is high in saturated fats, which make up nearly one-third of our fat consumption. It is recommended that Americans adjust their diets so that the total fat consumed is only 30 percent of our caloric intake. It is also recommended that we increase our carbohydrate intake from 46 percent to 58 percent of our total calories, and that we increase our ingestion of complex carbohydrates. Currently, only half of our carbohydrate intake is complex carbohydrate, with the remaining proportion being refined and processed sugars and a small amount of naturally occurring sugars. It is recommended that we increase our complex carbohydrate and naturally occurring sugar intake considerably so that only a very small percentage of our carbohydrate intake will be refined and processed sugars. Most of the currently available tube-feeding formulas that may be given to elderly individuals contain adequate and recommended amounts of fats and carbohydrates. Although the proportions of fat and carbohydrate may be altered in specialized diets, fats should never provide more than 60 percent of the total calories given to an individual.

While a regular house diet provided in nursing homes and most hospitals will provide patients with adequate calories and protein, frequently elderly individuals are unwilling or unable to consume this diet. Additionally, these patients or individuals may be receiving clear or full liquid diets, as these are frequently ordered for patients who may be undergoing various tests or for elderly individuals who are edentulous. Liquid or full liquid diets are inadequate in both calorie and protein content. Additional calories of up to 1,000–1,500 Cal/day may be provided by nutritional supplements given between meals or at bedtime. Also, when liquid diets are requested or required to administer medication, juices or other calorie-containing fluids should be given instead of water.

There are elderly individuals who have a functional gastrointestinal tract, but who are unable to tolerate an oral diet due to severe anorexia, nausea, or other conditions such as oropharyngeal obstruction, which may preclude taking a diet by mouth. These patients are best nourished by enteral feedings. Available tube feedings are safe, simple to use, and less expensive than other forms of nutritional therapy. Nasogastric feeding tubes are available which are very small (Nos. 8–10 French) and soft, as they are made of silastic. Many of these are mercury weighted at the tip to facilitate passage, and a stylet may be inserted to facilitate tube placement in the stomach or proximal jejunum. Patient tolerance is excellent, and many patients or individuals may learn to pass these tubes themselves at home and manage tube feeding successfully on an outpatient basis. Any elderly individual who has severe gastroesophageal reflux, or who is obtunded from previous cerebrovascular accident or other condition, should not receive tube feedings into their stomach in order to minimize the potential for reflux and aspiration of partially digested foods. These patients are candidates for nasojejunal tube feedings. These tubes are somewhat more difficult to position and, when necessary, placement is aided by fluoroscopic visualization and guidance of the tube with a rigid guidewire. Jejunal feedings may be instituted and administered slowly and continuously with the aid of pumps, thereby allowing for gradual absorption of nutrients through the intestinal tract and avoiding a bolus of hypertonic solution in the small intestine, which frequently causes cramping, diarrhea, and possible dehydration. On the other hand, gastric feedings may be given either continuously or by intermittent bolus.

Many elderly people are candidates for permanent tube placement to facilitate nutritional care. Patients who have suffered a cerebrovascular accident and who are semicomatose or obtunded, patients who are senile or bedridden, and patients with severe debilitating illness such as terminal cancer may be best handled by placement of a permanent feeding tube. If the patient is able to handle his own vomitus, and severe gastroesophageal reflux is not a problem, a gastrostomy tube is preferred, because the stomach may serve as a reservoir and allow the delivery of a bolus or large quantities of feedings at one time. Elderly patients who have significant oropharyngeal obstruction secondary to carcinoma or stricture may be good candidates and well handled by a gastrostomy tube. A feeding gastrostomy tube can be inserted under either local or regional anesthesia, thereby diminishing the risk of administration of a general anesthetic in this elderly population. Intermittent or bolus feedings of blenderized regular food at home or provision of a specific tube-feeding product will result in improved nutritional status over a period of time. Patients who are receiving gastrostomy feedings should have the head of their bed elevated 30° for at least one hour after each feeding to reduce the risk of aspiration. Residual gastric volume should be determined immediately prior to feeding, and if the aspirate is in excess of 100 mL, the feedings should be withheld or reduced for a period of time.

Table 17-1 Available Enteral Supplements and Defined Formula Diets

Product	Caloric Density g/L	Carbohydrate g/L	Fat g/L	Protein g/L	Osmolality m osm/kg water
Nutritionally complete formula (ideal p.o. supplement)					
Compleat-B	1.07	128.00	42.8	42.8	690
Ensure	1.06	145.00	37.2	37.2	450
Meritene	1.07	119.00	33.8	69.2	405
Sustacal	1.00	140.00	23.0	61.0	625
Defined Formula E/or low-residue diets					
Criticare HN	1.10	1.10	3.3	36.0	650
Isocal	1.06	132.00	44.0	34.0	350
Osmolyte	1.06	143.00	38.0	37.0	300
Precision-Isotonic	0.96	144.00	30.0	29.0	300
Precision LR	1.11	248.00	0.8	26.0	520
Renu	1.00	1.00	40.0	35.0	300
Travasorb	1.06	1.06	30.0	30.0	450
Travasorb HN	1.00	1.00	13.0	50.0	450
Vital	1.00	185.00	10.0	42.0	450
Vivonex	1.00	231.00	15.0	21.0	550–645
Vivonex HN	1.00	210.00	1.0	42.0	810

Table 17-2 Available Defined Diets of High-Calorie, High-Nitrogen Formula for Enteral Use

Product	Caloric Density g/L	Carbohydrate g/L	Fat g/L	Protein g/L	Osmolality m osm/kg of water
Ensure Plus	1.50	145	53.0	55.0	600
Isocal HCN	2.00	225	90.9	74.8	740
Isotein HN	1.20	156	33.9	67.8	300
Magna Cal	2.00	250	80.0	70.0	590
Stresstein	1.20	170	28.0	70.0	910
Sustacal HC	1.50	190	57.5	60.9	650
Trauma Cal	1.50	140	67.4	82.0	550
Travasorb MCT	2.00	254	66.0	98.0	475

For patients who are abtunded and cannot handle their own vomitus, a feeding jejunostomy can also be placed under local anesthesia. This procedure may also be done concomitantly if another intraabdominal operative procedure is anticipated. Although a gastrostomy tube allows the delivery of bolus feedings of 200–400 mL every two to three hours, jejunostomy feedings are best managed by continuous administration. In general, patients will be initiated at a rate of about 30–50 mL/hour and gradually increased to a total volume of 100–125 mL/hour. Initially, a dilute (½–¾ strength) formula should be administered slowly to assess patient tolerance, unless the tube feeding is isotonic. Isotonic tube feedings may be initiated at full strength. Diarrhea is the most frequent complication of tube feedings, and this can be managed by either reducing the osmolarity and volume of the feeding delivered or by providing antidiarrheal agents. Table 17-1 refers to commonly available nutritional supplements and defined diets available for tube-feeding use. More recently, high-calorie, high-nitrogen tube feedings have become available (Table 17-2). These products allow delivery of concentrated calories and protein, in a smaller fluid volume, and may be very beneficial for the elderly person with congestive heart failure, renal failure, or peripheral edema.

Parenteral Feeding

Elderly patients who cannot be fed oral diets, that is, whose intestinal tract is nonfunctional because of disease or its treatment, are candidates for parenteral feeding. Parenteral feedings may be delivered either by a peripheral vein or by central vein; the choice of peripheral or central venous nutrition will be determined both by patient requirements and by the venous access available in the patient. Peripheral vein nutrition allows the infusion of a carbohydrate source (dextrose), amino acids, fat emulsions, vitamins, and trace elements. However, the quantity of calories that can be delivered by peripheral venous route is limited by the tonicity of these solutions. In general, a solution with a tonicity of greater than 700 m osm should not be delivered by peripheral vein. Most commercially available peripheral vein solutions have tonicity between 600–700 m osm. Peripheral vein solutions allow a relatively low caloric intake to be delivered (1,200–1,800 Cal/day in 2,500–3,000 mL of fluid volume). This severely limits the use of peripheral vein solutions. In general, the indications for peripheral vein are summarized as follows:

1. Peripheral vein solution may provide enough calories and protein for weight maintenance in very small patients whose metabolic requirements are low or in patients who are not hypermetabolic (ie, patients whose basal energy expenditure does not exceed 1,600–1,800 Cal/day).
2. Peripheral vein feedings may also be used in the elderly who will require central vein feeding, but in whom central vein feeding has not yet been instituted. Thus, in the interim these patients may receive peripheral vein feedings and approximately 1,800 Cal/day in an effort to minimize protein depletion.
3. Peripheral vein feeding may be used as supplement when the quantity of enteral feedings are limited by dysfunction of the gastrointestinal tract.

Currently available peripheral vein solutions provide approximately 280–300 calories/L and 4.6–7.1 g nitrogen/L. These solutions are prepared by mixing 500 mL of a 10% dextrose solution with 500 mL of a 5.5% or 8.5% amino acid solution. Additional nonprotein calories may be provided by the use of fat emulsions. An additional 550 Cal will be provided by 500 mL of a 10% fat emulsion, and an additional 1,100 Cal will be provided by 500 mL of a 20% fat emulsion. These solutions should be administered through a large-bore peripheral vein, and the infusion catheter should be changed every 48 to 72 hours to avoid thrombophlebitis, which is a very frequent mechanical complication of peripheral vein feeding.

The fat emulsions may be delivered simultaneously by IV piggyback technique into the dextrose and amino acid solution. It should be kept in mind, however, that at least 2.5–3.0 L of fluid will have to be administered to provide approximately 1,800 Cal by peripheral vein feeding, which severely limits the use of this technique in many elderly patients. Elderly patients with a history of congestive heart failure, renal failure, or pulmonary edema may not be able to tolerate 2.5–3 L of fluid administered in a 24-hour period. Therefore, peripheral vein feeding should be delivered with extreme caution in the elderly, particularly those with superimposed illnesses that may limit their tolerance to the delivery of large amounts of intravenous fluid.

All patients who are fed by peripheral vein should be weighed daily, preferably on the same scale. It is essential that accurate intake and output records be maintained as well. Laboratory data that ought to be obtained in these patients at the initiation of peripheral vein total parenteral nutrition (TPN) include serum electrolytes, blood urea nitrogen (BUN), and serum glucose. These should also be obtained at least twice weekly after the patient is stabilized on peripheral vein TPN. Liver function tests, calcium, phosphate, magnesium, and triglyceride levels ought to be determined weekly if the patient is clinically stable (Table 17-3). Peripheral vein feeding is associated with a minimum number of mechanical and septic complications. Probably the most frequent complication associated with peripheral vein feeding is thrombophlebitis and phlebothrombosis. These complications can be minimized again by using a very

Table 17–3. Variables to Be Monitored During Intravenous Alimentation with Suggested Frequency of Monitoring*

Variables to Be Monitored	Suggested Frequency First Week	Later
Energy Balance		
Weight	Daily	Daily
Metabolic Variables		
Blood Measurements		
Plasma electrolytes (Na^+, K^+, Cl^-)	Daily	3 × weekly
Blood urea nitrogen	3 × weekly	2 × weekly
Plasma osmolarity†	Daily	3 × weekly
Plasma total calcium and inorganic phosphate	3 × weekly	2 × weekly
Blood glucose	Daily	3 × weekly
Plasma transaminases	3 × weekly	2 × weekly
Plasma total protein and fractions	2 × weekly	Weekly
Blood acid-base status	As indicated	As indicated
Hemoglobin	Weekly	Weekly
Ammonia	As indicated	As indicated
Magnesium	2 × weekly	Weekly
Triglyceride	Weekly	Weekly
Urine Measurements		
Glucose	4–6 × daily	2 × daily
Specific gravity or osmolarity	2–4 × daily	Daily
General Measurements		
V_lume of intravenous solution	Daily	Daily
Oral intake (if any)	Daily	Daily
Urinary output	Daily	Daily
Prevention and Detection of Infection		
Clinical observations (activity, temperature, symptoms)	Daily	Daily
WBC count and differential	As indicated	As indicated
Cultures	As indicated	As indicated

*Adapted from Wilmore DW (10).

†May be predicted from 2 × Na^+ concentration (mEq/L) + blood glucose (mg/dL) divided by 18.

large peripheral vein for the feeding, and changing the catheter site every two days. Strict attention to aseptic technic during line insertion, as well as care of the line, will further minimize these complications (2).

Metabolic complications are infrequently seen in patients receiving peripheral vein TPN, in large part because the tonicity of the solution limits the amount of dextrose and amino acids that can be delivered via peripheral vein. Fluid and electrolyte abnormalities that are seen are very similar to those seen in patients receiving standard intravenous electrolyte solutions, and can be corrected by altering the quantity of intravenous solutions or by manipulating the electrolyte concentration. Hyperglycemia and glucosuria are infrequent findings unless the elderly patient is diabetic. One of the more common metabolic complications noted in patients receiving peripheral vein feedings is mild uremia. In the absence of renal dysfunction, this usually indicates dehydration in the elderly patient; however, uremia may also be observed when large quantities of amino acids are administered without an appropriate nonprotein calorie source. In this situation, the amino acids are shunted through the urea cycle because the appropriate energy source for protein synthesis is not available. In this situation, the uremia is corrected by increasing the quantity of nonprotein calories delivered, thereby improving the calorie-to-nitrogen ratio or decreasing the amount of amino acids given to the patient. Both of these maneuvers improve the calorie-to-nitrogen ratio and provide more energy substrate for protein synthesis.

Fat Emulsion

As a nonprotein energy source, fat provides more energy per unit weight (9 Cal/g) than either carbohydrate or protein, which both provide 4 Cal/g. Intravenous fat is available as an emulsion with particles that are handled exactly as chylomicrons. Fat emulsions may be used to provide for essential fatty acids, and they may also be used to serve as a nonprotein calorie source. If fat emulsion is administered as a major calorie source during parenteral nutrition, that is, for example, during peripheral nutrition, then positive nitrogen balance and weight gain may be achieved in both adults and children. In this situation, fat may comprise between 40% and 60% of the toal nonprotein calories delivered.

Fat may also be delivered as a source of essential fatty acids. These essential fatty acids are linoleic, linolenic, and oleic acid. Fatty acid deficiency in adults is prevented by supplying at least 4% to 10% of the total daily caloric requirements as essential fatty acids. In most adult elderly patients, this will necessitate administering two to three 500-mL bottles of a 10% fat emulsion weekly, or one to two bottles of a 20% fat emulsion weekly.

Since fat emulsions provide 1.1 calorie/mL in a 10% solution or 2 calories/mL in a 20% solution, fats can provide high energy in a low volume. Fats should never add up to more than 60% of the nonprotein calories delivered, and adult elderly patients should not receive more than 2.0–2.5 g of fat per kilogram body weight per day. Fat has several advantages, including a high caloric value and a low osmolarity. A 10% fat solution has an osmolarity of 280 m osm/L, and a 20% solution an osmolarity of 350 m osm/L. This permits easy delivery by peripheral vein with a low incidence of thrombophlebitis. Additionally, fat does not alter lipid profiles in adult patients unless patients have primary hyperlipoproteinemia. Patients with adult respiratory distress syndrome, hepatic failure, and coagulopathy need to have serum triglyceride levels monitored while they are receiving fat emulsion. Because of their high phosphate content, fat emulsions should be used with caution in patients with renal failure as well. Patients who receive fat emulsion should have a baseline fasting triglyceride level drawn prior to initiating therapy. Triglyceride levels should then be monitored weekly, and a sample should be drawn six hours following the infusion of fat emulsion. If the triglyceride level is elevated, the quantity of the fat infused should be reduced, or the rate of fat administration lowered.

Central Vein Nutrition

Elderly individuals may have diseases that increase their energy expenditure as well as urinary nitrogen output. The elderly patient who is traumatized or septic may meet the need for increased glucose by breaking down lean body mass to provide gluconeogenic amino acids. As visceral protein production falls, anergy and other manifestations of altered immune function may result. As visceral and structural breakdown continues, wasting of intercostal and diaphragmatic muscles occurs. Respiratory function is compromised and respiratory infection or failure may result. The increased protein and energy substrate required by these individuals cannot be provided safely by peripheral vein nutrition. The amount of fluid that would need to be delivered to provide adequate calories and protein would be prohibitive. Central vein nutrition, however, allows the delivery of a large amount of calories and protein in a relatively low fluid volume.

Glucose or dextrose is the primary calorie source used in central vein nutrition. The six carbon compound is broken down to three carbon fragments, which enter the Krebs cycle, providing substrate for generation of more glucose and energy. Although other carbohydrate sources have been used for this, glucose is preferred, as fructose may cause elevated lactate and pyruvate production and consequent metabolic acidosis, and Xylitol is associated with hepatoxicity (3).

Central vein solutions are infused through a catheter that has been placed into the internal jugular or subclavian vein. The hypertonicity of these solutions necessitates that the catheter tip be located either in the superior vena cava or the right atrium. Delivery of hypertonic solutions of this nature into a vein of smaller caliber is associated with a high incidence of venous thrombosis and possible superior vena cava syndrome (4–7). Standard central vein solutions commonly are a combination of 500 mL of 50% dextrose with 500 mL of 8.5% or 10% amino acid solution. The final solution contains 250 g of carbohydrate and over 7 g of nitrogen per L, which provides approximately 1,000 Cal/L. Electrolytes, trace minerals, and vitamins can then be added as needed. Two and one-half to three liters of this solution daily will then provide 2,500–3,000 Cal and over 130 g of protein. This will meet the energy needs and protein requirements of most stressed elderly individuals.

Elderly individuals may have concomitant disease states that complicate the delivery of either enteral or parenteral nutrition. For elderly individuals with congestive heart failure or renal failure, administration of excessive fluid volumes may be contraindicated. In these instances, 500–750 mL of 70% dextrose may be used to provide adequate calories in a more compact fluid volume.

Elderly patients with renal failure will require a parenteral formula that provides a relatively high calorie-to-nitrogen ratio, ideally 450:one, in an effort to support protein synthesis from amino acids rather than allowing the amino acids to contribute to excessive urea production. Additionally, specialized parenteral renal failure formulas are available that provide a high ratio of essential to nonessential amino acids, which should further lower urea production. Amino acid solutions for renal failure should also contain relatively low amounts of arginine, as this amino acid is crucial in the urea cycle to utilize ammonia (NH_3) and consequently produce urea. Enteral formulas are also available for use in renal failure, and similar to their parenteral counterparts, contain a high proportion of essential amino acids and low amounts of arginine, with a high calorie-to-nitrogen ratio.

Hepatic failure in the elderly may require specialized nutritional support, particularly if the hepatic dysfunction is severe enough to cause altered mental status. These patients have impaired protein synthesis with decreased levels of albumin, transferrin, and clotting factors. Vitamin metabolism may be affected in hepatic failure as evidenced by an inability to convert vitamin D_3, an inert compound, to a more active form. There may also be depletion of pyridoxine (vitamin B_6) and thiamine (vitamin B_1) in these individuals. Since the liver is the storage site for folate, thiamine, pyridoxine, nicotinamide, and pantothenic acid, the concentration and availability of all of these may be decreased. The mechanism of altered mental status and encephalopathy in these people is complex but is related to an increase in plasma aromatic amino acids (phenylalanine, tyramine, and tryptophan), an increase in methionine, glutamine, and aspartate, and a decrease in plasma branched chain amino acids (leucine, isoleucine, and valine). Efforts to feed persons with serious hepatic disease have been directed at offering a diet that provides:

1. An adequate carbohydrate substrate
2. A large proportion of the total amino acid content (50%) as branched chain amino acids
3. A decrease in the aromatic amino acids
4. A decrease in ammonia-generating amino acids (especially glycine)
5. An increase in the ammonia-processing amino acid, arginine.

Both enteral and parenteral formulas are available to achieve these effects and can be used in patients with liver disease who require specialized support.

Vitamins

There are relatively little data available on the vitamin requirements in various disease states. Requirements of the water-soluble B and C vitamins do increase with stress and injury and may be given liberally. These vitamins are supplied daily to patients receiving total parenteral nutrition. More caution shoud be exercised with delivery of the fat-soluble vitamins. Excesses of vitamins A, D, and E have been reported with deleterious side effects. For this reason, fat-soluble vitamins are usually added to a regimen of parenteral nutrition on a weekly or biweekly basis (3).

Trace Metals

Trace metal deficiencies may be seen in the elderly who receive no food orally for longer than 2 to 3 weeks, or who are very cachectic. The aged with gastrointestinal fistulas may have marked zinc deficiency from loss of zinc in enteric fluid. Zinc deficiency is associated with poor wound healing, dermatitis and skin rash, hair loss, alterations in ability to taste, and disturbances in immune function. Zinc is a vital trace element in protein and muscle metabolism. The zinc requirement for patients receiving total parenteral nutrition is 2–6 mg zinc/day (3, 8, 9). Patients with excessive nasogastric drainage, fistula drainage, or severe diarrhea may have parenteral zinc requirements as high as 10–20 mg/day.

Copper deficiency may be associated with megaloblastic anemia in patients being fed intravenously for long periods. However, this deficiency is rare and copper requirements are usually met by supplying 0.5–2 mg copper/day (9). Copper is metabolized in the liver, however, and ought to be used with caution if at all in patients with hyperbilirubinemia.

Chromium deficiency may cause peripheral neuropathy, or produce an abnormal glucose tolerance. Fortunately, chromium deficiency is also rare, and the daily requirement is approximately 15 μg chromium/day.

Manganese is also supplied on a daily basis to the elderly receiving TPN (0.15 mg–0.8 mg manganese/day), although manganese deficiency like chromium is quite rare (8).

References

1. Herrmann VM, Osteen RT, Wilmore DW: Cancer and the kidney, in Rieselbach RE, Garnick MB, et al (eds) *Nutritional Consideration.* Philadelphia, Lippincott, 1982, pp 234–235.
2. Harvey KB, Bothe A, Blackburn GL: Nutritional assessment and patient outcome during oncological therapy. *Cancer* 1979; 43:2065.
3. Fischer JE, Freund HR: Surgical nutrition, in *Central Hyperolimentation.* Boston, Little, Brown & Co, 1983, p 663.
4. Henzel JH, DeWeese MS: Morbid and mortal complications associated with prolonged central venous cannulation: Awareness, recognition and prevention. *Am J Surg* 1971; 121:600.
5. Ryan JA, Abel RM, Abbott WM, et al: Catheter complications in total perenteral nutrition: A prospective study of 200 patients. *N Eng J Med* 1974; 290:757.
6. McDonough JJ, Altemeier WA: Subclavian vein thrombosis secondary to indwelling catheters. *Surg Gyn-Obst* 1971; 133:397.
7. Fabri PJ, Mirtallo JP, Ruberg RL, et al: Incidence and prevention of thrombosis of the subclavian vein during total parenteral nutrition. *Surg Gyn-Obst* 1982; 155:238.
8. Expert Panel, AMA Department of Food and Nutrition: Guidelines for essential trace element preparation for parenteral use. *JAMA* 1979; 241:2051.
9. Lowry SF, Goodgame JT, Smith JC, et al: Abnormalities of zinc and copper during total perenteral nutrition. *Ann Surg* 1979; 189:119.
10. Wilmore DW. *The Metabolic Management of the Critically Ill.* New York, Plenum Press, 1977, p 231.

18

Problems in Nutritional Management of the Elderly

Margaret A. Flynn

The preceding chapters have identified many of the nutritional issues that create special problems in health care of the elderly. This chapter reviews some approaches to management of selected problems. The management of nutritional problems in the elderly requires reliable assessment of food in the diet and their nutrients. Too often, health professionals don't recognize the difference in the use of "nutrient," "food," and "diet" in their messages to clients. Nutrients are specific organic substances used by body cells for growth and maintenance of health and reproductive function. Foods contain nutrients. Diets contain food eaten by people or animals.

Information about nutrients will be plagued with problems of inaccuracy unless the dietary intake is constant and measured, and aliquots are chemically analyzed. Even under these circumstance, individual variability in digestion and absorption does not guarantee the same nutrient circulation in the blood and their subsequent availability to metabolizing cells of all persons. Our studies in young healthy men have demonstrated different efficiencies of digestive-absorptive functions (1). In the aged gut, these efficiencies could be highly variable, depending on digestive enzymes, hormonal changes, food intolerances, polypharmacy, etc.

Measurement of Nutrient Intake

How do we acquire nutrient intake data from individuals in a free-living or institutionalized population? The most frequently used methods of acquiring this information have been 24-hour recall of food eaten, a check of food frequency intake, or three- to seven-day food records kept by the client. Once the client's food intake is documented, there is the additional problem of determining the character and quantity of nutrients therein. This information can be derived from food composition tables, but this process is of limited value in evaluating dietary intake. Not only are there wide variations in nutrient content of foods in raw state due to soil, harvest methods and storage, but the processing and cooking also provide many avenues for nutrient losses. Data about food nutrients are averages of chemical analyses of raw and cooked food samples drawn from various parts of the United States. The data should be recognized as average estimates, not as specific always reproducible values. One has to remember also that all dietary information obtained from a client is subjective. Despite these drawbacks, food composition tables are used widely in computer banks as well as published handbooks from the U.S. Department of Agriculture. Studies have shown that calculated nutrient data from food records compare well with chemically analyzed aliquots of the food records for energy, protein, and calcium but not for other nutrients. For this reason food composition tables are the routine tools used by dieticians, just as handbooks of blood and urine values are routine references for physicians and nurses.

It is difficult to estimate the percent of transfer of food nutrients to blood nutrients, but skinfold measurements and formulas for estimating body composition, for deriving muscle mass via creatinine excretion, and for estimating nutritional assessment are no more certain. Humans are indeed variable and any management of nutritional problems has to be individualized to life style, financial burden, ethnic background, and desire to comply.

Nutritional Problems in the Aged

As man ages, the most prevalent chronic health problems are cardiovascular disease, cancer, diabetes mellitus, and degenerative joint disease. In adults, these problems may result from affluence and life style interacting with age, sex, and genetic contributions. Atherosclerosis, for instance, has been with mankind for centuries and yet it is an enigma because no one can be sure what is its exact cause, its certain cure, or its prevention. Risk factors involved include cigarette smoking, hypertension, diabetes, obesity, diet, and emotional stress. No single agent such as diet causes atherosclerotic disease. Yet the populace often views diet as causal and changes in diet as preventive. Specifically, they believe dietary cholesterol and saturated fats are the culprit. It is unfortunate that many health professionals encourage this view. In fact, because calorie intake in the United States is often overabundant, everyone has multiple opportunities to manufacture cholesterol and saturated fatty acids, which circulate in blood and can form atheromata.

Therefore, in the elderly, strict control of dietary cholesterol and saturated fat is much less important than control of obesity and total calories. As Andres has stated, few data support the argument that switching to a diet high in polyunsaturated fat changes serum cholesterol (2). In the Baltimore longitudinal study, a middle-class, highly educated population was surveyed for dietary status between 1961 and 1975, using a seven-day dietary diary technique. In this study Andres and colleagues found there was a tendency among their clients to eat less saturated (S) fat and more polyunsaturated (P) as years passed (2). There was also a tendency for cholesterol levels to increase in early adulthood, but to stabilize and decrease in later years. Andres (2) stated:

> . . . it is one thing to look at a population and say that serum cholesterol fell during a certain time period in the same *population* in which P/S ratio increased. But when we examined the same *individuals* to see whether those whose P/S ratios changed the most were the same people whose cholesterol levels changed the most, and whether those whose P/S ratio changed in the wrong direction (ie, decreased when those whose cholesterol values had the opposite kind of change), we found we could not explain the changes in serum cholesterol in our population from the change in P/S ratio. (p 12)

In longitudinal studies in Missouri, investigators found similar results when men who ate eggs, beef, and pork were compared with those who did not eat them (3–5).

Persons 65 years old and older may not benefit by rigid restrictions of diet in which specific nutritious foods such as eggs, whole milk products, beef, and pork are advised to be strongly limited because of their cholesterol and saturated fat content. They will benefit by total caloric intake restrictions only if they are obese and/or have diabetes mellitus or joint problems.

Hypertension

Another cardiovascular problem, which may be nutrition related, is hypertension. In a special edition of the *Annals of Internal Medicine* on hypertension, Kaplan (6):

> ... the current definitions of hypertension have led to falsely high estimates of its prevalence, inexact assessments of risk and overly aggressive use of antihypertensive drug therapy. An analysis of available data show that at least one-third of persons found to be hypertensive on initial screening will not have elevated blood pressure subsequently, that persons with mild hypertension (diastolic blood pressure 90 to 104 mm Hg) are not at high risk of cardiovascular disease, and that many patients with mild hypertension should be treated with nondrug therapies unless their diastolic blood pressure remains above 100 mm Hg. (p 705)

A tendency for increases in blood pressure accompanies aging and many elderly will have blood pressure readings in the 90–100 mm Hg range. Besides Kaplan's admonitions, decisions regarding therapy should be tempered by the knowledge that side effects, such as hypokalemia and hyperlipidemia, often accompany the use of diuretics and other hypertensive agents. As mentioned previously, a low sodium, high potassium diet is an alternative treatment. Clinicians should be advised that in prescribing low sodium diets they should inform their patients that the three food groups, grains, meat/fish, and milk/dairy products, must be controlled since these contribute about 50% of average sodium intake from food. These foods also contribute significant amounts of dietary calcium, iron, magnesium, and vitamin B_6 (7).

McCarron et al (8) recently reviewed nutrition correlates of blood pressure. Defining high blood pressure as 160/95 mm Hg or greater, he presented the nutritional data from 24-hour food recall in hypertensive men and women aged 55 to 74 years, showing that their sodium intake was not excessive, but their calcium and potassium intakes were low. Laragh and Pecker (9) stated that rigorous sodium deprivation can lower blood pressure of 30% to 50% of patients with essential hypertension. In the rest, sodium depletion is ineffective and can raise blood pressure in some instances. They stated that there is no evidence that widely applied moderate salt intake reduction could prevent development of hypertension. Evidence is lacking to show that in sodium-sensitive hypertensive patients, moderate salt restriction would lower blood pressure.

Several investigators have cited intake of potassium as being significant in nutritional management of hypertension. Langford (10), looking at epidemiologic data, stated that an acute increase of potassium intake lowers blood pressure probably by negating blood-pressure-raising effects of sodium. In a more cautious fashion, Tannen (11) stated that a potassium intake of 120–175 mEq daily in humans results in a modest lowering of blood pressure of 3% to 10%. He warned that although intake of this amount of potassium is not hazardous in persons with normal renal function, it poses a definite risk in those with compromised renal function. He does not recommend wide use of high potassium therapy for hypertension at this time.

Estimates of sodium and potassium intake by humans are usually designated as discretionary (consumer controlled) and nondiscretionary (naturally occurring and commercially controlled). Fregly (12), using data from 12 different studies dating from 1970 to 1982 involving food intake, salt production, and salt sales, stated that urinary excretion of sodium showed an average daily nondiscretionary intake of sodium chloride (NaCl) by males aged 1 to 74 was 6.3 g, and by females, 4.6 g. Fregly stated that total (discretionary plus nondiscretionary) daily NaCl intake was 10–14.5 g per person. Nondiscretionary potassium chloride intake ranged from 4 to 11 g daily per person. Although individual data were not available to analyze, the mean data suggest a negative correlation between sodium and potassium intake and percent of persons with hypertension.

Cancer

Health professionals are intently aware of the debilitating effects of cancer, with weight loss and its possible beginnings of malnutrition. There is a logical desire to use nutritional intervention because it has proved successful in other forms of malnutrition and because modern available commercial enteral and parenteral feedings are available as an adjunct in efforts to treat the usual accompanying anorexia of patients with cancer. Chemotherapeutic agents often create disorder with nausea, emesis, diarrhea, ulcerations in mucosa during ingestion, digestion, and absorption of nutrients from dietary foods. Radiation treatments are accompanied by stomatitis, enteritis malabsorption. Surgical procedures may remove entire digestive–absorptive surfaces.

All of these treatments for cancer would be better tolerated if the patient were in good nutritional status. Often, when clients are malnourished, nutritional repletion is used prior to therapy, with liquid supplements for clients who are outpatients or with tube feedings or intravenous hyperalimination for hospitalized patients. If the gastrointestinal tract is functional, the oral route is preferred for maintaining mucosal integrity of the tract. Dietary counseling is necessary during oral supplementation because of poor patient compliance. For patients who are at maintenance, a good prescription has been 35 kcal/kg body weight/day. For improved wound healing or anabolism during or posttreatment, 45 kcal/kg day and 1–1.5 g of protein/kg/day are recommended (13). If the gut cannot be depended on, Daly has suggested parenteral nutritional support via peripheral or central vein. The peripheral method can supply up to 2,500 kcal/day. His central venous total parenteral nutrition infusion has a solution that is 20%–30% dextrose, 3.5%–5% amino acids plus supplementation with vitamins, electrolytes, and minerals. In addition, Goodgame et al (14) recommended that 500 mL of 10% or 20% fat emulsion be infused two to three times weekly for prevention of essential fatty acid deficiency (14).

Parenteral nutrition in cancer patients may be problematic if patients have depressed platelet levels. If there is a possibility of hemorrhage due to thrombocytopenia, platelets can be transfused. Additionally, the precise indication for nutritional intervention as adjunct to cancer therapy must be more realistically defined. Whereas retrospective studies show that improved nutritional status may renew immunocompetence, improve antineoplastic therapy, reduce postoperative morbidity, and increase survival, prospective clinical trials have not confirmed these results. Daly (13) bases his decision to prescribe nutritional support for cancer patients only when malnutrition may interfere with required therapy and when severe malnutrition must not develop following treatment. Further, "only those patients with disease states not so extensive as to preclude any hope for a meaningful therapeutic response should be considered candidates for nutritional support."

Diabetes Mellitus

The evaluation and management of elderly patients with diabetes mellitus is beset by difficulties. Not everyone defines diabetes mellitus as only aberrant carbohydrate metabolism. Some define it as a disorder of protein, fat, and carbohydrate metabolism wherein an absolute or relative deficiency of insulin is secreted by the pancreas. Terminology used to describe the disease is equally confusing. "latent," "chemical," "juvenile," "adult onset," "gestational," "insulin dependent," and "noninsulin dependent" are terms that are commonly used. Also, diagnostic testing for diabetes mellitus has previously involved oral glucose loading followed by half-hour plasma levels extending through three hours to ascertain rise and fall of glucose influx. Certainly this procedure yields data for intolerance to simple carbohydrates. However, many elderly who have age-related changes in glucose tolerance may be erroneously declared to have diabetes mellitus by such testing.

Recently the National Diabetes Data Group of NIH proposed new diagnostic criteria and another classification of diabetes mellitus. These criteria are not universally accepted, but do appear to do away with age adjustment. They state that in nonpregnant adults, elevated *fasting* glucose (venous plasma) of 140 mg/dL or more is diagnostic if it is present on more than one occasion. When an Oral Glucose Tolerance Test (OGTT) is done, the two-hour sample *and* some other sample taken between administration of a 65-g glucose dose and an interval of two hours *must* be 200 mg/dL or greater (venous plasma), using a standardized

OGTT format. Earlier standards had made an age adjustment for OGTT by adding 10 mg/dL per decade of age after the fifth decade to the two-hour limit of 140 mg/dL.

Role of the Nutritionist

From a standpoint of nutritional problems in the elderly, simple carbohydrate intolerance as well as diabetes mellitus have dire effects on kidneys, eyes, and arteries. Therefore, the dietary aims have been the attainment of body weight judged to be ideal for height and close control of plasma glucose acceptable for good health. The role of a dietitian or nutritionist in this management is not only educational, but can also be persuasive. Dietitians know food and nutrients and can individualize diet plans to suit the client, making better compliance possible. Acceptable dietary distribution of calories allows 50% to 60% carbohydrate, 15% protein, and the rest fat calories. A recent study examined whether the form of dietary carbohydrate influences glucose and insulin responses in 12 patients who had insulin-dependent diabetes mellitus with mean age of 26 years (range 19 to 35), 10 patients who had noninsulin-dependent diabetes mellitus with mean age of 62 years (range 44 to 82), and 10 healthy subjects with mean age 39 (range 22 to 69). The mean duration of diabetes mellitus was eight years (15). A 700-kcal test breakfast was composed of common foods containing the same amounts of carbohydrate, protein, and fat, but a different test carbohydrate that accounted for 25% of total caloric value of the meal. The subjects tested glucose, fructose, sucrose, potato starch, and wheat starch. The breakfast contained two eggs, bacon, margarine, and milk. The results showed that the sucrose meal did not produce significantly greater peak increments in the plasma concentration of glucose or greater increments in the area under the plasma-response curves than meals containing potato, wheat, or glucose. A cautionary observation must be made about this study: The carbohydrates were within a *meal* of 33% calories as fat, 18% as protein, and 49% as carbohydrate. The news media heralded the results as "diabetics may consume sugar, physicians reveal," hardly a true presentation of the constraints of the study.

Basic principles of diet therapy for persons who have diabetes are the same for all ages: Keep blood glucose under control without risk of serious hypoglycemia. Self-administered insulin becomes difficult in elderly persons because of poor eyesight and stiffening joints. Compliance with diet is often poor. Coexisting diseases may mandate sodium restriction, abstinence from lactose-containing food, and changes in fat ingestion.

Drugs commonly taken by older persons may modify nutrients or can be modified by them. Elderly people who have used certain drugs over a long time or who use multiple drugs or patients who are malnourished and are prescribed drugs may be at risk. Certain drugs such as tetracycline and penicillin are better absorbed in a fasting state. Propranolol, hydralazine, and griseofulvin are better absorbed with food or after eating. Patients should be given oral and written instructions as to when the drug should be taken. The effect of drugs on nutrient absorption, drug/food and drug/alcohol incompatibilities, as well as drugs that alter food intake are well discussed and documented by Roe (16).

References

1. Flynn MA, Gehrke C, Maier BR, et al: Effect of diet on fecal nutrients. *J Am* Diet Assoc 1977; 71:521–526.
2. Andres R: in Redfern DE (ed): *Assessing the Nutritional Status of the Elderly—State of the Art. Roundtable discussion on medical issues.* Columbus, Ohio, Ross Laboratories, 1982, p 12.
3. Flynn MA, Nolph GB, Flynn TC, et al: Effect of dietary egg on human serum cholesterol and triglycerides. *Am J Clin Nutr* 1979; 32:1051–1057.
4. Flynn MA, Heine B, Nolph GB, et al: Serum lipids in humans fed diets containing beef or fish and poultry. *Am J Clin Nutr* 1981; 34:2734–2741.
5. Flynn MA, Naumann HD, Nolph GB, et al: Dietary "meats" and serum lipids. *Am J Clin Nutr* 1982; 35:935–942.
6. Kaplan NM: Hypertension: prevalence, risks and effect of therapy. *Ann Intern Med* 1983; 982:705–709.
7. USDA Nationwide Food Consumption Survey: Food and Nutrient Intake of Individuals in One day in the U.S. (1977–78 Preliminary Report No. 2) Science and Education Administration, 1980.
8. McCarron DA, Stanton J, Henry H, Morris C: Assessment of nutritional correlates of blood pressure. *Ann Intern Med* 1983; 98:715–719.
9. Laragh JH, Pecker MS: Dietary sodium and essential hypertension: some myths, hopes and truths. *Ann Intern Med* 1983; 98:735–743.
10. Langford HG: Dietary potassium and hypertension: epidemiologic data *Ann Intern Med* 1983; 98:770–772.
11. Tannen RL: Effects of potassium on blood pressure control. *Ann Intern Med* 1983; 98:773–780.
12. Fregly MJ: Estimates of sodium and potassium intake. *Ann Intern Med* 1983; 98:792–799.
13. Daly JM: Nutritional support and the cancer patient. Clin Consult Nutr Support 1983; 3:1–5.
14. Goodgame JT, Lowry SF, Brennan MF: Essential fatty acid deficiency in total parenteral nutrition: time course of development and suggestions for therapy. *Surgery* 1978; 84:271–277.
15. Bantle JP, Laine DC, Castle GW, et al: Postprandial glucose and insulin responses to meals containing different carbohydrates in normal and diabetic subjects. *N Engl J* 1983; 309:7–12.
16. Roe D: *Clinical Nutrition for the Health Scientist.* West Palm Beach, FL, CRC Press, 1979.

19

Interrelationship of Exercise and Nutrition in the Elderly

John W. Shepard, Jr.

Although there is both truth and humor in the statement "We are what we eat," a more comprehensive description of ourselves would be, "We are both what we eat and what we do." The genetically determined components of body composition are known to be importantly modified by both nutritional status and physical activity levels throughout the human life span. This chapter is intended to provide a broad overview of how alterations in substrate consumption (nutrition) and combustion (energy production) throughout adult life affect the composition and functional capacities of the human body.

Body Composition

From extensive anthropometric studies of the composition of the human body, Behnke (1) developed the concept of the reference man and woman. The average height, weight, and body composition in terms of muscle and fat for Behnke's reference young healthy adults are presented in Figure 19-1. It is against these "ideal" body compositions that we will discuss the changes that occur with alterations in caloric intake and levels of physical activity throughout the aging process.

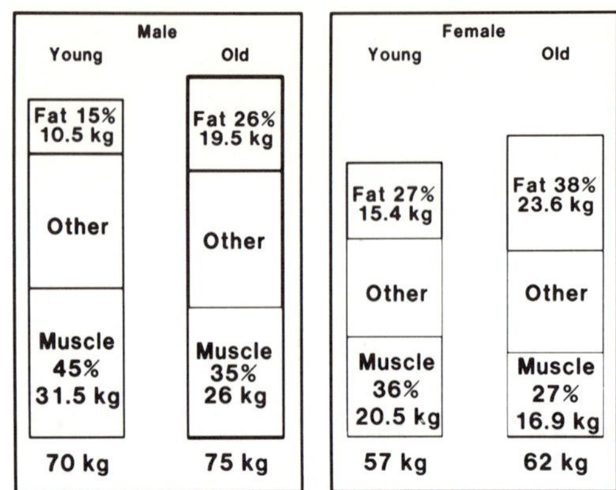

Figure 19-1. Average body compositions for young (20–25 years old) and elderly (60–65 years old) men and women.

Effects of Exercise on Body Composition (Muscle)

Although exercise has protean effects on multiple organ systems within the human body, the changes in skeletal muscle structure and function are perhaps the most dramatic. Skeletal muscle is composed of numerous individual fibers oriented parallel to one another along the axis of contraction. There exist two major fiber types. Slow-twitch (type I) fibers contain abundant mitochondria and generate energy predominantly via oxidative metabolism. They are resistant to fatigue and ideally adapted for the performance of prolonged aerobic exercise (2,3). In contrast, fast-twitch (type II) fibers, which have been further subdivided into types II-A and II-B, contain high levels of myosin ATPase, along with the glycolytic enzymes necessary for energy production via anaerobic metabolism. These fibers are functionally important to the performance of short-duration high-intensity work, but are more susceptible to fatigue. The ratio of slow- to fast-twitch muscle fibers varies considerably between individuals as well as between different muscle groups.

Both types of fibers are in actuality multinucleated muscle cells, which have developed from the fusion of myoblasts during gestation. Because the number of these postmitotic cells (fibers) probably remains constant after birth, changes in muscle size result from hypertrophy and/or atrophy of the component fibers. Exercise performed against heavy resistive loads (strength training) is considerably more effective than prolonged exercise at low resistive loads (endurance training) in producing muscular hypertrophy (4,5). Muscle biopsies performed before and after eight weeks of progressive resistance training have demonstrated selective hypertrophy of the fast-twitch fibers (6). If strength training is discontinued, prolonged bed rest is imposed or an extremity is immobilized in a cast, muscular atrophy will eventually occur (7,8). Figure 19-2 schematically depicts the effects that extremes in levels of physical activity can have on body composition, assuming a caloric intake adjusted to maintain a constant store of body fat.

Effects of Caloric Balance on Body Composition (Adipose Tissue)

Just as the level of physical activity is a major determinant of muscle mass, caloric balance is the primary determinant of body fat content. In fact, the response of the adipose system at the cellular level to an excessive or deficient caloric balance is similar to the response of skeletal muscle to varying levels of physical activity. Although the total number of fat cells increases throughout infancy and adolescence, once adulthood is reached the total number of fat cells is considered to remain relatively constant. In nonobese adult male volunteers, Salans et al (9) have demonstrated that a weight gain of 15% to 25% is achieved by an increase in fat-cell size (hypertrophy) with no significant change in fat-cell number. Subsequent weight reduction was associated with a decrease in fat-cell size to control values, with no change in cell number. Figure 19-3 schematically depicts the effects of excessive and deficient caloric balance on body composition where the physical activity level and muscle mass have been held constant. In comparison, obesity developing during childhood and adolescence is characterized by substantial increases in the number of fat cells (hyperplasia) as well as fat-cell size (10,11). Because the upper limit for adipocyte lipid content is approximately 1.0 μg of lipid per cell, massive weight gain in adults is also associated with fat-cell hyperplasia accompanying hypertrophy (12).

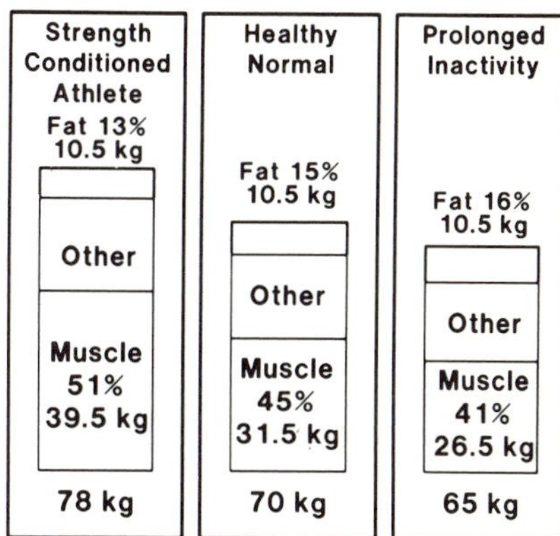

Figure 19-2. Effects of extremes in physical activity on body composition with caloric intake adjusted to maintain a constant store of body fat.

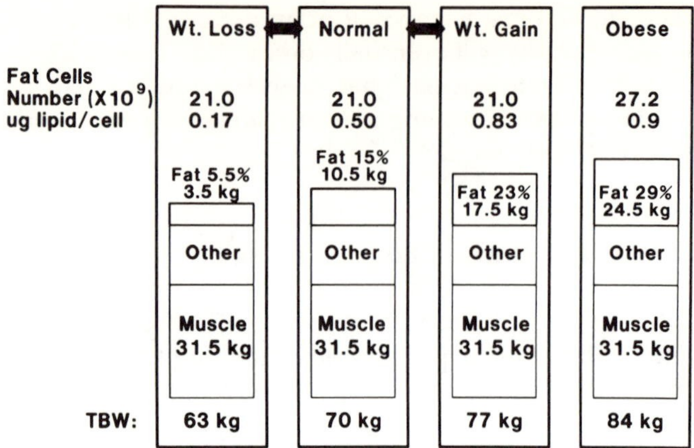

Figure 19-3. Effects of exercise and deficient caloric intake on body composition with physical activity level adjusted to maintain a constant muscle mass.

Changes in Body Composition with Age

From studies of body weight as a function of age in developed countries, body weight increases about 10% from early adulthood through middle age and thereafter progressively declines (13). While increasing stores of body fat are responsible for the initial increase in body weight, decrements in lean body mass, predominantly muscle, contribute to the reversal of this trend. Studies utilizing hydrostatic weighing and measurement of total body water have indicated that percent body fat increases from approximately 15% to 26% in men and from 27 to 38% in women between young adulthood and old age (13,14).

Over the same age range, total body potassium stores have been observed to decrease by 15% to 25%, reflecting a decrease in body cell mass (13,15). Because muscle has the highest intracellular concentration of potassium and is the largest organ system by weight, these findings imply significant reductions in muscle mass, as do the reductions in creatinine excretion which occur with age (16). Muscle fibers have also been demonstrated to decrease in size with age by direct morphologic measurement (17). Figure 19-1 graphically illustrates the differences in body composition which occur with age. The direct implications of these changes in body composition are: (1) Physical work will have to be performed with reduced muscle mass functioning under the added burden of transporting excess stored fat. (2) A combination of caloric limitation and exercise will be required to reduce fat stores and rebuild muscle, thereby returning body composition to "ideal." While caloric restriction can reduce fat stores to youthful proportions, there are major unresolved questions regarding the extent to which exercise training can reverse age-related muscular atrophy and cardiovascular functional deterioration.

Substrate Requirements for Physical Activity

Good nutrition is necessary not only to provide substrates for cellular growth and development, but also to provide the chemical energy required for the performance of physical work. The basic metabolic fuels required for the generation of this chemical energy under aerobic conditions are shown in Figure 19-4. Under anaerobic conditions, the energy available to support muscle contraction is limited to regional stores of adenosine triphosphate (ATP), creatine phosphate, and the ATP that can be generated by the metabolic conversion of glucose to lactate via the glycolytic pathway. In the presence of oxygen and aerobic conditions, tremendously greater quantities of energy can be generated via Krebs cycle activity coupled to mitochondrial oxidative phosphorylation. Although nutritionists have traditionally focused on the nutrients delivered via the gastrointestinal tract, and exercise physiologists have concentrated on the delivery of oxygen via integrated cardiopulmonary function, the holistic overview presented in Figure 19-4 recognizes the mutual importance of both systems in providing the biologic fuels required to perform physical work.

The combustion of a standard quantity of each of these metabolic substrates generates a relatively specific amount of energy. These values are given in Figure 19-5, along with the approximate total body store of each substrate and the energy potentially available from the combustion of the respective body stores. Because basal oxygen (O_2) consumption averages about 0.25 L/minute, corresponding to an energy production of 1.25 kcal/minute, body stores of O_2 are only sufficient to sustain basal metabolic activity for about eight minutes. At the 10- to 15-fold higher levels of O_2 consumption associated with vigorous exercise, body O_2 stores would be exhausted within 60 seconds, emphasizing the critical role of continuous O_2 delivery in maintaining energy generation to support physical activity.

In comparison to O_2 stores, the potential energy available from stored carbohydrate is two orders of magnitude greater, and therefore capable

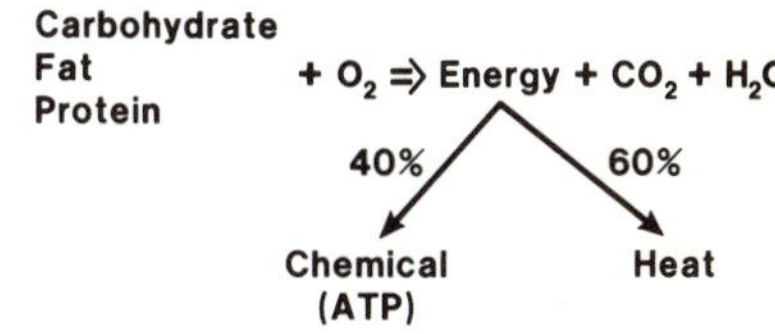

Figure 19-4. Biologic fuels for energy production.

	Body Stores	Potential Energy (kcal)
Oxygen (5 kcal/L)	2L	10
Carbohydrate (4 kcal/g)		
Muscle Glycogen	375 g	1,500
Liver Glycogen	105 g	420
Extracellular Glucose	20 g	80
	500 g	2,000
Protein (4 kcal/g)	6,300 g	25,200
Fat (9 kcal/g)	10,500 g	94,500

Data are for 70 kg σ 15% Fat, 45% Muscle

Figure 19-5. Total body stores of substrates and potentially available energy to support physical activity.

of supporting energy production during exercise for more extended periods of time. In addition, metabolic pathways permit the interconversion of proteins and the glycerol portion of storage fat (triglycerides) to carbohydrate; these pathways act to buffer the depletion of carbohydrate stores. Despite these supplemental pathways and relatively abundant carbohydrate stores, muscle fatigue at heavy workloads has been documented by Bergstrom et al (18) to coincide with muscle glycogen depletion. In this study, nine healthy subjects underwent quadriceps muscle biopsy before and after exercising to exhaustion at 75% of their maximal O_2 consumption ($\dot{V}O_2max$) on a cycle ergometer. The exercise studies were performed following three days of ingesting a normal "mixed" diet, a 2,800-kcal carbohydrate-deficient diet and a 2,800-kcal high-carbohydrate diet. On the normal mixed diet, work duration averaged 114 minutes and muscle glycogen content decreased from 1.75 to 0.17 g/100 g muscle. Following three days of the carbohydrate-deficient diet, work duration was decreased by 50% and muscle glycogen fell from a markedly reduced control value of 0.63 to 0.13 g/100 g muscle postexercise. In contrast, the high-carbohydrate diet boosted pre-exercise muscle oxygen content to 3.31 g/100 g muscle, which had the beneficial effect of extending work duration by 46%.

Blood glucose is known to play an increasingly important role in providing energy for exercising muscle as work duration is extended and local glycogen stores become progressively depleted (19). It has also been shown that glucose infusion and carbohydrate feeding during strenuous exercise can respectively delay muscle glycogen depletion and extend endurance time (20,21). In addition, histochemical staining technics have documented that muscle glycogen depletion occurs selectively within the muscle fiber type predominantly responsible for performance of the activity. In long distance running, a high-intensity but predominantly aerobic form of exercise, glycogen depletion has been found to be greatest in the slow-twitch fibers (22). In contrast, high-intensity largely anaerobic exercise predominantly depletes glycogen stores from fast-twitch fibers (23). These studies clearly indicate the importance of diet and muscle glycogen stores to high-intensity exercise. At work rates below 40% of maximal O_2 consumption, exercise is not associated with severe muscle glycogen depletion and can be maintained for greatly extended periods of time.

Because of the large body stores of protein and the fact that protein catabolism plays only a minor indirect role in providing energy for muscular contraction, the selective elimination of protein from the diet has been observed to have little impact on exercise performance for a period of up to several weeks (24,25). Eventually protein elimination from the diet will result in muscular atrophy, weakness, and development of nutritional edema.

In contrast to protein, free fatty acids released from triglyceride stores represent a major fuel source for exercising muscle (26). Despite this fact, the selective elimination of fat from the diet has been shown to have minimal effects on physical work performance for periods lasting several months (25). This ability of the human body to maintain exercise capacity for extended periods in the absence of dietary fat intake is accounted for by the large body fat stores as well as the metabolic pathways that exist to convert carbohydrates and protein into fat. In the complete absence of caloric intake, exercise capacity is impaired within two or three days.

Aging and Oxygen Delivery

Although prolonged high-intensity exercise can be limited by the depletion of muscle glycogen stores, the major factor establishing an upper limit to physical work capacity is the ability of the oxygen delivery system to sustain aerobic metabolism. The transfer of O_2 from the atmosphere to exercising muscle with the corresponding elimination of CO_2 is recognized to depend on the coordinated functioning of the pulmonary, blood, and cardiovascular systems. Both cross-sectional and longitudinal aging studies have documented reductions in maximal oxygen consumption ($\dot{V}O_2max$) with age (27–34). While genetic factors undoubtedly have a major effect in determining $\dot{V}O_2max$ (35), the rate of decline with age is significantly influenced by the level of physical conditioning at the time of measurement (28,30,34,36). The approximate 35% reduction in $\dot{V}O_2max$, which occurs between ages 25 and 65, Figure 19-6, is predominantly caused by the decline in cardiovascular and not pulmonary function. Since $\dot{V}O_2max$ equals the product of maximal cardiac output and

$$\text{Oxygen Consumption} = (\text{Cardiac Output})\ (\text{a-}\bar{v}O_2\ \text{Difference})$$

$$\underset{(ml/min)}{\dot{V}O_2} = \underset{(beats/min)}{(HR} \times \underset{(ml/beat)}{SV)} \quad (\underset{(ml/dl)}{CaO_2} - \underset{(ml/dl)}{CvO_2})\ (10^{-2})$$

Young (25y)	3,400 =	195 x	118	x	(19.1 -	4.3)
Old (65y)	2,200 =	160 x	106	x	(18.9 -	5.9)
% Change	-35%	-15%	-10%		-1%	+37%

$\Delta CO = -26\%$ $\Delta(a\text{-}\bar{v}DO_2) = -12\%$

Figure 19-6. Differences in maximal O_2 consumption and its components (cardiac output and arterial to mixed venous O_2 content difference) between young and elderly male subjects.

maximal arterial to venous oxygen content difference, the 25% to 30% decrement in maximal cardiac output is responsible for the major portion of the reduction in $\dot{V}O_2max$ with age. The decrease in maximal cardiac output in turn predominantly results from reductions in maximal heart rate and, to a lesser extent, from decreases in maximal stroke volume (28,29,32,37–40). Recent studies have indicated that left ventricular ejection fraction decreases with maximal exercise as a function of increasing age (41). Experimental studies have indicated that the increased impedance to left ventricular ejection imposed by the decreased compliance of the aged arterial vasculature likely plays a major role in limiting stroke volume during exercise in old animals (36,42).

In addition to reductions in maximal cardiac output, the magnitude of the arterial to mixed venous oxygen content difference at maximal exercise has also been found to decrease with advancing age (43–45). Although there tends to be a small decrease in arterial oxygen content (CaO_2) with age, the major effect is the inability of the older individual to extract as much oxygen from the blood, thereby leaving a larger content of oxygen in the mixed venous blood (CvO_2). A decreased capacity of the aged systemic vascular bed to distribute blood flow selectively to the exercising muscle is the most likely, but unproven, mechanism responsible for this finding.

Although the partial pressure of oxygen in arterial blood (PaO_2) decreases with age (46,47), this decrease occurs on the relatively horizontal portion of the oxyhemoglobin dissociation curve. Consequently, arterial oxyhemoglobin saturation (SaO_2) is minimally reduced in older persons free of pulmonary disease. This factor, combined with the fact that hemoglobin concentrations remain normal with aging is responsible for the near constancy of CaO_2 with age. However, the development of anemia, for which there are multiple nutritional causes, is known to limit maximal exercise by reducing the oxygen-carrying capacity of arterial blood (48).

Physical Activity and Exercise Capacity with Aging

In industrial societies there are multiple reasons for the well-documented decline in physical activity that occurs with advancing age. Several studies have indicated that the average daily caloric intake or energy requirement decreases from approximately 2,900 to 2,100 kcal/day between the third and seventh decades of life for men and from 2,000 to 1,500 kcal/day for women over the same age span (49). This approximately 25% decrease in caloric (energy) requirement results from decreased physical activity as well as basal metabolic rate (BMR). The decrease in BMR with age is proportional to the decrease in metabolically active tissue, primarily muscle, which occurs with aging (16,50). In active young adults, greater than 50% of total caloric intake may be utilized to support physical activity, whereas elderly individuals may use less than 40%. Figure 19-7 shows the effects of varying intensities and durations of physical activity on daily energy requirements expressed in terms of both oxygen consumption and caloric expenditure. As illustrated, eight hours of light exercise will require an O_2 consumption of 360 L, an amount equivalent to the total daily resting O_2 consumption. If the remaining 16 hours are spent at the resting level of O_2 consumption, total daily O_2 consumption would be increased by 240 to 600 L, which would correspond to a daily caloric requirement of 3,000 kcal. This level approximates the energy requirements of a normally active young adult male. For an older man in whom resting O_2 consumption has decreased by 10%, it is easily calculated that only 3 hours of light exercise per day would be sufficient to achieve the normative elderly males' daily energy expenditure of 2,100 kcal. From consideration of these caloric data alone, one would estimate that the physical activity of the elderly would be decreased by approximately one half. Other studies employing more direct methodologies and recently reviewed by Shephard (14) have further documented the substantial decrease in physical activity which occurs in the elderly, especially in those who have been institutionalized. In comparison, highly conditioned athletes may train six hours per day at O_2 consumptions averaging

	$\dot{V}O_2$ (L/min)	Exercise Duration (h/d)	$\dot{V}O_2$(L/d) Rest	$\dot{V}O_2$(L/d) Exercise	Energy Expenditure kcal/d
Rest	0.25	0	360	-	1,800
Exercise Level					
Light	0.75	8	240	360	3,000
Moderate	1.25	4	300	300	3,000
Heavy	2.25	2	330	270	3,000

Figure 19-7. Effects of physical activity level and duration on daily caloric (energy) expenditure.

2.0 L/minute. At this level of physical activity 5,000 kcal/day would be required to meet total energy needs, of which 3,600 kcal (72%) would be used to support physical activity.

Multiple variables contribute to the general decrease in physical activity with age. Of major importance to a constantly increasing percentage of the aging population are the limitations imposed by the development of age-related disease processes. The protean medical consequences of systemic atherosclerosis, including coronary heart disease, stroke, and peripheral vascular insufficiency, commonly limit physical activity as does the frequent development of musculoskeletal disorders including degenerative joint disease, back pain, osteoporosis, and fractures, especially of the hip. Physical activity is restricted by the progressive development of chronic obstructive lung disease in a significant proportion of the cigarette-consuming segment of society. Massive obesity also tends to restrict physical activity because of difficulties encountered in performing specific activities as well as the unpleasant sensation of dyspnea, which accompanies exertion.

In addition to age-related disease processes, the physiologic changes accompanying aging progressively limit exercise capacity via the decrements in cardiovascular function and muscle mass previously discussed. It is important to realize that aging is associated not only with a decrease in $\dot{V}O_2max$, but also with deconditioning secondary to decreased physical activity. Deconditioning results in the onset of anaerobic metabolism (anaerobic threshold) at a lower percentage level of $\dot{V}O_2max$ than occurs in well-conditioned subjects (51,52). Because workloads exceeding the anaerobic threshold can be tolerated for only short periods of time, the actual reduction in workload which can be tolerated by deconditioned elderly subjects is greater than would be predicted on the basis of percentage reductions in $\dot{V}O_2max$ alone. Representative values for young and old subjects are presented in Figure 19-8. These data illustrate why an activity like jogging, which requires an O_2 consumption of 1,800 mL/minute, can be performed for a relatively unlimited time by a conditioned athlete, for a substantial duration by an active young adult, but only transiently by a sedentary elderly individual whose anaerobic threshold is only 1,200 mL/minute. Even walking cannot be tolerated for prolonged periods by the sedentary elderly because it requires an O_2 consumption greater than 40% $\dot{V}O_2max$.

In addition to the limitations imposed by physiologic aging and age-associated disease processes, there also exist a number of important social, psychologic, and economic reasons for the decline in physical activity with age. The general attitude in most societies, which fortunately appears to be changing, is that older people have worked hard and should take it easy in their retirement years. Unless recreational activities requiring physical exertion are incorporated into the life style of individuals retiring from occupations demanding physical work, a decrease in

	$\dot{V}O_2$ max. (ml/min)	40% $\dot{V}O_2$ max.* (ml/min)	Anaerobic Threshold (ml/min)
Young (25y)			
Active	3,400	1,360	2,210 (65% $\dot{V}O_2$ max.)
Athlete	4,600	1,840	3,450 (75% $\dot{V}O_2$ max.)
Old (65y)			
Sedentary	2,200	880	1,200 (50% $\dot{V}O_2$ max.)
Trained	2,500	1,000	1,500 (60% $\dot{V}O_2$ max.)

* Level of oxygen consumption which can be maintained for an extended period of time

	$\dot{V}O_2$ (ml/min)
Walking 2.5 mph	1,000
Jogging 5 mph	1,800
Running 10 mph	3,500

Figure 19-8. Effects of level of conditioning on maximal O_2 consumption and anaerobic threshold in young and elderly male subjects.

physical activity and caloric expenditure will occur. Without a concomitant reduction in caloric intake, obesity will likely develop. Even before retirement, older workers are frequently transferred or promoted into jobs requiring limited physical exertion. However, for these individuals retirement may actually provide an opportunity to increase physical activity through the additional time made available to pursue recreational activities.

Exercise Training and the Elderly

The effects of exercise training have been extensively studied in young and middle-aged adults and evidence exists that most of these effects can be achieved in the elderly. The effects obtained with any training program are dependent upon several variables, which include the pretraining level of fitness as well as the frequency, intensity, duration, and type of training activity performed. In general, activities generating high muscle tensions at low frequencies of repetition are employed for strength (anaerobic) training while endurance (aerobic) training is accomplished by high-frequency, low-tension muscular contractile activity. Because endurance activities rely on aerobic metabolism for energy production, many of the effects observed with endurance training are functionally related to improved oxygen delivery and utilization. Improvement in $\dot{V}O_2$max with endurance training predominantly results from an increase in maximal cardiac output, with increased oxygen extraction contributing in young, but not older subjects (52–54). Because maximal heart rate does not increase with training, increases in cardiac output result from increased stroke volume as a result of augmented left-ventricular end-diastolic volume with constant ejection fraction (55). With endurance training, skeletal muscle shows hypertrophy of slow twitch (oxidative) muscle fibers, increased mitochondrial and myoglobin content, as well as increased activity of the mitochondrial enzymes involved in oxidative metabolism (56–60).

Although the results of several early studies suggested that older individuals were not likely to benefit from exercise training (61,62), more recent studies have clearly documented improvements in work capacity, $\dot{V}O_2$max, and/or reductions in heart rate at submaximal workloads (63–69). While the reported increases in $\dot{V}O_2$max have ranged from 5% to 38%, it is reasonable to expect a 15% increase $\dot{V}O_2$max along with an increase in anaerobic threshold. Figure 19-8 presents representative values for $\dot{V}O_2$max, 40% of $\dot{V}O_2$max, and anaerobic threshold for a sedentary elderly male and the estimated improvements that can be anticipated with training. In this example, the 14% increase in $\dot{V}O_2$max with training augments 40% $\dot{V}O_2$max from 880 to 1,000 mL/minutes. Despite the relatively small magnitude of this response, the functional result may be more significant. This results from the fact that walking, which requires an O_2 consumption of approximately 1,000 mL/minute, now utilizes only 40% of maximal capacity and activities requiring this percentage or less of maximal oxygen consumption can usually be performed for extended periods of time without fatigue. The associated improvement in anaerobic threshold which occurs with training will additionally extend functional work capacity.

It is important to remember that the extent of gain in aerobic capacity will depend on the frequency, intensity, and duration of training as well as pretraining fitness. Sidney and Shephard (69) observed a 33% increase in $\dot{V}O_2$max in previously sedentary older adults who trained frequently (3.3 times per week) at high intensity (heart rates 140–150 beats/minutes), whereas individuals training infrequently (1.5 times per week) at low intensity (heart rates 120–130 beats/minute) showed no improvement. Subjects training infrequently but at high intensity showed an intermediate 10% increase in $\dot{V}O_2$max.

Although endurance training has been shown to increase $\dot{V}O_2$max in the elderly, care must be taken to increase physical activity gradually to avoid musculoskeletal injury. In general, training sessions should be conducted three to four days per week, with individual sessions lasting from 30 to 60 minutes. Following an adequate warmup period, each session should be designed to expend 200 to 300 kcal of energy at an intensity equal to or greater than 60% of $\dot{V}O_2$max. Because each pound of adipose tissue contains approximately 3,500 kcal, it is easily calculated that this quantity of stored energy would be sufficient to power an exercise program conducted three days per week, expending 292 kcal per session for four weeks.

A number of studies have directly focused on the effects of training on body weight and composition in the elderly (63,64,67,70,71). Even when no restrictions are placed on caloric intake, exercise training produces consistent reductions in body fat content (64,67,70,71), but minimal reductions in total body weight. These findings imply an increase in lean body mass, which has been substantiated by the report of a 4% increase in total body ^{40}K in one study (70). These results are consistent with those obtained in numerous studies of young and middle-aged subjects (72,73). On average, an aerobic exercise program of four months' duration can be expected to decrease body fat stores by 4% to 10%, increase lean body mass by 1%, and decrease total body weight by 1%.

Summary

Aging is a biologic process associated with important changes in the composition and functional capacity of the human body. Under conditions of essentially unrestricted caloric intake, total body weight increases throughout early adult life, plateaus during late middle age, and begins to decline in the seventh decade of life. Throughout most of the adult life span, there is progressive hypertrophy of adipose tissue and atrophy of lean body mass. This necessitates increased work on the part of the decreased muscle mass to move the stored fat during physical work. Caloric intake decreases in a relatively linear pattern throughout adult life and is related to the decrease in metabolically active lean body mass as well as adoption of a more sedentary life style. The extent to which decreased physical activity with aging contributes to the decrease in lean body mass is not known. However, it is clear that physical work capacity declines with age, as related to a progressive decline in cardiovascular function. Exercise has been shown to improve work capacity and cardiovascular function in the elderly when training is undertaken with sufficient frequency, intensity, and duration. While the relative gains are similar to those reported for younger subjects, they cannot ultimately prevent the progressive decline in function with age. Although basic research in molecular biology may some day provide methods to delay or even arrest the aging process, it is presently within the power of every healthy aging individual to delay the physiologic decline and body compositional changes associated with aging by integrating exercise into his or her daily routine and adjusting caloric intake to maintain a youthful proportion of body fat.

References

1. Behnke AR, Wilmore JH: *Evaluation and Regulation of Body Build and Composition.* Englewood Cliffs, New Jersey, Prentice-Hall, 1974.
2. Saltin B, Henriksson J, Nygaard E, Andersen P: Fiber types and metabolic

potentials of skeletal muscles in sedentary man and endurance runners. *Ann NY Acad Sci* 1977; 301:3–29.

3. McArdle WD, Katch FI, Katch VL: *Exercise Physiology: Energy, Nutrition, and Human Performance.* Philadelphia, Lea & Febiger, 1981, pp 234–248.
4. Edstrom L, Ekblom B: Differences in sizes of red and white muscle fibres in vastus lateralis of musculus quadriceps femoris of normal individuals and athletes. Relation to physical performance. *Scand J Clin Lab Invest* 1972; 30:175–181.
5. MacDougall JD, Ward GR, Sale DG, Sutton JR: Biochemical adaptation of human skeletal muscle to heavy resistance training and immobilization. *J Appl Physiol* 1977; 43:700–703.
6. Thorstensson A: Muscle strength, fibre types and enzyme activities in man. *Acta Physiol Scand (Suppl)* 1976; 443.
7. Booth FW, Gollnick PD: Effects of disuse on the structure and function of skeletal muscle. *Med Sci Sports Exerc* 1983; 15:415–420.
8. Greenleaf JE, Bernauer EM, Juhos LT, et al: Effects of exercise on fluid exchange and body composition in man during 14-day bed rest. *J Appl Physiol* 1977; 43:126–132.
9. Salans LB, Horton ES, Sims EAH: Experimental obesity in man: Cellular character of the adipose tissue. *J Clin Invest* 1971; 50:1005–1011.
10. Bjorntorp P, Carlgren G, Isaksson B, et al: Effect of an energy-reduced dietary regimen in relation to adipose tissue cellularity in obese women. *Am J Clin Nutr* 1975; 28:445–452.
11. Hirsch J, Knittle JL: Cellularity of obese and nonobese human adipose tissue. *Fed Proc* 1970; 29:1516–1521.
12. Hirsch J, Batchelor BR: Adipose tissue cellularity in human obesity. *Clin Endocrinol Metab* 1976; 5:299–311.
13. Rossman I: Anatomic and body composition changes with aging, in Finch CE, Hayflick L (eds): *Handbook of the Biology of Aging.* New York, Van Nostrand Reinhold, 1977, pp 189–221.
14. Shephard RJ: *Physical Activity and Aging.* London, Croom Helm, 1978.
15. Meneely GR, Heyssel RM, Ball COT, et al: Analysis of factors affecting body composition determined from potassium content in 915 normal subjects. *Ann NY Acad Sci* 1963; 110:271–281.
16. Tzankoff SP, Norris AH: Effect of muscle mass decrease on age-related BMR changes. *J Appl Physiol* 1977; 43:1001–1006.
17. Parizkova J, Eiselt E, Sprynarova S, Wachtlova M: Body composition, aerobic capacity, and density of muscle capillaries in young and old men. *J Appl Physiol* 1971; 31:323–325.
18. Bergstrom J, Hermansen L, Hultman E, Saltin B: Diet, muscle glycogen and physical performance. *Acta Physiol Scand* 1967; 71:140–150.
19. Wahren J: Glucose turnover during exercise in man. *Ann NY Acad Sci* 1977; 301:45–55.
20. Coyle EF, Hagberg JM, Hurley BF, et al: Carbohydrate feeding during prolonged strenuous exercise can delay fatigue. *J Appl Physiol* 1983; 55:230–235.
21. Bergstrom J, Hultman E: A study of the glycogen metabolism during exercise in man. *Scand J Clin Lab Invest* 1967; 19:218–228.
22. Costill DL, Gollnick PD, Jansson ED, et al: Glycogen depletion pattern in human muscle fibres during distance running. *Acta Physiol Scand* 1973; 89:374–383.

23. Gollnick PD, Armstrong RB, Sembrowich WL, et al: Glycogen depletion pattern in human skeletal muscle fibers after heavy exercise. *J Appl Physiol* 1973; 34:615–618.
24. Felig P: Amino acid metabolism in exercise. *Ann NY Acad Sci* 1977; 301:56–63.
25. Young DR: *Physical Performance Fitness and Diet.* Springfield, Ill, Charles C Thomas, 1977, pp 11–49.
26. Gollnick PD: Free fatty acid turnover and the availability of substrates as a limiting factor in prolonged exercise. *Ann NY Acad Sci* 1977; 301:64–71.
27. Astrand P-O: Physical performance as a function of age. *JAMA* 1968; 205:729–733.
28. Dehn MM, Bruce RA: Longitudinal variations in maximal oxygen intake with age and activity. *J Appl Physiol* 1972; 33:805–807.
29. Astrand I, Astrand P-O, Hallback I, Kilbom A: Reduction in maximal oxygen uptake with age. *J Appl Physiol* 1973; 35:649–654.
30. Robinson S, Dill DB, Tzankoff SP, et al: Longitudinal studies of aging in 37 men. *J Appl Physiol* 1975; 38:263–267.
31. Hossack KF, Bruce RA: Maximal cardiac function in sedentary normal men and women: Comparison of age-related changes. *J Appl Physiol* 1982; 53:799–804.
32. Robinson S, Dill DB, Robinson RD, et al: Physiological aging of champion runners. *J Appl Physiol* 1976; 41:46–51.
33. Sidney KH, Shephard RJ: Maximum and submaximum exercise tests in men and women in the seventh, eighth, and ninth decades of life. *J Appl Physiol* 1977; 43:280–287.
34. Heath GW, Hagberg JM, Ehsani AA, Holloszy JO: A physiological comparison of young and older endurance athletes. *J Appl Physiol* 1981; 51:634–640.
35. Klissouras V, Pirnay F, Petit J-M: Adaptation to maximal effort: Genetics and age. *J Appl Physiol* 1973; 35:288–293.
36. Gerstenblith G, Lakatta EG, Weisfeldt ML: Age changes in myocardial function and exercise response. *Prog Cardiovasc Dis* 1976; 19:1–21.
37. Strandell T: Circulatory studies on healthy old men. *Acta Med Scand (Suppl)* 1964; 414:1–44.
38. Granath A, Jonsson B, Strandell T: Circulation in healthy old men, studied by right heart catheterization at rest and during exercise in supine and sitting position. *Acta Med Scand* 1964; 176:425–446.
39. Granath A, Strandell T: Relationships between cardiac output, stroke volume and intracardiac pressures at rest and during exercise in supine position and some anthropometric data in healthy old men. *Acta Med Scand* 1964; 176:447–466.
40. Strandell T: Cardiac output in old age, in Caird FI, Dall JLC, Kennedy RD (eds): *Cardiology in Old Age,* New York, Plenum Press, 1976, pp 81–100.
41. Port S, Cobb FR, Coleman RE, Jones RH: Effect of age on the response of the left ventricular ejection fraction to exercise. *N Engl J Med* 1980; 303:1133–1137.
42. Yin FCP, Weisfeldt ML, Milnor WR: Role of aortic input impedance in the decreased cardiovascular response to exercise with aging in dogs. *J Clin Invest* 1981; 68:28–38.
43. Julius S, Amery A, Whitlock LS, Conway J: Influence of age on the hemodynamic response to exercise. *Circulation* 1967; 36:222–230.

44. Conway J, Wheeler R, Sannerstedt R: Sympathetic nervous activity during exercise in relation to age. *Cardiovasc Res* 1971; 5:577–581.
45. Kanstrup I-L, Ekblom B: Influence of age and physical activity on central hemodynamics and lung function in active adults. *J Appl Physiol* 1978; 45:709–717.
46. Sorbini CA, Grassi V, Solinas E, Muiesan G: Arterial oxygen tension in relation to age in healthy subjects. *Respiration* 1968; 25:3–13.
47. Mellemgaard K: The alveolar-arterial oxygen difference: its size and components in normal man. *Acta Physiol Scand* 1966; 67:10–20.
48. Ekblom B, Goldbarg AN, Gullbring B: Response to exercise after blood loss and reinfusion. *J Appl Physiol* 1972; 33:175–180.
49. Bray GA: The energetics of obesity. *Med Sci Sports Exerc* 1983; 15:32–40.
50. Shock NW: Systems integration, in Finch CE, Hayflick L (eds): *Handbook of the Biology of Aging*. New York, Van Nostrand Reinhold, 1977, pp 639–665.
51. Astrand P-O, Rodahl K (eds): *Textbook of Work Physiology*. New York, McGraw-Hill, 1977.
52. Davis JA, Frank MH, Whipp BJ, Wasserman K: Anaerobic threshold alterations caused by endurance training in middle-aged men. *J Appl Physiol* 1979; 46:1039–1046.
53. Saltin B, Blomqvist G, Mitchell JH, et al: Response to exercise after bed rest and after training. A longitudinal study of adaptive changes in oxygen transport and body composition. *Circulation* (Suppl VII) 1968; 38:1–78.
54. Hartley LH, Grimby G, Kilbom A, et al: Physical training in sedentary middle-aged and older men. III. Cardiac output and gas exchange at submaximal and maximal exercise. *Scand J Clin Lab Invest* 1969; 24:335–344.
55. Rerych SK, Scholz PM, Sabiston Jr DC, Jones RH: Effects of exercise training on left ventricular function in normal subjects: A longitudinal study by radionuclide angiography. *Am J Cardiol* 1980; 45:244–252.
56. Gollnick PD, Armstrong RB, Saubert IV CW, et al: Enzyme activity and fiber composition in skeletal muscle of untrained and trained men. *J Appl Physiol* 1972; 33:312–319.
57. Gollnick PD, Armstrong RB, Saltin B, et al: Effect of training on enzyme activity and fiber composition of human skeletal muscle. *J Appl Physiol* 1973; 34:107–111.
58. Fournier M, Ricci J, Taylor AW, et al: Skeletal muscle adaptation in adolescent boys: Sprint and endurance training and detraining. *Med Sci Sports Exerc* 1982; 14:453–456.
59. Gillespie AC, Fox EL, Merola AJ: Enzyme adaptations in rat skeletal muscle after two intensities of treadmill training. *Med Sci Sports Exerc* 1982; 14:461–466.
60. Young JC, Chen M, Holloszy JO: Maintenance of the adaptation of skeletal muscle mitochondria to exercise in old rats. *Med Sci Sports Exerc* 1983; 15:243–246.
61. Benestad AM: Trainability of old men. *Acta Med Scand* 1965; 178:321–327.
62. Roskamm H: Optimum patterns of exercise for healthy adults, in Proceedings of the International Symposium on Physical Activity and Cardiovascular Health. *Can Med Assoc J* 1967; 96:895–899.
63. Barry AJ, Daly JW, Pruett EDR, et al: The effects of physical conditioning on older individuals. I. Work capacity, circulatory-respiratory function, and work electrocardiogram. *J Gerontol* 1966; 21:182–191.

64. deVries HA: Physiological effects of an exercise training regimen upon men aged 52 to 88. *J Gerontol* 1970; 25:325–336.
65. Stamford BA: Physiological effects of training upon institutionalized geriatric men. *J Gerontol* 27:451–455.
66. Tzankoff SP, Robinson S, Pyke FS, Brawn CA: Physiological adjustments to work in older men as affected by physical training. *J Appl Physiol* 1972; 33:346–350.
67. Adams GM, deVries HA: Physiological effects of an exercise training regimen upon women aged 52 to 79. *J Gerontol* 1973; 28:50–55.
68. Niinimaa V, Shephard RJ: Training and oxygen conductance in the elderly. II. The cardiovascular system. *J Gerontol* 1978; 33:362–367.
69. Sidney KH, Shephard RJ: Frequency and intensity of exercise training for elderly subjects. *Med Sci Sports Exerc* 1978; 10:125–131.
70. Sidney KH, Shephard RJ, Harrison JE: Endurance training and body composition of the elderly. *Am J Clin Nutr* 1977; 30:326–333.
71. Pollock ML, Dawson GA, Miller Jr HS, et al: Physiologic responses of men 49 to 65 years of age to endurance training. *J Am Geriatr Soc* 1976; 24:97–104.
72. Wilmore JH: Body composition in sport and exercise: Directions for future research. *Med Sci Sports Exerc* 1983; 15:21–31.
73. Misner JE, Boileau RA, Massey BH, Mayhew JL: Alterations in the body composition of adult men during selected physical training programs. *J Am Geriatr Soc* 1974; 22:33–38.

Index